JAPAN[ESE]
ACUPUNCTURE

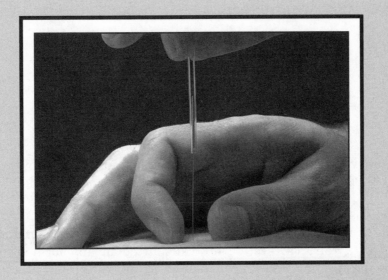

A Clinical Guide

STEPHEN BIRCH

JUNKO IDA

 Paradigm Publications

Japanese Acupuncture: a Clinical Guide

by

Stephen Birch and Junko Ida

©1998, 2010 Paradigm Publications

ISBN 0-912111-42-9

ISBN-13: 9780912111421

Library of Congress Card Number: 94-18574

Library of Congress Cataloging-in-Publication Data from the
National Library of Medicine is available for this title

Printed in the United States of America

Published by

PARADIGM PUBLICATIONS

Publisher: Robert L. Felt

http://www.paradigm-pubs.com

Distributed by

REDWING BOOK COMPANY, TAOS, NEW MEXICO, USA

http://www.redwingbooks.com

Cover Design by Laura Shaw Design

Photos by Stanley Rowin Photography

Table of Contents

Dedication and Acknowledgements

We dedicate this book to our teachers, the late Yoshio Manaka and the late Kodo Fukushima, who envisioned bringing Japanese acupuncture traditions to the West.

Many friends and fellows supported our work and contributed to our efforts to bring it to fruition. Among them we would in particular extend our appreciation to Yoshio Manaka, Kazuko Itaya, Kōdō Fukushima, Akihiro Takai, Toshio Yanagishita, Shozo Takahashi, Koryo Nakada, Denmei Sh do, Soichiro and Yuichiro Tobe, and Martin Feldman.

Additionally, we would thank our editors, Jack Lincoln and Martha Fielding, and our publisher, Robert Felt, for their continuous support of our efforts.

Introduction

Acupuncture is generally believed to have originated in China over two thousand years ago. Practiced almost continuously since its inception, it remains a significant component of the Chinese medical system, and is undertaken in most of the countries around the world, having become part of the accepted or mainstream medical practice in several of these countries.

Currently, the most popular methods and theories of acupuncture are those of the modern Chinese. Non-Asian countries have paid attention primarily or exclusively to what the Chinese are doing or have done in the field of acupuncture. But acupuncture has been practiced in other Asian countries for quite a long time, and has legitimate claims to traditions of practice and serious lineages. In Japan, for example, it has been part of the practice of medicine for about 1400 years. Yet the scope, history, and variety of acupuncture and moxibustion practice in countries like Japan are virtually unknown in the West. It is to this end that we offer this current volume to our readers.

Japanese Acupuncture: A Clinical Guide is the foundation volume in a series on Japanese clinical practice of acupuncture. It explores the history and nature of current practices in Japan and offers an in-depth study of commonly used techniques of needling, moxa, and so forth, that are either uniquely "Japanese" or clearly of Japanese origin.

This current text initiates a presentation of Japanese "root" treatment patterns[1] and shows how to employ them in conjunction with the techniques and approaches described. It is intended as a "materials and methods" guide to serve both as a complement to the existing books in English on Japanese root acupuncture approaches and as a starting point for further volumes that focus on explicit aspects of practice. Extensive research and translation has made it

---

[1]Described in previous works co-authored by Stephen Birch: *Five Elements and Ten Stems, Extraordinary Vessels, Hara Diagnosis,* and *Chasing the Dragon's Tail* (see Bibliography).

possible for us to present some of the important aspects of clinical practice in modern Japan which we feel typify the practice of acupuncture in Japan. While the extremely wide scope of practice in Japan and the vast number of different techniques used requires far more discussion than is possible in this work, we hope that the breadth and depth of the material we have included will give the reader a good sense of modern practice as well as the background and tools necessary to successfully undertake the clinical techniques presented.

Traditionally, acupuncture was used to treat the diseases described by the conceptual framework of the classical literature (yin-yang, five phases, channels, *zang-fu*, and so forth). Modern Japanese acupuncture techniques have been used and combined for the treatment of biomedical (Western-classified) disorders, as well as conditions described by traditional concepts.

Much of the information offered in this text stems from the experience of specialists whose works we have translated and Japanese teachers with whom we have studied. Where appropriate, we have contributed from our own experiences, especially where cross-cultural clarification seemed necessary, or where we felt that we had valuable examples or experiences of our own.

A number of texts and papers have been used as references for Chapters 3 through 11 in this text. Many of these are specialized books or papers that describe a single technique, such as moxibustion, bloodletting, cupping, *kyūtōshin* (moxa on the handle of the needle), intradermal needles, and press-tack needles. Many are more general texts that have chapters or sections on the subject being described, such as the uses of the needle and insertion tube, non-inserted needles, the *teishin*, press-spheres, or the wooden hammer and needle.

The focus of the current text is to describe as completely as we can, the techniques, recommendations, and prohibitions of the selected methods. There is only secondary emphasis on the uses of these methods for the treatment of specific symptoms. We recommend studying and practicing each technique before applying it in therapy.

Chapter 1

A Brief History of Acupuncture and Moxibustion in Japan[1]

While some dissent appears in the literature, most authors agree that knowledge of acupuncture, moxibustion, and herbal medicines arrived in Japan from China with a Chinese monk-physician named Chisō (Chinese, Zhicong) in 562 C.E. This physician is reputed to have brought about 160 volumes of Chinese medical treatises with him, including the then-famous book, the *Ming Tang Tu,* which is no longer extant. The material was studied and rapidly assimilated, as was much that came from China during that time. The Japanese of that period believed that Chinese culture was far more advanced than their own. With the initial influx of books, language, science, medicine, and so forth, Japan rapidly assimilated all it could from China. The introduction of Chinese medical techniques was part of this vast importation and rapidly gained popularity. The government of Japan built free public hospitals attached to Buddhist temples and asked that envoys to China return with more medical literature following each visit.

In 701 C.E. the first legal system was introduced in Japan, and with this, acupuncture and moxibustion were given priority in the practice of medicine and the first regulations governing their practice were formulated. In 718 C.E., a free, government-sponsored medical school was established where the study of acupuncture was a seven-year program, and the study of *anma* massage was a three-year program. Until the mid-ninth century all medical knowledge from China was rapidly and openly assimilated, but then, because of various political problems, contact with China was curtailed, which forced Japanese physicians to begin refining and developing their own ideas and methods.

---

[1]The following is an edited version of a paper originally written by Stephen Birch and serialized in the journal *Review*.

In 984 C.E., the emperor of Japan commissioned Yasuyori Tamba to compile and publish a large work on traditional medicine. This was published in 30 volumes as *I Shin Pō,* which dealt with many different subjects including acupuncture and moxibustion.

During the period 1185-1574, complex political, social, and cultural changes caused traditional medical techniques to fall into disrepute and acupuncture and moxibustion declined with little new development. However, from the mid 1500s onward, there was a flourishing of traditional medical literature and techniques in Japan. There was a notable increase in the number of books on traditional medicine written in the sixteenth through nineteenth centuries. There were, for example, more than fifty commentaries on the *Nan Jing* written between 1550 and 1900.[2] This period was a time of prolific output in the study and description of traditional medicine in Japan.

In the late 1500s, Isai Misono, a court physician, developed a new method of treatment with gold and silver needles that were used in the abdominal region and lightly tapped with a small wooden mallet. He not only had a unique method of treatment, but he employed a unique diagnostic method, based solely on abdominal palpation, using a pattern quite unlike any that had preceded it.[3] This Mubunryū style remains in use today, though practiced by only a few acupuncturists.

In the 1680s, a blind acupuncturist named Waichi Sugiyama developed the *shinkan* (insertion tube) which allowed relatively painless insertion. This innovation rapidly became popular, sparking a revival of interest in acupuncture. Employed by virtually every acupuncturist, the insertion tube was influential on nearly all forms of acupuncture practice in Japan. Some have called Waichi Sugiyama "the father of acupuncture in Japan." He established the first acupuncture school for the blind, thus beginning two trends still current today: acupuncture administered by blind practitioners; and a simpler, more pragmatic approach to the literature. In general, theory is de-emphasized while point location and practice are heavily emphasized. This latter trend is very apparent in the modern literature written by blind acupuncturists and in the curricula of acupuncture schools in Japan today.

In 1712, Ryoan Terashima published his massive work, *Wakan Sansai Zue.* Like the *I Shin Pō,* it was a multivolume compilation of current knowledge.

During the Edo period (1602-1868), increasing Western influence in Japan inspired some practitioners to experiment with integrating

---

[2]P. Unschuld, *Medicine in China: Nan Ching, The Classic of Difficult Issues,* pp. 665-669.

[3]K. Matsumoto and S. Birch, *Hara Diagnosis, Reflections on the Sea,* p. 29.

traditional ideas with modern anatomical and physiological knowledge. A pivotal point in this development was the publication of
Sugita Gempaku's translation of a Dutch anatomical text.[4] This
influenced, for example, Sōtetsu Ishizaka, who wrote an important
book, *Shinkyū Setsuyaku,* in the early 1800s. It is also worth not-
ing that during the Edo period, in particular in the 1670s to 1690s,
Japanese acupuncture and moxibustion practice had a reciprocal
influence on Western physicians. In 1674 for example, the Dutch
physician W. ten Rhijne studied in Japan and took medical ideas
back to Europe, as did the German physician E. Kaempfer in 1690.
These exportations are among the earliest known in Europe.[5]

During the nineteenth century the influence of Western ideas
in Japan increased, culminating in a major governmental policy
shift known as the Meiji Restoration. The government was des-
perately trying to modernize and reform Japan. In the field of
medicine the consequences were dramatic. In 1876 and again in
1883, early in the Meiji Restoration, it was decreed that traditional
medicine could be practiced only by those trained in Western medicine. This put acupuncture, moxibustion, and herbal medicine in
a status lower than that which they had previously enjoyed, and
this decree virtually outlawed the professions of traditional practitioners. While the impact on acupuncture and moxibustion was
negative and significant, the effect on herbal medicine was worse.
In 1895 the "medical practitioner's law" was passed, formalizing the
earlier decrees; only Western physicians or blind people were able
to study and practice acupuncture and moxibustion, and only Western physicians or pharmacists were allowed to practice herbal medicine.

In effect, the Meiji restoration brought the practice of medicine
in Japan closer to modern Western medical standards. It also antic-
ipated by about half a century the changing of traditional medical
practices in China. At the end of the nineteenth century the government permitted the remarkable social policy, unique to Japan,
which allowed the continued study of acupuncture and moxibustion
by blind non-physician practitioners. This is still a strong trend in
Japan today, where the visually handicapped are encouraged to
study and practice either acupuncture, *anma,* or *shiatsu* massage
therapies.[6]

The strong role that blind practitioners assumed in Japanese
acupuncture, starting with Waichi Sugiyama in the late 1600s,
which was solidified by the laws passed at the end of the nineteenth

[4]See S. Birch and R. Felt, *Understanding Acupuncture,* Churchill Livingstone, 1998.
[5]Lu Gwei-Djen and J. Needham, *Celestial Lancets,* p. 270 *passim.*
[6]This was reported to the authors by several blind practitioners in Japan.

century, not only made it a respectable profession for the blind, but brought about some entirely unique changes, influences, and developments in the field of acupuncture in Japan.

In another surprising decree, parallel to what would later happen in China, provisos in Meiji Restoration policy stripped acupuncture and herbal medicine of their traditional theories and nomenclatures, allowing only "scientific" terminology and concepts to be used. Acupuncture was defined as a form of "stimulation" therapy, and the ideas of channels and channel acupoints were replaced by a more pragmatic concept of discreet, unconnected *kōketsu* (Chinese *kongxue*), "acuholes," points with specific effects, which could be combined into groups and used to treat specific biomedical diseases. These changes, while reducing the traditional theories to more scientifically acceptable concepts, did preserve acupuncture and moxibustion as allowed, or even preferred, professions for the blind.

By 1905, a movement began to elucidate the mechanisms of acupuncture and moxibustion in scientific terms. Considerable research was conducted. For example, between 1912 and 1940 the pharmacological effects of moxibustion were studied. The findings from these studies are still virtually unknown outside Japan but are taught as basic information in Japanese acupuncture schools today. Since the Second World War, research into the effects and mechanisms of acupuncture and moxibustion has continued at medical schools and acupuncture schools almost without interruption.

In the mid 1920s a movement began to research and revive the study and practice of traditional acupuncture and moxibustion. One of the famous leaders of this movement was Sorei Yanagiya, a practitioner and scholar of great renown. He is credited with having written so many books on acupuncture and moxibustion that when stacked together their height exceeded his own. Proponents of this movement, such as Sōdō Okabe, Keiri Inoue, and Shōhaku Honma, focused on detailed studies and analyses of concepts from the oldest traditional literature which was primarily Chinese. Their belief was that one should not blithely follow or believe all the traditional concepts and ideas; after all, the traditional authors were not infallible. Only through careful scholarly and clinical research could one proceed.

After the surrender of the Japanese government which ended the Second World War, American occupation forces under General Douglas MacArthur tried to ban traditional medicines such as acupuncture and moxibustion altogether. A number of reputable practitioners and scholars resisted. Following a Tokyo demonstration by the blind, the new Japanese government designed laws governing the system of education and examination in Japan. In 1947, the government passed laws redefining the study of acupuncture and moxibustion, laying down a universal curriculum for all acupuncture and moxibustion schools. This curriculum, though strongly influenced by Western medical knowledge, nonetheless established separate licensing procedures for acupuncture, moxibustion, and massage therapies such as *anma* and *shiatsu*. *Anma* and *shiatsu* are taught in most acupuncture schools where students obtain separate licenses in massage, acupuncture, and moxibustion. These regulations were further refined and revised in 1970 and are currently being studied in regard to further revision. (See Appendix 1 for a discussion of school curricula and training.)

Throughout Japan's 1400-year history of acupuncture and moxibustion practice, herbal medicine (known as *kampō* since the late nineteenth century), *anma,* and *shiatsu* coexisted and underwent distinct and individual evolutions. The Meiji-era legislative restrictions and additional commercial pressures virtually assured that in Japan acupuncture would be affected by secondary influences coming from the practice of massage techniques such as *anma, shiatsu,* and *ampuku*. For example, the use of palpation described in the *Nan Jing* and the *Shang Han Lun* was studied, researched, and further developed in Japan. In China it was ignored or replaced with newer theories or techniques. The Japanese saw herbal medicine as a discipline separate from acupuncture and moxibustion, driven by its own theories. As a consequence, there was little interaction or confluence of acupuncture and moxibustion with herbal medicine. Again, the Japanese situation was distinctly different from China where for centuries these medical systems had been closely aligned.

Currently, acupuncture in Japan can be practiced only by licensed acupuncturists and physicians. Moxibustion is practiced by licensed moxibustionists, physicians, priests, and nuns; it is also used as a home remedy among family members. No medical schools in Japan currently teach acupuncture or moxibustion, though there are a number of specialized colleges. (See Appendix 1 for an overview of who practices, and an overview of the structure of the profession in modern Japan.) Herbal medicine *(kampō)* can be prescribed only by Western physicians or Western-trained pharmacists. While experiencing an increased use since the national health insurance system included it as an acceptable drug therapy, it is practiced as a complete system by very few physicians. Yet it is a billion-dollar industry in Japan, frequently advertised on national television, often bought as a non-prescription remedy,[7] and

---

[7]E. Ohnuki-Tierney, *Illness an Culture in Contemporary Japan*, p. 107. See also K. Sonoda, *Health and Illness in Changing Japanese Society.*

prescribed in a simple allopathic manner, according to recent estimates, by up to 80% of physicians in Japan, who are bowing to
increasing demands.[8]

Thus we can begin to gather a clearer perspective on the development of acupuncture and traditional medicine in Japan. The political
restrictions that compelled Japanese medical students to learn Chinese medical systems primarily through the classical literature contributed to rendering a uniquely Japanese contribution to East Asian
medicine, firmly based in the Chinese tradition itself. By trying to
understand the oldest literature in the context of their own culture
and relative to their own social upheavals and changes, the Japanese
evolved techniques and ideas that differed from those of the Chinese.
This process of assimilation, integration, and development is very
important if we are to understand the nature of acupuncture and moxibustion practice in Japan today. Paul Unschuld has written a thorough analysis of the influence of political and social climates on the
evolving medical systems in China; it would not be unreasonable to
expect similar processes have been at work in Japan.[9]

It is important that we not ignore the cultural, sociological, and
political pressures put on the practice of acupuncture and moxibustion in the countries where they are practiced. China has gone
through major upheavals in the last few decades, with major governmental policy shifts concerning the scope, nature, education,
and practice of acupuncture and moxibustion. The health care
needs of China have been immense, and it is remarkable that the
government has included traditional medical practices as part of its
modernized medical system. But one should not overlook the fact
that life in China is very different from life in the West. The majority of China's population live in rural areas. In the West the urban
population is proportionately much greater. Consequently the
health problems and needs are different. Some of the adaptations
made in China to meet the needs there will not successfully transplant to Western countries. Further, traditional medical systems
such as acupuncture, moxibustion, and herbal medicine have been
of necessity merged with Western allopathic techniques in China to
create a new medicine. And, while competition exists between the

---

[8]K. Tsutani, 1993. Tsutani states that as well as having one of the highest per
capita consumptions of Western drugs in the world, Japan has perhaps the highest
per capita consumption of traditional herbal products.

[9]P. Unschuld, *Medicine in China, A History of Ideas.* See also S. Birch and R. Felt,
Understanding Acupuncture (at press).

[10]S. M. Hillier and J. A. Jewell, *Health Care and Traditional Medicine in China
1800-1982;* M. M. Rosenthal, *Health Care in the People's Republic of China: Moving
Toward Modernization;* N. Sivin, *Traditional Medicine in Contemporary China;* P.
Unschuld, *Medicine in China: A History of Ideas;* S. Birch and R. Felt,
Understanding Acupuncture.

traditional and allopathic medicines in China, it is more at a political and ideological level. Patients have free access to either kind of medicine, though at times access is limited to traditional techniques.

On the other hand, Japan is a major industrial nation, with a primarily urban population. It is comparable in many respects to Western nations such as the U.S. and the U.K. While it too has gone through major changes in the last few decades, these have been more in line with the changes that Western countries have experienced. As a consequence, health care needs in Japan are not dissimilar to those in the U.S., the U.K., and much of Europe. Diseases and disorders in industrialized nations show similar tendencies, and competition between Western medicine and traditional methods such as acupuncture and moxibustion is similar. In Japan, less than five percent of the public take advantage of traditional techniques such as acupuncture, moxibustion, and massage, with the great majority utilizing Western medicine and *kampō*[11]. This is comparable to the situation in the U.S. and U.K., where acupuncture and moxibustion are utilized by a very small percentage of the population.

The fact that Japan has already had to contend with these issues, and that acupuncturists and moxibustionists there have been molded and have successfully adapted to a very competitive climate, suggests that many of the changes and adaptations may be applicable to other industrialized countries where similar processes of assimilation are under way. This gives credibility to the proposal that the scope and variety of acupuncture and moxibustion practice in Japan are suitable to the U.S., U.K., and other similar countries.

In practical terms, it is likely that not only the variety of techniques and treatment approaches in acupuncture and moxibustion in Japan are suitable to Western countries, but also the nature of the techniques used, which are often gentler, more subtle, and less painful than the techniques used in China, are more appropriate.[12] In fact, the Chinese themselves state that the more superficial, gentler needle techniques are more appropriate for people who do not perform hard physical labor.[13] This does not necessarily mean that the Chinese approach using the stronger needle techniques, where the needles are more deeply inserted (the predominant practice in the U.S. and U.K.) will be displaced; rather that there will be an expansion and proliferation of the Japanese approaches alongside

---

[11]K. Tsutani, 1993.

[12]Y. Manaka, K. Itaya and S. Birch, *Chasing the Dragon's Tail;* S. Birch and R. Felt, *Understanding Acupuncture;* D. Shūdo, *Japanese Classical Acupuncture: Introduction to Meridian Therapy.*

[13]J. Bischko, *Intermediate Acupuncture vol II,* p. 41.

the Chinese approaches. It should be remembered that modern Chinese acupuncture (T.C.M.) is a popular therapy in Japan as well. The tendencies towards a greater pluralistic medical system will increase, both in the East Asian and Western arenas.

Several authors who have studied medical practices in Japan have reached the conclusion that the pluralistic nature of medicine in Japan is an important facet of health care there.[14] This pluralism allows a highly functional approach to the complexities of medical issues that in advanced industrial nations are constantly evolving beyond the scope of current medical technologies. This outcome may yet obtain in the U.S. and U.K., where recent government, academic, and biomedical research into herbs have spawned new structures and programs. At the least, traditional medicines such as acupuncture and moxibustion will probably gain in strength and popularity as they fill a need unmet by Western medical practices.

Historically, acupuncture and moxibustion therapies in China and Japan have been diverse in nature and scope, with a tendency towards a pluralistic approach. It is difficult to trace a single tradition continuously for more than a few decades in either of these countries; variation and diversity have been the norm.[15] Thus it would be neither untraditional nor contradictory to have a modern flourishing of ideas and techniques in the West. Our personal feelings are that as this trend occurs, many of the Japanese approaches and techniques will enjoy a boom in the U.S., the U.K., and Europe as more information becomes available and a broader range of ideas becomes the norm.

---

[14]M. M. Lock, "Organization and Practice of East Asian Medicine in Japan: Continuity and Change," *Social Science and Medicine* 148:245-253, 1980; and T. Matsunaga, "Socio-cultural transformation of Japanese medical systems," Ph.D. thesis, Western Michigan University, 1983.

[15]M. Lock, *Ibid.* pp. 148:245-253, 1980; N. Sivin, *Traditional Medicine in Contemporary China;* P. Unschuld, *Medicine in China: A History of Ideas;* P. Unschuld, *Medicine in China: Nan Ching, the Classic of Difficult Issues;* and P. Unschuld, *"Traditional Chinese Medicine: Some Historical and Epistemological Reflections,"* *Social Science and Medicine* 24, 12:1023-1029, 1987.

Chapter 2
Traditional Correspondences and Treatment Systems

According to the traditional literature, acupuncture treatment is delivered in two different steps, the "root" or "general" treatment method, termed *honchihō,* and the "local" or "symptom control" treatment method, termed *hyōchihō.* Root treatment seeks to address the basic imbalances in the patient, utilizing the theories of yin-yang the and five phases, and the techniques of radial pulse palpation, abdominal palpation, and other inspection methods to discover problems of qi circulation (vacuity, repletion, and/or stagnation) in the twelve principal channels. Local treatment addresses symptomatic relief of patient complaints.

In theory, once these primary channel problems have been identified and corrected, the whole "system" self-corrects; i.e., the various complaints or symptoms in the body are healed. This simplified description essentially reflects the underlying concept of traditionally-based systems of acupuncture: once the problems of vacuity, repletion, and/or stagnation of the twelve primary channels are corrected, normal *zang-fu* functions are restored, various other traditionally described physiological processes are restored, and the body's innate healing abilities—arguably the focus of all traditional models of acupuncture—are activated.

The primary methods in our focus that represent this model are the Keiraku Chiryo meridian/channel therapy system developed since the 1920s by Sorei Yanagiya, Sōdō Okabe, and others; the related system of Tōyōhari developed by Kōdō Fukushima and others; and the "yin-yang channel balancing therapy" system developed by Yoshio Manaka. To understand how these systems generally use channel theory as described, it is useful to examine the essential components of the *Nan Jing* model and later additions that developed over the next millennium and a half.

As with everything in Chinese medicine and acupuncture, theories are not monolithic. They have been stated, restated, interpreted, re-interpreted, modified, compiled, and evolved, and can be found at virtually any period in the history of acupuncture in many forms. Sometimes these forms are contradictory, at other times complementary, depending on the interests, backgrounds, and biases of those who use them clinically and those who discuss them theoretically.

The descriptions that follow represent a compilation of ideas from the historical literature as seen through the lenses of modern practitioners and colored by the background, preferences, and interests of the authors.

VARIETIES OF CHANNEL SYSTEMS AND THEIR BASIC THEORIES

The early literature on the channel systems describes the following:
- The 12 principal channels *(jing mai)* *(Ling Shu 10, Nan Jing 1).*
- The 15 network vessels *(luo mai)* *(Ling Shu 10, Nan Jing 26).*
- The 12 channel sinews *(jing jin)* *(Ling Shu 13).*
- The 12 channel divergences *(jing bie)* *(Ling Shu 11).*
- The 8 extraordinary vessels *(qi jing ba mai)* *(Su Wen 44, 60; Ling Shu 2, 10, 11, 17, 21, 33, 38,62, 65; Nan Jing 27 ,28, 29).*
- The water channels *(jing shui)* *(Ling Shu 12).*

Some of these channel systems have been extensively discussed in later texts (e.g., *Zhen Jiu Jia Yi Jing* (282), *Huang Di Nei Jing Tai Su* (700s), *Tong Ren Shu Xue Zhen Jiu Tu Jing* (1027), *Shi Si Jing Fa Hui* (1341), *Zhen Jiu Da Quan* (137), *Zhen Jiu Ju Ying* (1529), *Qi Jing Ba Mai Kao* (c. 1570), *Zhen Jiu Da Cheng* (1601), where continuous (and often contradictory) elaborations of the earlier descriptions have been made. Other channel systems have been ignored (e.g., water channels) or discussed rarely by other authors (e.g.,*jing jin, jing bie*).

The primary channel systems that practitioners have attempted to utilize are the twelve principal channels and the eight extraordinary vessels, following the focus that is found in the historical literature. While texts such as the *Tong Ren Shu Xue Zhen Jiu Tu Jing* and the *Shi Si Jing Fa Hui* helped formalize and flesh out the earlier descriptions of the primary channels to approximately what we recognize today, the extraordinary vessels did not really gain focus and depth in practice until the fifteenth to sixteenth centuries, evolving considerably beyond the earlier descriptions

(Zhen Jiu Da Quan, Zhen Jiu Ju Ying, Qi Jing Ba Mai Kao, Zhen Jiu Da Cheng).[1] In the current practice of traditional acupuncture in Japan, the twelve channels and eight extraordinary vessels have become the primary focus for achieving the basic goals of acupuncture treatment.

THE PRIMARY CHANNELS

The twelve channels have a series of basic correspondences through which they influence each other or interact:

- Each is an arm or leg channel, each a yin or yang channel, in one of three yin and three yang pairings: *tai yin-yang ming, shao yin-tai yang,* and *jue yin-shao yang).*
- Each has a five-phase correspondence.
- Each has a connection to at least two internal organs or functional systems.
- Qi is said to flow through them in a continuous circuit.
- The channels manifest a natural cycle of ebb and flow throughout the course of a single day.

The following table illustrates most of these relationships:

ARM/LEG	YIN/YANG	ORGAN	PHASE	CHANNEL
arm	*tai yin*	lung	metal	LU
arm	*yang ming*	large intestine	metal	LI
leg	*yang ming*	stomach	earth	ST
leg	*tai yin*	spleen	earth	SP
arm	*shao yin*	heart	fire	HT
arm	*tai yang*	small intestine	fire	SI
leg	*tai yang*	bladder	water	BL
leg	*shao yin*	kidney	water	KI
arm	*jue yin*	pericardium/ heart master	fire	PC
arm	*shao yang*	triple burner	fire	TB
leg	*shao yang*	gallbladder	wood	GB
leg	*jue yin*	liver	wood	LR

Ling Shu 15 and *Nan Jing 1* describe the continuous circulation of qi in these channels. Starting at CV-12, the qi circulates through the channels starting at the lung, then passing through the channels of the large intestine, stomach, spleen, heart, small intestine, bladder, kidney, triple burner, gallbladder, liver, and back to CV-12.

---

[1]See K. Matsumoto and S. Birch, *Extraordinary Vessels*, pp. 4-137.

The circuit also exhibits the following biorhythm, where each channel has an ebb and flow, peaking in a two-hour period, and ebbing in the opposite two-hour period:

CIRCADIAN RHYTHM PEAKING HOURS			
11 PM—1 AM	GB	11 AM—1 PM	HT
1 AM—3 AM	LR	1 PM—3 PM	SI
3 AM—5AM	LU	3 PM—5 PM	BL
5 AM—7 AM	LI	5 PM—7 PM	KI
7 AM—9 AM	ST	7 PM—9 PM	PC
9 AM—11 AM	SP	9 PM—11 PM	TB

In this fashion, each of the twelve channels maintains a series of relationships to other channels. For example, within the pair of metal channels, arm *tai yin* lung (LU) and arm *yang ming* large intestine (LI), there is a yin-yang relationship whereby each is affected by and exerts natural regulatory effects on the other. If the lung channel is weak, the large intestine channel tends to be too strong, but at the same time, the large intestine channel tries to correct the lung channel weakness. This is like a see-saw effect, a complex of antagonistic-syntagonistic relationships. This extends to the other channels in the *tai yin-yang ming* set, so that the lung channel is also related to leg *tai yin* spleen (SP) and leg *yang ming* stomach (ST). A change in any of the four channels in the *tai yin-yang ming* set can create change, exert influence on, or be influenced by each of the other three channels in the set. This principle also holds for each of the other four channel sets, *shao yin-tai yang* and *jue yin-shao yang*.

The five-phase cycles also describe how each channel maintains a relationship with and is influenced by other channels. There are engendering, restraining, counter-engendering, and counter-restraining cycles:

Earth engenders metal, metal engenders water, water engenders wood, wood engenders fire, fire engenders earth.

Earth restrains water, water restrains fire, fire restrains metal, metal restrains wood, and wood restrains earth.

A change in any channel could create change in, and by feedback be influenced by, any other channel. If the lung channel increased, the kidney channel might tend to increase, the liver, heart, and pericardium channels might tend to decrease, and the spleen channel might tend to decrease.

The *zi wu* (Japanese *shigo*) midday-midnight relationships of the channels implicit in the circadian rhythm of the channels involve a complex set of rhythmical relationships. For example, between 3–5 AM when the LU channel is at its peak or maximum, the BL channel is at its nadir or minimum. Between 3–5 pm when the BL channel is at its peak or maximum, the LU channel is at its nadir or minimum. These rhythmical cycles hold for each pair of channels, but their relationships are somewhat complex, involving interesting yin-yang pairings, where an arm yin channel is paired with a leg yang channel or an arm yang channel is paired with a leg yin channel.

TIME	CHANNEL	TIME	CHANNEL
3–5 AM	LU (arm-yin)	3–5 PM	BL (leg-yang)
5–7 AM	LI (arm-yang)	5–7 PM	KI (leg-yin)
7–9 AM	ST (leg-yang)	7–9 PM	PC (arm-yin)
9–11 AM	SP (leg-yin)	9–11 PM	TB (arm-yang)
11–1 PM	HT (arm-yin)	11–1 AM	GB (leg-yang)
1–3 PM	SI (arm-yang)	1–3 AM	LR (leg-yin)

These yin-yang, five-phase, and *zi-wu* relationships appear to describe a complex of possible interactions that each channel maintains with the other channels. The following shows the possible interactions each channel theoretically maintains with the other channels according to the relationships described above.

CHANNEL RELATIONSHIPS					
LU→LI	ST→LU	HT→LU	BL→LU	PC→LU	GB→LI
→ST	→LI	→SP	→LI	→ST	→ST
→SP	→SP	→SI	→ST	→SP	→HT
→HT	→SI	→BL	→HT	→HT	→SI
→BL	→BL	→KI	→SI	→KI	→BL
→KI	→PC	→PC	→KI	→TB	→PC
→PC	→TB	→GB	→TB	→GB	→TB
→LR	→GB	→LR	→GB	→LR	→LR
LI →LU	SP→LU	SI →LI	KI →LU	TB→LI	LR→LU
→ST	→LI	→ST	→LI	→ST	→SP
→SP	→ST	→HT	→SP	→SP	→HT
→SI	→HT	→BL	→HT	→SI	→SI
→BL	→KI	→KI	→SI	→BL	→KI
→KI	→PC	→TB	→BL	→PC	→PC
→TB	→TB	→GB	→PC	→GB	→TB
→GB	→LR	→LR	→LR	→LR	→GB

It is instructive to examine how this chart is composed by detailing the relationships noted. Taking the SP channel for example, we have SP → LU= *tai yin* + five-phase, SP →LI = *tai yin* + *yang ming,* SP → ST = within-phase yin-yang + *tai yin-yang ming,* SP → HT = five phase, SP → KI = five phase, SP → PC = five phase, SP → TB = *zi-wu,* and SP → LR = five phase.

We can see then, in terms of diagnosis, that a problem of the spleen channel may result in symptoms in any of eight other channels (LU, LI, ST, HT, PC, KI, PC, TB, LR). This could even manifest as a patient with a primary SP channel problem who has no symptoms associated with the SP channel, but only symptoms in the other channels. There are of course typical patterns and symptoms that occur, but many seemingly unrelated symptoms can occur.

It is important to understand this because in a clinical setting the principal signs used to determine the selection of the primary channel problem can be chosen based solely upon finding certain palpable reactions associated with that channel (e.g., radial pulse and abdominal palpation). This emphasis has developed because the primary focus of treatment is to correct the disturbance in qi circulation (thought to have caused the patient symptoms), and which have, over time, been associated with key signs and reactions in the body. If symptoms can theoretically develop in any of a number of channels that are not clearly associated with the channel that is the primary focus of treatment, detailed analysis of those symptoms can be confusing and even misleading. However, this does not mean that symptoms should be ignored, and it should be remembered that most patients show a pattern of signs and symptoms that typically match the primary target channel.

The relationships described above are also important in treatment selection. Many of the basic treatment principles or methods are based on utilization of one or more of the above relationships. Many treatment methods have developed that take explicit advantage of these relationships to both correct the disturbances in the qi system (channels), or to relieve specific symptoms.

These relationships can be even more complex, further reinforcing the focus on primary signs rather than symptoms in selecting the primary focus of treatment. For example, each channel passes through two organs (the yin-yang, within-phase pairing), but some channels pass through other channels as well. For example, the SP also passes through the heart organ, the LR through the ST and LU.[2] Additionally, in the model just developed, every channel is interacting with at least eight other channels in a complex rhythm of

---

[2]Details of these internal trajectories can be found in K. Matsumoto and S. Birch, *Hara Diagnosis, Reflections on the Sea,* pp 49-65.

push-pull, antagonistic-syntagonistic and feedback mechanisms, For all practical purposes, any change in one channel could initiate changes in any of the other channels, and in turn be influenced by those other channels. In mathematical terms, this describes a "complex dynamical system," where the twelve channels interact with each other so as to be the medium both for transmission and regulation of disturbances within the whole system, capable of holding the whole system in a more steady, stable state.

In addition to the basic theories and relationships of the twelve channels, there is the system of eight extraordinary vessels. The classical literature shows almost continuous variation in how the theories, pathways, and utilization of the extraordinary vessels have been described.[3] The extraordinary vessels, their pairings, and their treatment points are given in the following table.

VESSEL	MASTER POINT	COUPLED POINT	PAIRED VESSEL
ren mai	LU-7	KI-6	*yin qiao mai*
yin qiao mai	KI-6	LU-7	*ren mai*
du mai	SI-3	BL-62	*yang qiao mai*
yang qiao mai	BL-62	SI-3	*du mai*
chong mai	SP-4	PC-6	*yin wei mai*
yin wei mai	PC-6	SP-4	*chong mai*
dai mai	GB-41	TB-5	*yang wei mai*
yang wei mai	TB-5	GB-41	*dai mai*

The extraordinary vessels are generally thought to influence the primary twelve channels as they exert their effects. Several models have been proposed.[4]   Generally the extraordinary vessels were thought of as reservoirs rather than as channels for the flow of qi. We find concepts such as the *ren mai* as the "ocean of yin," the *du mai* as the "ocean of yang," and the *chong mai* as the "ocean of the twelve channels," the "ocean of the *zang-fu*," and the "ocean of blood."[5] They are thought to play an auxiliary role to the primary channels, helping in the general redistribution of qi.

[3]See K. Matsumoto and S. Birch, *Extraordinary Vessels*, pp. 4-137 for further discussion.

[4]See e.g., S. Birch, "Dr. Yoshio Manaka's Yin-Yang Balancing Treatment; An Overview of His Life and the Development of his Unique System," *North American Journal of Oriental Medicine 1, 1:4-8,* 1994; S. Birch, "Dr. Yoshio Manaka's Yin-Yang Balancing Treatment (Part 2)," *North American Journal of Oriental Medicine 2, 3:4-6,* 1995; S. Birch, "Dr. Yoshio Manaka's Yin-Yang Balancing Treatment (Part 3)," *North American Journal of Oriental Medicine 2, 4:5-7,* 1995; and Y. Manaka, K. Itaya and S. Birch, *Chasing the Dragon's Tail.*

[5]K. Matsumoto and S. Birch, *Extraordinary Vessels*, pp 27, 30, 41.

Another idea is that when treating each pair of vessels, all the primary channels that intersect with those vessels or that are influenced by or intersecting with those vessels can be influenced so as to aid in a general redistribution or harmonization of qi among those channels. For example, when treating SP-4 and PC-6, the *yin wei mai-chong mai* pair, the channels thought to be on the pathway of the *chong mai* (SP, KI, LR, ST) and those thought to be on the pathway of the *yin wei mai* (KI, SP, LR, *ren mai*) are affected, helping in a general redistribution of qi among those channels.[6]

We can also consider that treatment effects of needling extraordinary vessel pairs can be brought about by stimulation of the channels on which the treatment points lie, for example TB and GB for the *yang wei mai-dai mai* pair, PC and SP for the *yin wei mai-chong mai* pair. Thus the extraordinary vessels can be seen through a number of models to bring about general and broad redistributions of qi among the primary channels, thereby achieving the primary goal of acupuncture treatment: to restore more normal circulation of qi in the channels.[7]

The biorhythmic cycle components of the channel and extraordinary vessel systems offer further avenues of theoretical exploration. Beyond the daily or circadian cycle mentioned earlier, the historical literature on acupuncture contained much more elaborate biorhythm models. Principal among the texts that described these biorhythm models were the *Zi Wu Liu Zhu Zhen Jing* (circa 1300), the *Zhen Jiu Da Quan, Zhen Jiu Ju Ying,* and the *Zhen Jiu Da Cheng.* These texts described a complex cycle of the twelve channels and points on those channels that were "open" at particular times of day on a ten-day cycle *(nai jia fa),* based on the ten stems,[8] and a cycle of the eight extraordinary vessel treatment points that were "open" at particular times on a 60-day cycle *(ling gui ba fa),* based on certain ideas from the *Yi Jing.*[9] Further models were developed based on Ming dynasty era concepts, among these the *nai zhi fa* based on a daily bihourly cycle.

These are the basic models and concepts that underlie the Japanese acupuncture systems which we describe in this text.

---

[6]The pathways of the extraordinary vessels are most completely described in K. Matsumoto and S. Birch, *Extraordinary Vessels,* pp 25-67.

[7]See the discussions in *Extraordinary Vessels,* and Manaka's octahedral model of the extraordinary vessels for more in-depth presentation of these concepts.

[8]See Liu Bian Que, *Optimum Time for Acupuncture;* Manaka Y., K. Itaya and S. Birch, *Chasing the Dragon's Tail,* pp. 103-105, 168-169; and Matsumoto K. and S. Birch, *Hara Diagnosis: Reflections on the Sea,* pp 398-402.

[9]See Liu Bian Que, *Ibid.;* Y. Manaka, K. Itaya, and S. Birch, *Chasing the Dragon's Tail,* pp. 105-106, 170-175; and K. Matsumoto and S. Birch, *Hara Diagnosis: Reflections on the Sea,* pp. 403-408.

ACUPUNCTURE AND MOXIBUSTION TREATMENT OPTIONS

The following is a partial listing of the varieties of acupuncture and moxibustion treatment options available throughout Japan. It would take a considerable effort to document all the options available, especially since new techniques and ideas are spawned with great regularity, but the list that follows covers the primary techniques, those most commonly known, and a few of the less well-known techniques.[10]

NEEDLE THERAPIES

• Root treatment based on traditional channel theory and pulse diagnosis, utilizing needle techniques where the needles can be inserted or not inserted, depending on the practitioner, for supplementation and draining. Needles are usually made of stainless steel, silver, or gold, but there are varieties of other types of needles available, such as cobalt and molybdenum needles. There are several schools of thought in this category.

• Needle therapy based on empirical uses of the acupoints, relative to patient symptoms. There are many schools of thought in this category.

• Needle therapy based on scientific ideas and principles, e.g., needling points that lie on nerve routes and muscle structures. There are many schools of thought in this category.

• Needle therapy based on principles described in China today (T.C.M.). In Japan, since herbal medicine can only be practiced by physicians or specially trained pharmacists, most practitioners in this category do not combine acumoxa therapy with herbal medicine, but use only acumoxa therapy, which is different from the trend in China. A school in Tokyo, the Gotō College of Medical Arts and Sciences, specializes in the study and practice of T.C.M. acupuncture, with instructors from China, notably Beijing and Tianjin. Dr. Akira Hyōdō of the Gotō College estimated that there are as many as 1000 T.C.M.-style practitioners, and up to 2000 including physician T.C.M.-style practitioners in Japan.

• Needle therapy based on electrodermal diagnosis and predictions, for example, Ryōdōraku, A.M.I. There are several schools of thought in this category.

SPECIALIZED NEEDLE THERAPIES

• Electroacupuncture: Needles are inserted and then stimulated with electric current, for the relief of patient symptoms; there are

---

[10]Appendix 1 lists some of the foremost practitioners in Japan of the better-known systems and methods.

many schools of thought in this category and many different electrostimulating devices.

• Ion-Pumping Cords: These are wires with a diode in them and are attached to needles shallowly inserted in the body. They are used mostly as a form of root treatment, but can be used to treat specific symptoms. There are several schools of thought regarding their use.

• Intradermals: These are used for the Akabane channel balancing techniques, for the relief of specific symptoms, and to support root treatment. Many practitioners throughout Japan use intradermals.

• Minus-Plus Needles: For example, copper and zinc needles are used both for root treatment and to treat specific symptoms. There are several schools of thought.

• Bloodletting: This technique is used by different practitioners as root treatment, as a support for root treatment, or to relieve specific symptoms.

• Non-insertion needles: These include blunted and rounded needles such as the *teishin*, the *zanshin*, and the *enshin*, used for stimulating the flow of qi in the channels without actually having to pierce the skin. They are often used for children, but also used by some practitioners for the treatment of adults. There are several schools of thought on the uses of these instruments.

MOXIBUSTION THERAPIES

• Direct moxa therapy that includes scarring and non-scarring methods for root treatment.

• Direct moxa therapy that is applied to treat specific symptoms. There are several schools of thought concerning this technique.

• Indirect moxa therapy that includes moxa therapy to support both root treatment and to treat specific symptoms. There are several schools of thought in this category.

• Direct and indirect moxa therapies including methods for home therapy, administered by family members or friends.

OTHER COMMON TREATMENT METHODS[11]

• Cupping: Used as support for root treatment and to relieve specific symptoms, often used with bloodletting.

• Bloodletting: Used by lay practitioners as a form of folk remedy.

---

[11]Some brief preliminary discussions of a number of these different techniques and tools can be found in the literature. See e.g., Y. Manaka, K. Itaya, and S. Birch, *Chasing the Dragon's Tail;* and K. Serizawa and M. Kusumi, *Clinical Acupuncture.*

- Magnets for home therapy: These are sold in most pharmacies in Japan and advertised on national television in Japan.
- Magnets for root treatment: There are several schools of thought on their use.
- Magnets for treatment of specific symptoms: Used both on their own and in combination with electrical stimulation. There are several schools of thought on their use.
- *Shonishin:* Children's needle methods; there are probably more than fifty different instruments that are used to treat children with rubbing, scratching or pecking type techniques. Insertion techniques are generally not used, and treatment is very quick— usually less than five minutes. There are several schools of thought concerning these techniques.
- Stimulation devices: Used on points based on traditional theory, and including various electrical "moxa-stimulation" instruments or devices used to stimulate areas of the body.
- Other techniques and tools: These include devices which can be commonly obtained to give mild stimulation to specific points or areas, such as Manaka's wooden hammer and needle.

Only a few of these techniques are actually taught in the acupuncture or moxibustion schools. For example, only the second and third categories of the needle therapy techniques and the second and third categories of the moxa therapy techniques are taught in most schools. All schools teach basic needle and moxa techniques and most teach the uses of these techniques on a more empirically based or scientifically based approach. Very few teach root treatment approaches. Intradermals, minus-plus needles, bloodletting, ion-pumping cords, cupping, and magnets are rarely if ever taught in any of the schools, but some schools teach the use of intradermal needles, some teach the *shonishin* techniques, and some teach the use of electroacupuncture. Of the vast assortment of techniques that are available and widely practiced, many are not taught in school and must be learned in the clinics with practitioners or at the numerous seminars or association meetings that occur routinely and regularly around Japan.

We cannot point to any one of these techniques and say, "This is Japanese acupuncture." The nature of acupuncture in Japan is pluralistic, and in a sense, there is no such thing as "Japanese acupuncture." Instruction offered by Japanese teachers coming to the West can only be a representative part of "Japanese acupuncture." This may confuse some Western students who are taught to believe there is only one "right way" to practice acupuncture–a misconception that renders them intolerant of unresolved or unresolvable contradictory ideas.[12]

[12]See e.g. P. Unschuld, "Traditional Chinese Medicine: Some Historical and Epistemological Reflections." *Social Science and Medicine* 24, 12:1023-1029, 1987.

The broad nature of the study and practice of acupuncture and moxibustion in Japan, and the pluralistic approach that is also characteristic of the overall health care system in Japan, permits the individual practitioner to develop and refine techniques continuously. There are few ideas or techniques that cannot be studied. Strong-minded clinicians routinely study, absorb, test, and assimilate what they come across, to the betterment of their clinical skills and their patients. These processes are deeply ingrained in the Japanese system and have allowed a veritable flourishing of acupuncture and moxibustion, despite the immense pressures from biomedicine.

JAPANESE ACUPUNCTURE SYSTEMS

Clearly, there are many styles, methods, and techniques in the practice of acupuncture in Japan. Some are are uniquely or typically Japanese. Others are similar to the styles and methods that come from other countries.

For example, methods of practice utilizing thicker needles, inserted somewhat deeply to obtain the *de qi* sensation, or methods utilizing electroacupuncture stimulation, are practiced widely in Japan and around the world today. While such techniques and methods when used in Japan exhibit a typically Japanese flair because they have been adapted and modulated by Japanese practitioners, they are not uniquely Japanese.

Our focus in this text must be limited to those techniques which we define as "representative" of Japanese practice, and thus will include methods that fall into one or more of the following three categories:

- Those uniquely Japanese, by virtue of their having been invented by Japanese practitioners.
- Those uniquely Japanese by virtue of having been developed and refined by Japanese practitioners.
- Those typical of a method or approach that is more common in Japan than elsewhere.

In the first sense, representative techniques include the uses of the *shinkan* (insertion tube) invented by Waichi Sugiyama; the uses of *hinaishin* (intradermal needles) invented by Kōbei Akabane; and the uses of the wooden hammer and needle, a simple form of therapy invented by Yoshio Manaka as a refinement of the sixteenth century treatment methods of the Mubunryū school.

Representative techniques in the second sense are those developed to a greater degree by Japanese practitioners than by practitioners from other countries. We discussed above the degrees of specialization that have occurred in Japan. Many practitioners use their specialized techniques for almost all their patients, adapting the techniques for treatment of virtually all disorders. Each method of treatment utilizes a variety of approaches. Different practitioners select from among this range to compose their root and local treatment, developing a nearly unique combination of techniques.

There are several classes of techniques in Japan where this has happened, with unique developments in the utilization of those techniques. One obvious example is the use of moxibustion. Japan is, as far as we know, the only country with separate licenses for moxibustion and acupuncture. This has encouraged and supported unique extensions, refinements, and developments in the field of moxibustion therapy. Specialists such as Isaburo Fukaya, Seiji Irie, and Takeshi Sawada, for example, almost never used needles and relied instead on the use of moxibustion for the treatment of disorders where moxibustion was often contraindicated by other non-specialists. Their extended examination and refinement of techniques and uses of moxibustion surpassed the work of the non-specialist practitioners, thereby greatly extending the range of therapeutic applications. This is a refinement of moxibustion usage that is uniquely Japanese. While it is true that there is a legacy of moxibustion therapeutic manuals in the historical literature of China, this degree of specialization does not appear to have survived in China.

Another good example is the use of bloodletting. Most systems of acupuncture around the world either do not use bloodletting or employ it in a limited manner, more as an adjunct to their usual forms of therapy. However, there were specialists in Japan, for example, Drs. Masao Maruyama and Kunimasa Kudō, who used bloodletting on virtually all their patients. In order to do this they had to adjust their techniques and study the correct dosages, limitations, and contraindications to a far greater degree than any other practitioners before them. Adjusting their methods in this manner allowed the development of bloodletting techniques for many more diseases than previously described.

The use of the intradermal needles saw a uniquely Japanese specialization as well. Both Kōbei Akabane and Matsuo Takaoka used them extensively in their practice. Detailed and specialized cupping techniques were developed and refined by groups of Japanese lay-practitioners and administered to all patients who came to them for therapy.

Techniques and methods utilizing much thinner or smaller needles that are typically shallowly inserted or not inserted at all, and techniques giving very small stimulation to the treatment points are not so common around the world, but are quite common in Japan today. The selection of treatment methods that generally use smaller stimulation techniques, or that embody what we have called the "less is better" approach, are, we feel, representative of acupuncture in Japan because they are unique in both the first and second senses.

Examples of the third class of representative techniques again includes the use of the insertion tube for needle application. While the insertion tube is now used by many practitioners around the world, it is used by almost all Japanese practitioners, and the technique is thus a characteristic trademark of Japanese acupuncture. The use of the intradermal needles in Japan is also so widespread that we can classify their use as a characteristic trademark of acupuncture practice in Japan. Likewise, the use of palpation for diagnosis, point selection, point location, and treatment assessment is so widespread in Japan that we feel that it too is characteristic of acupuncture practice in Japan.

The techniques included in our discussions generally, but not exclusively, utilize smaller doses of stimulation. These include:

- General needling techniques characteristic of acupuncture in Japan that use thinner needles shallowly inserted using an insertion tube, with little or no manipulation.

- General moxibustion techniques, where very small moxa punk are burnt on the acupoints, to give very small stimulation which is a characteristic difference between the Japanese usages of moxibustion and the Chinese usages.

- Intradermal needling, used by most practitioners in Japan today to deliver very small stimulation to the points.

- Use of the small "press-tack" needles, specifically on body points, again to deliver small stimulation to the acupoints.

- Use of the "metallic-grain" or "press-spheres" to apply tiny pressure to the acupoints and deliver small doses of stimulation to the acupoints.

- Cupping therapy where pumps (rather than the "fire-cupping" method) are used to regulate the dosage of pressure-stimulation, thus allowing for the delivery of very small to larger amounts of stimulation to the treated areas.

- Bloodletting techniques utilizing individualized variations in needling techniques and quantities to achieve very small to larger amounts of bloodletting appropriate to the condition of each patient.

•Use of Manaka's wooden hammer and needle to deliver very small to somewhat stronger stimulation to a point or area, depending on the needs of each patient.

These techniques, and a description of Japanese palpation techniques for diagnosis and assessment, comprise the majority of textual presentation in this book.

There is another important trademark of acupuncture in Japan, especially when the "less is better" approach is adopted. While specialists utilize their refined techniques for virtually all their patients, the majority of the practitioners in Japan select from among the papers and texts published by these specialists and add those techniques to augment their usual treatment protocols.

KEIRAKU CHIRYŌ PRACTICE IN JAPAN

Our focus is to describe the works of practitioners who have typically used a "less is better" approach to treatment. The different groups that fall under the heading of *keiraku chiryō* make the most extensive references to the "less is better" approach to treatment which we feel is most "representative" of Japanese acupuncture.

There are actually many schools of thought and a number of different associations that fall under this heading. The traditional literature provides the theoretical basis of treatment, specifically the conceptual systems that utilize the "qi-circulation" model of the channel system.[13]

The term *keiraku chiryō* is most aptly used to describe the systems of practice of a number of traditional associations such as the Toyohari group founded by Kōdō Fukushima and currently headed by Akihiro Takai or the Keiraku Chiryō groups headed by Meiyu Okada, Denmei Shūdo, and others. It is also used in a slightly extended sense to include groups such as the Shinkyū Topology group that was headed by Yoshio Manaka.

However, the most "representative" school of thought in Japan that explicitly adheres to the "less is better" principle is the Keiraku Chiryō (meridian therapy) school. Generally this school is more traditional in its outlook. Other practitioners, including Yoshio Manaka and Kōdō Fukushima, developed logical and systematic treatment protocols utilizing and combining different techniques and methods, while still adhering to the "less is better" principle.

---

[13]For publications in English describing this model, see e.g., *Five Elements & Ten Stems, Extraordinary Vessels, Hara Diagnosis, Chasing the Dragon's Tail, Introduction of Meridian Therapy,* and *Meridian Therapy: A Hands-on Text for Traditional Japanese Hari Based on Pulse Diagnosis.*

When we look at how specific practitioners integrate different treatment methods available in Japan, we find that it is impossible to describe how every practitioner does this. The following are two practitioners with whose work we are familiar: Yoshio Manaka and Kōdō Fukushima. Describing their treatment methods shows the often eclectic, research-based but very clinically oriented methods of each.

Both Manaka and Fukushima undertook a several-step treatment protocol. The techniques described in this text can be used for the application of the root treatment methods or the local treatment methods developed by these practitioners and taught in the groups which they established.

DR. YOSHIO MANAKA'S WORK

Dr. Yoshio Manaka practiced and researched acupuncture and moxibustion for more than 40 years. His practice was more diverse than many other practitioners in Japan because he was a physician and often treated unusual or very difficult cases.

His root treatments were most often based on abdominal diagnostic findings and performed with the ion-pumping cords, which he designed in the 1950s. As alternatives for the ion-pumping cords, he also used his ion beam device and his electrostatic adsorbers, both of which he designed, and, while having different "hardware" than the ion-pumping cords, have similar "software" effects. He would sometimes use the *zi wu liu zhu* treatment methods, the biorhythm treatments to achieve the goals of the root treatment. Likewise, just prior to his demise he was using *Yi Jing* signals that were specially coded to stimulate specific acupoints as a root treatment.

Sometimes he used colors or sounds to stimulate the acupoints as a root treatment. Sometimes he used moxa for root treatment, and sometimes zinc-copper needles or north-south magnets, though he used the latter more often in research investigations. After Step One of his root treatment method, he would use as many as three more steps depending on the needs of the patient. Some of the techniques he employed in these steps were moxa on the handle of needles (typically on back-*shu* points); *danōkyū,* a rather strong form of moxa that purifies the blood; moxibustion; needling; *sōtai* exercises; intradermals on body points, auricular points, and special hand points; electrical stimulation; bloodletting; cupping; and the Manaka wooden hammer and needle.

Each technique was thoroughly explored theoretically, experimentally, and then clinically to determine how effective it could be and for what purposes it was most useful. Based on his findings and clinical experiences, Dr. Manaka designed a very flexible treatment methodology with which he obtained remarkable results even with the most recalcitrant conditions.[14]

MANAKA'S TREATMENT METHOD

In Manaka's treatment method, Steps One, Two, and Three comprised his root treatment approach, and Step Four the local treatment. He used the needles and insertion tube as tools in his unique treatment approach for completion of both Steps One and Two of his treatment protocol. Occasionally, he used direct moxa for Steps One or Two, but more often, direct moxa was used for Steps Three and Four. Indirect moxa in the form of moxa on the handle of the needle was commonplace as a Step Two treatment protocol. Intradermals were a mainstay of Manaka's Step Four treatment method. Occasionally the press-tack needles, and less often the press-spheres, were utilized for Step Four. Both cupping and bloodletting were used for Step Four protocols. The wooden hammer and needle was occasionally used for Steps One and Three, though mostly for Step Four and home-therapy.

Manaka's approach is essentially a four-step treatment process:[15]

Step One

•Diagnosis by palpation of abdominal and other regions.

•Shallow needling with ion-pumping cords attached, based on patterns of treatment points selected by palpation.

•Application of alternative methods using color, sound, moxa, and open points.

Step One typically uses shallow needling with the ion-pumping cords on patterns of treatment points selected by palpation diagnosis of the abdominal and other regions. Alternative treatment methods at this stage include the use of colors, sounds, moxa, and open points.

Step Two

•Moxa on the handle of the needle on back-*shu* points.

•Shallowly inserted needles to other reactive points, especially on the neck and shoulder regions.

•Alternative treatment methods including moxa with channel-stretching exercises, moxa or needling of other points, *danōkyū* blood purifying moxa techniques.

---

[14]For further details of the treatment methods and combinations of techniques that he used, see Y. Manaka, K. Itaya, and S. Birch, *Chasing the Dragon's Tail.*

[15]*Chasing the Dragon's Tail* gives more details of the treatment flow charts.

Step Two usually involves the use of moxa on the handle of the needle on related back-*shu* points, sometimes with shallowly inserted needles to other reactive points, especially in the neck and shoulder regions. Alternative treatment methods include moxa with channel-stretching exercises, moxa or needling of other points, and *danōkyū*–blood purifying moxa techniques.

Step Three

•Simple structural exercises to release physical constrains in the musculoskeletal system, e.g., *sōtai* exercises; often combined with moxa treatment.

Step Three involves the use of simple structural exercises to release physical constraints in the musculoskeletal system. These exercises are usually *sōtai* exercises and are often combined with moxa.

Step Four

•Intradermal needle placement, especially on the auricles, but also on the body and on hand points.

•Direct moxa therapy.

•Home therapy recommendations including moxa and wooden hammer and needle.

Step Four frequently involves the use of intradermal needles, especially in the auricles, but also on the body, as well as Korean hand acupuncture points. Other methods include moxa, cupping, bloodletting, and wooden hammer and needle. The press-tack needles and press-spheres are less often used; patients are sometimes sent home with procedures for home therapy such as moxa therapy or and wooden hammer and needle therapy.[16]

KŌDŌ FUKUSHIMA'S WORK

Kōdō Fukushima practiced acupuncture for over fifty years. His main method of performing root treatment was to use silver or stainless steel needles for supplementation and draining techniques based on his pulse and touch diagnosis. The silver needles were usually not inserted to produce the therapeutic effects. The stainless needles were often inserted, but usually only shallowly.

---

[16]Yoshio Manaka and Kazuko Itaya, who used the ion-pumping cords extensively for root treatment, along with a number of alternative approaches and supplementary techniques for different steps of therapy, have had their work published and described in English. Extensive discussions of their work can be found in Y. Manaka, K. Itaya, and S. Birch, *Chasing the Dragon's Tail.* Further discussions can be found in K. Matsumoto and S. Birch, *Hara Diagnosis: Reflections on the Sea.*

His treatments were highly refined, requiring considerable sensitivity, and, like Manaka's methods, were routinely and continuously explored conceptually, experimentally, and clinically so that he might better understand and implement them. He used a variety of techniques and tools as support for the root treatment, including direct and indirect moxa, intradermals, and zinc and copper needles, all of which are used as treatment for specific symptoms, too. Various non-inserted needles such as the *teishin* and *enshin* were also used, as well as bloodletting and cupping.

The organization of which he was president, the Toyohari Igakukai, continues to investigate and refine different treatment techniques. Each of the 60 branches is assigned areas of research and investigation, and reports of investigative and clinical findings are routinely presented at meetings or written up in the monthly journal.

FUKUSHIMA'S TREATMENT METHOD

Kōdō Fukushima used the needle and tube for all steps of his root treatment, and for some of his local treatment methods. Moxa was used mostly as a local treatment step, as were intradermals, press-tack needles, press-spheres, cupping, and bloodletting, though each was used on occasion as a supportive approach in the root treatment. He did not use the wooden hammer and needle.[17]

Fukushima's treatment method was not so clearly defined in terms of steps used. However, the first part of treatment used silver needles to supplement the most vacuous yin channel; then supplementation or draining techniques were used according to the pulse reading of vacuity or repletion of a yin channel on the restraining cycle of the five phases. The next part of treatment involved the use of supplementation or draining techniques on vacuous or replete yang channels.

These steps represent his essential root treatment. Use of supplementation techniques on related back-*shu* points supports the root treatment, as does the use of non-insertion needles, such as the *enshin* and *zanshin* on the back. When the radial pulses and abdominal reactions are sufficiently improved, the symptom control part of treatment begins. Needles are used in the neck and groin regions for upper half and lower half body problems, respectively. Bloodletting, cupping, zinc-copper needling of the extraordinary vessels, use of gold needles based on midday-midnight relationships, moxa, intradermals, or press-spheres are used for the rest of the symptom control portion of treatment.

---

[17]See K. Fukushima, *Meridian Therapy: A Hands-on Text on Traditional Japanese Hari Based on Pulse Diagnosis,* for details of the nature of his acupuncture practice. The Toyohari "meridian therapy" approach is used by other distinguished practitioners including Katsuyuki Kozato, Toshio Yanagishita, and Akihiro Takai.

Part One

•Silver needles to supplement vacuous yin channels.

•Supplementation or draining techniques applied according to the pulse reading of vacuity or repletion of a yin channel on the controlling cycle of the five phases.

Part Two

•Supplementation or draining techniques on vacuous or replete yang channels.

•Supplementation techniques on related back-*shu* points.

•Non-insertion needling (*enshin* and *zanshin*) on the back, sufficient to improve radial pulses and abdominal reactions.

Part Three

•Needles applied to neck and groin regions for the upper half of the body and the lower half of the body (termed *naso* and *muno* treatments respectively).

•Bloodletting, cupping, zinc-copper needling of the extraordinary vessels, supplementation with gold needles based on midday-midnight relationships, moxa, intradermal needles, press-spheres.

OTHER KEIRAKU CHIRYŌ PRACTITIONERS

Denmei Shūdo is a Keiraku Chiryō practitioner made prominent in the West through publication of his book, *Japanese Acupuncture, Introduction to Meridian Therapy*.

SHŪDO'S TREATMENT METHOD

Shūdo's treatment protocol is also not so clearly defined in terms of steps of treatment, but the basic approach is as follows: Supplementation and draining techniques are applied by shallow insertion of needles on the vacuous and replete channels, focussing first on the vacuous yin channels. Often at the same time shallow needles are applied to points related to the patient's symptoms. Further techniques used as the symptom-control part of therapy include the uses of intradermal needles in the auricles and on body points, as well as moxa, and bloodletting.

Part One

•Supplementation and draining techniques using shallow insertion of needles first on vacuous channels and then on replete channels.

•Shallow needling at points related to the patient's symptoms.

Part Two

•Intradermal needling at auricle points and body points, moxa, and bloodletting.

All three channel-focused treatment methods utilize *hyōchihō* (local) procedures after the *honchihō* (root) portions of treatment. If you use these techniques purely for symptom relief, you should add them at the end of your regular treatment. Always remember that "less is better." Try to select what you think is the best technique and sites of application so that you need apply less rather than more. Assess the effects of the technique by checking reactions such as pressure pain and range of motion.

Chapter 3

Palpation

Palpation as a diagnostic method, a method of locating acupoints, and a method to assess treatment strategies, has been strongly endorsed by practitioners of both acupuncture and herbal medicine *(kampō)* in Japan. Much of the original source material from which these methods were designed and developed comes from classical Chinese sources such as the *Nan Jing* and *Shang Han Lun*.[1]

In *honchihō* (root) treatment, palpation is a predominant technique, being, perhaps, the major diagnostic technique. The methods of general treatment that we have referenced in this text use palpation as a very significant part of diagnosis.[2]

The use of palpation in finding acupoints or just sensitive points for treatment is highly developed in Japan. Each different treatment method, whether it utilizes needles, moxa, or intradermal needles, has specific methods and interpretations of palpation. Since the treatments undertaken generally employ mild stimulation, maximum effect comes from the most exact point location possible.

In the Tōyōhari Association, students of the monthly or near-weekly meetings, both beginners and highly experienced practitioners practice point location with simple feedback methods to

---

[1]See K. Matsumoto and S. Birch, *Hara Diagnosis: Reflections on the Sea,* Chapter 2 for some details of the history and uses of palpation.

[2]The use of palpation in the "general" treatment methods has been covered quite thoroughly in other texts. (See K. Matsumoto and S. Birch, *Hara Diagnosis: Reflections on the Sea* (Chapters 11, 15 and 16 particular), where abdominal palpation in the five-phase and Manaka approaches is covered. For further details of Manaka's methods, see Y. Manaka, K. Itaya, and S. Birch, *Chasing the Dragon's Tail.* For further details of the meridian therapy- five phase approach, see D. Shūdo, *Introduction to Meridian Therapy,* and K. Fukushima, *Meridian Therapy: A Hands on Text for Traditional Japanese Hari Based on Pulse Diagnosis.*

determine the most correct point location. In the moxibustion tradition, when members of an association meet in a study group, much of the study time is spent practicing point location. With Manaka's methods, having the needle be as little as 1mm off the exact point can have clearly observable differences in effect. In nearly all these systems, when the point is located and treated accurately, very specific effects can be observed. If treating pain, the pain immediately diminishes in intensity or simply disappears; if working with a limited range of motion, the range immediately increases. The effects of treating the correct point with an appropriate method at the exact point location can be quite dramatic.

Palpation is the most commonly used method of finding the correct and exact points, but, since the points are usually extremely small, and the finger pads are relatively big, it takes unrelenting practice to reliably find and treat the exact points. As a novice, it is possible to locate points accurately and obtain sufficient effects, but to acquire the ease of greater skill demands persistent study, practice, and a few clear pointers.

It is important to have an idea where to start looking for the acupoint that needs treating. If, in a specific treatment formula, a specific acupoint is listed, this generally means going to the standard anatomical location for that point and then palpating around it to find the reactive point which is defined by the presence of pressure pain or a small knot or indentation. This is explicitly discussed by some authors, such as the moxibustionist Seiji Irie.[3]

Sometimes the reactive point is some distance from the standard anatomical location, but as long as this point is not located closer to another standard anatomical acupoint, there are no difficulties. Many practitioners report that the most reactive point tends to be located in recurring typical positions. For example, Manaka stipulated that when he used SP-4 in his ion-pumping cord extraordinary vessel treatments, he usually found it to be more proximal and inferior to the standard anatomical location of point. Sometimes practitioners will describe typical reactions that are to be found at that specific acupoint when it is palpated. Manaka stipulated that SP-4 has a distinctive knot, and that LR-14 will show clear pressure pain and/or muscle stiffness.

Given these stipulations in the literature, it is important to have a standard acupoint location reference guide and a list of the typical reactions that can be found when palpating acupoints. For a standard acupoint location reference guide, we recommend *Illustration of Acupoints* by Haruto Kinoshita, which clearly describes most locations according to the Japanese tradition. On

---

[3]See S. Irie, *Fukaya Kyūhō (The Method of Fukaya)*, p. 8.

occasion, the indications for points that should be treated may be no more than "palpate on the shoulder and treat the most reactive point." In such cases, what is really important is knowing what to look for when palpating to find the points to be treated. In Chinese acupuncture, these points are called *ashi* points, but in the Japanese approaches, many more clinical details are given as to how these points feel.[4]

FINDING THE CORRECT ACUPOINT FOR TREATMENT

There are certain visual clues that can indicate a point needing treatment. These include signs of swelling, tight underlying musculature, and depressions in the skin or musculature. When you first touch the point, there might be very subtle signs, primarily at the skin level, such as sponginess of the skin, dryness or roughness of the skin, stickiness of the point, or a palpable "hole" at the point.

As a little pressure is applied to the point, there is some resistance, hardness, a knot, a very subtle response of the tissues that can feel like a non-symmetric compression of the tissues, a "ratchet-like" compression rather than a smooth compression of the tissues, or a feeling which almost appears to be "avoidance."

With still more pressure, the patient will usually start reacting to the pressure. The patient might have sensations of pressure pain, discomfort, soreness, achiness, or radiating sensations. The tissues might be clearly felt to respond to the pressure almost in a defensive or avoidance reaction where the tissues underneath feel like they are "jumping." The practitioner might feel a clear hardness or tightness at the point, and sometimes a clearly definable and palpable knot at the point. Close observation of the patient reveals other visual clues that often accompany this degree of pressure. The patient might squirm a little on the table; laugh or smile, or report ticklishness. In cases of ticklishness, always compare left and right equivalent points; if one side is ticklish and the other not, this is not really ticklishness, but instead merely called that for lack of a more appropriate term. If both sides are ticklish, this is more likely true ticklishness, but this, too, has its own significance.[5]

During palpation with additional pressure, the patient might also manifest a number of subtle facial feature changes. Often these cues are significant. The patient's frowns, grimaces, or blank featureless expression can indicate the presence of a good treatment point. Usually when any of the above visual or behavioral cues manifest, the practitioner should be aware of some reaction in

---

[4]For a full description of the different kinds of palpatory responses that can be found, see K. Matsumoto and S. Birch, *Hara Diagnosis: Reflections on the Sea,* Chapter 11.

[5]See *Ibid.,* p. 394.

the point, whether it is a clear hardness or resistance, or a more subtle response of the underlying tissues.   Beginners using this approach will likely get better results by using mild to deeper pressure to find reactions at the points. As the practitioner becomes more experienced, the points can be located with less pressure.

A few patients manifest hyposensitivity to pressure, which might be caused by their condition or from consumption of medication for hypertension, pain, depression, etc. Regardless of palpation style, these patients are unable to tell you if anything is sore or painful. In such cases the practitioner must rely more on what is felt, which of course makes the process more difficult. Look for the clear tight, tense, or knotty reactions, and pay special attention to the visual clues and tissue responses under your fingertips.[6]

Some practitioners believe that once they have defined the approximate location of the point to be treated, they need to focus even more specifically in that area to find the exact point. Some use a small probe such as a *teishin* to palpate and look for this exact point, while others use an electrodermal instrument to measure the exact point. When working in small densely packed areas such as the microsystems of the auricles and hands, it is actually a good idea to use instruments such as a *teishin* to facilitate locating the exact point more precisely.

On the body, however, reliance on the sensitivity of the fingertips will in the long run have better results in finding the correct points. The density of acupoints on the body itself is much less than on the auricles. Treating too far from the reactive point will have little effect; treatment closer to the real point will have a stronger effect. Palpating for the points using only the pads of the fingers can define an area the size of the pad of the finger within which the point lies. After finding the general area of the point using the fingerpad, turn the finger slightly and use the side or tip of the finger, to locate a reactive area that is much smaller and more precise. With practice, the more precise point can be found more and more often.

The proof of point location accuracy can be established in several ways. For *honchihō* root treatment in T y hari, a sufficient grasp of radial pulse diagnosis enables detection of changes of the pulse following application of a needle to verify to the correctness of the point location.

Another method is to select a point that was reactive before needle application and palpate it again to see if the reaction at the point is different. If the reaction is dramatically reduced, this is an indication of the accuracy of the location and the appropriateness of

---

[6]This issue is described in some detail in Y. Manaka, K. Itaya, and S. Birch, *Chasing the Dragon's Tail*, pp. 141-142.

the technique used on the point. We recommend this method when using *okyū* (direct moxa) and *hinaishin* (intradermal needles).

The other obvious way of assessing the accuracy of point location is to see how the patient's symptom(s) change following needle application. In cases of pain or restricted range of motion, this is easily assessable. For problems more internal in nature, assessment of improvement takes longer. In such cases, the luxury of immediately reassessing, except perhaps that of palpating reflex points elsewhere on the body, such as on the abdominal region, is not available. The use of this kind of feedback system is very typical of Japanese acupuncture and moxibustion practice, and it provides invaluable and immediate information about the status of the treatment strategies. By having immediate feedback concerning the treatment's effects, subtle adaptations and alterations of the treatment are possible.

There are three important points to stress as we conclude this chapter.

1. Variations and unusual circumstances require constant honing of point location skills.

2. The points to be treated almost **always** show some kind of palpable reaction.

3. The significance of palpation in the practice of Japanese acupuncture and moxibustion therapies can rarely be overstated.

Chapter 4
Hari to Shishin—Needles and Needling

TRADITIONAL NEEDLES

The early Chinese authors described nine different types of needles, some of which were not inserted. These nine needles were described in the first chapter of the *Huang Di Nei Jing Ling Shu,* one of the earliest and most important acupuncture treatises. Their importance, distinctions, and general uses were described further in the 7th and 78th chapters of the *Ling Shu.* These passages clearly stated how the practitioner must learn to distinguish which needle to use for which conditions.

According to the first chapter of the *Ling Shu,* these nine types of needles are used for a variety of purposes, such as lancing boils, bloodletting, shallow insertions, deep insertions, rubbing, scraping, and pressing. The following table lists the needles and their dimensions.

CHINESE	JAPANESE	ENGLISH	LENGTH/WIDTH
chan zhen	*zanshin*	arrow-headed needle	1.6 *cun*
yuan zhen	*enshin*	round-headed needle	1.6 *cun*
shi zhen	*teishin*	blunt needle	3.5 *cun*
feng zhen	*hōshin*	sharp three-edged needle	1.6 *cun*
pi zhen	*hishin*	sword-shaped needle	4 *cun* long, .25 *cun* wide
yuan li zhen	*enrishin*	round-sharp needle	1.6 *cun* long
hao zhen	*gōshin*	filiform needle	3.6 *cun* long
chang zhen	*chōshin*	long needle	7 *cun* long
da zhen	*taishin*	large needle	4 *cun* long

Unfortunately, no specimens remain of the original needles. Over the centuries different authors have speculated about the shapes of these different needles. The following illustrations are speculations from a traditional Chinese source, the *Zhen Jiu Da Cheng* of 1601, and two Japanese sources, the *Sugiyama Ryū Sambusho,* circa 1700, and the *Shinkyū Chō Hoki* of 1726, the last being commonly referenced in Japan today.

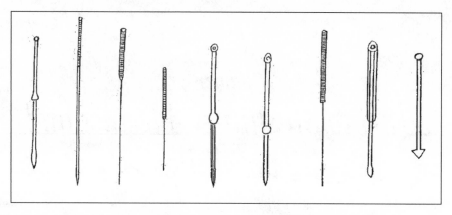

The Nine Needles from the *Zhen Jiu Da Cheng*

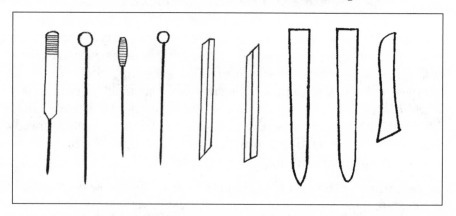

The Nine Needles from *Sugiyama Ryū Sambusho.*

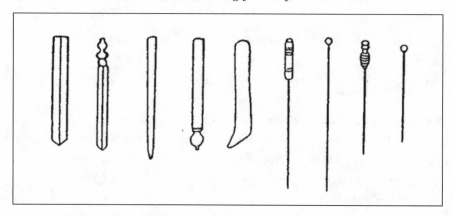

The Nine Needles from *Shinkyū Chō Hoki.*

The following table summarizes much of what was said in Chapters 1, 7, and 78 of the *Ling Shu* about these needles, their uses and characteristics.

NEEDLE	INSERTION	USES	CORRESPONDENCE
zanshin	shallow	remove evil qi[1] at surface	heaven
enshin	none	remove evil qi at borders of the flesh	earth
teishin	none	circulate blood and qi	person
hōshin	shallow	bloodletting	four seasons
hishin	shallow	remove pus	five sounds
enrishin	insert	remove fulminant qi	six tones
gōshin	insert	strengthen *zheng qi*, treat painful *bi*	seven orifices
hōshin	insert	remove chronic *bi* or deep problems	eight winds
taishin	insert	remove water qi of joints	nine fields

MODERN NEEDLES

There are a wide variety of different needles and tubes used in practice today. These range from ultra-thin to relatively thick needles, made of numerous different metals, and plastic or glass disposable tubes to stainless steel or even silver or gold tubes.

Since the export to the West of acupuncture from East Asia and especially China which followed President Nixon's visit to China in 1972, acupuncture needles have gone through a revolution both in their manufacture and usage. Needles and tubes were, until recently, almost always made of metal; the needles had a metal handle and the tubes are mostly made of stainless steel. But, with the rise of dangerous infectious diseases in the West, such as the AIDS virus, Japanese needle manufacturers responded to the demand for a safer, single-use needle. These companies started manufacturing disposable needles. As these needles grew in popularity in the West, several of the Japanese companies refined their manufacturing processes to cut the costs to practitioners. This gave rise to needles with plastic handles, plastic insertion tubes, glass insertion tubes, and individually packaged and sterilized needles with or without insertion tubes. A Japanese needle manufacturer, the Seirin company, pioneered the use of the "disposable" needle and even the "disposable" tube. Now many companies in Japan manufacture disposable needles which are used extensively in the West. Chinese and Korean companies have begun manufacturing disposable needles. Because of these developments, not only are there a number of different lengths and gauges of needles, made of a variety of metals, but there is also quite a variety in the types of needles.

---

[1]The term "evil qi" is a literal translation of the Chinese term *xie qi,* in Japanese *jaki.* It refers to normal qi in the body that is disrupted, has lost its normal function, and is causing symptoms.

Most needles are made of stainless steel. This metal has virtually replaced the older gold, silver, and bronze needles. In traditional times, gold and silver needles were common. They were found in the Mawang-dui graves which date from 168 B.C. and are some of the oldest acupuncture needles yet discovered. The stainless steel needle is stronger and easier to sterilize. Many traditional practitioners in Japan, especially the Keiraku Chiryō practitioners, prefer to use silver or gold needles because of their greater supplementing qualities. Since the 1950s gold and silver needles have also been used together in order to create small electrical currents; zinc and copper needles are now used in the same way. Recent investigations of different properties and values of different metals used in the needles, and the properties and effects of using two different kinds of needles together (i.e., the "minus-plus" needle approach or the "two-metal contact" approach), have contributed to a knowledge base that allows for a wider variety of needle types and techniques tbat are used in Japan. Different types of needles have advantages and disadvantages.

STAINLESS STEEL NEEDLES

Stainless steel needles, by nature more tensile, are accordingly stronger. This quality allows for easy needle insertion and very sharp thin points that do not blunt easily. For the simple stimulation of acupoints in order to relieve symptoms, the stainless steel needle is the most recommended. Stainless steel needles can be readily sterilized with either heat or autoclave apparati which makes them the ideal candidate if you choose to reuse needles. However, stainless steel needles are not as effective as silver or gold for supplementing type procedures. In the Keiraku Chiryō root treatment approaches, this is a significant limitation. Many practitioners use silver for supplementation and stainless steel for draining techniques.

Aside from the energetic quality of the metal itself, a further problem that makes it hard to achieve good supplementing effects is that the needle tends to insert too easily, possibly causing the inexperienced practitioner to insert the needle too deeply for appropriate supplementation techniques. A further, albeit minor, problem is that with the needle being a harder metal, it will tend to penetrate and injure tissues more easily than other needles.

SILVER NEEDLES

Silver needles are good for supplementation, being by their energetic nature more able to supplement. With greater control over the depth of insertion, less damage to local tissues occurs and supplementing techniques are more manageable. However, silver is a soft metal which makes it a little more difficult to insert. On the one hand, this allows greater control over the depth of insertion, but, on the other hand, it may contribute to more difficulty inserting because the needle tip will tend to blunt more easily.

Additionally, the silver needle cannot readily be sterilized. It cannot be heat- or autoclave-sterilized because these procedures tend to injure the needle. The silver also tends to tarnish, creating a non-silver coating which naturally has slightly different properties from the pure silver. Because of these properties and problems, the silver needle is used almost exclusively in the Tōyōhari root treatment procedures of supplementation where needles are either inserted to a very small depth or not at all. For the purposes of performing local or symptom control treatments, the silver needle is not very appropriate. The best method of sterilizing the silver needle is to use a gas sterilization system, such as ethylene dioxide gas; in the United States this usually requires access to a hospital sterilization center.

GOLD NEEDLES

Gold needles are probably the best for applying supplementation techniques because gold has very good supplementing properties. However, gold needles are expensive, very soft, more likely to cause injury (especially at the point), harder to insert, and cannot be heat- or autoclave-sterilized. Most practitioners today consider the disadvantages to outweigh the advantages, though many Keiraku Chiryō practitioners routinely use gold needles for root treatment. In Manaka's approaches, gold needles are recommended in some special treatments, such as the treatment of hepatitis.[2]

Gold and silver needles may be used together, especially on the extraordinary vessel master–coupled points as a form of "two-metal contact" or "minus-plus needle" therapy.[3] Gold needles can only be sterilized with the gas sterilization method, and are not recommended for the local or symptom control treatments except in a very specialized Tōyōhari method.[4]

GOLD-PLATED NEEDLES

Gold-plated needles are also available. They have the same problems with sterilization as gold needles, but are cheaper than the solid gold needles. In general, though, the gold is plated onto steel; thus you need to be careful about exceeding proper insertion depth.

[2]See K. Matsumoto and S. Birch, *Hara Diagnosis: Reflections on the Sea,* pp. 385-387.

[3]One practitioner we observed in Japan using these needles exclusively in this manner was Masahiro Nawafune of Kobe. Nawafune diagnosed and treated pairs of the extraordinary vessels exclusively, using only gold and silver needles.

[4]See K. Fukushima, *Meridan Therapy, A Hands-on Text for Traditional Japanese Hari Based on Pulse Diagnosis,* p. 238-243.

COPPER AND ZINC NEEDLES

Copper and zinc needles are used together based on their electro-chemical valence properties. Copper is relatively positive compared to zinc which is of negative electrochemical valence. When they are used together a small battery-like effect is thought to be produced which drives a small current and which has specific effects depending on the points selected for treatment. Copper needles are either made of solid copper or are electroplated. Solid copper needles are hard to use because copper is a soft metal and loses its point easily. The electroplated needles are better for insertion because the copper plating is on a stainless steel needle. Usually copper needles are used only in the "two-metal contact" or "minus-plus needle" methods along with zinc needles. The zinc needles are either solid or electroplated, like the copper; they have the same problems as the copper needles. These needles cannot be heat- or autoclave-sterilized; they require gas sterilization. These two needles are used together for root treatments, primarily of the extraordinary vessel master–coupled points.[5]

OTHER SPECIALIZED NEEDLES

Tin and tin-plated needles, molybdenum needles, cobalt needles, platinum and platinum-plated needles, and nickel alloy needles are other kinds of needles that are used in Japan. These specialized needles have very little literature pertaining to their use.

The properties of the different metals can, to some extent, be explained by an exploration of the electrochemical valency of the different metals. For instance, stainless steel needles are not used in the "two-metal contact" methods because different grades of steel have different electrochemical valency depending on the relative charge of the iron atoms in the steel. The table on page 45 shows some of the common metals and the relative valency.

The more positive metals have proven more effective for supplementing techniques, while the more negative metals are better for draining techniques. Based on these ideas and clinical experience, supplementation and draining techniques are enhanced by the use of the appropriate metals.

---

[5]See for example the treatments of Michi Tokitō described in K. Matsumoto and S. Birch, *Extraordinary Vessels*, pp. 143-157; and for local or symptom control treatments, see for example the work of Nagatomo in *Ibid.*, pp. 196-200. For the Tōyōhari treatment methods, see for example K. Fukushima, *Meridian Therapy: A Hands-on Text for Traditional Japanese Hari Based on Pulse Diagnosis*, pp. 243-250.

VALENCE	METAL
more negative	aluminum (AL)
	zinc (ZN)
	chromium (CR)
	ferrous iron (FEII)
	cobalt (CO)
	nickel (NI)
neutral	tin (SN)
	lead (PB)
	ferric iron (FEIII)
	copper (CU)
	silver (AG)
more positive	gold (AU)

TRADITIONAL NEEDLE USAGE AND MODERN ADAPTATIONS

Today, the most commonly used needle in the world is the *gōshin* or the filiform needle. The *zanshin, enshin, teishin,* and *enrishin* are used to varying degrees by some of the traditional schools such as the Keiraku Chiryō Association, the Meishin Association, the Tōyōhari Association, the Tōhō Association, and the Shinkyū Keiraku Kenkyū Kōshin Association. The *hōshin* is now adapted and used extensively around the world. Chapter 10 describes bloodletting methods which are now a specialty in Japan. The *hishin* is not so commonly used in acupuncture, at present primarily under the purview of the Western-trained physician. The *chōshin* and *taishin* needles are used, but again less commonly. Non-inserted needles, such as the *enshin, teishin,* and an adapted *zanshin* can be considered the basis for the practice of *shōnishin* pediatric acupuncture methods in Japan. In *shōnishin,* needles are usually not inserted, and a large number of different tools have been designed specifically for pediatric therapy.

In Japan there are practitioners who use these nine types of needles as part of their regular practice. These techniques are characteristic of Japanese practice, and as such distinguish it from acupuncture practice in other countries where the focus is on one or two of the nine types of needles. In fact, the term "acupuncture" tends to foment controversies among different schools because the practice of acupuncture in most parts of the world, following the Chinese tradition, relies on the use of needle insertion to accomplish therapy.

The term "acupuncture" may refer to either of two Japanese terms: *shin,* which is the same as the Chinese *zhen* and usually rendered as acupuncture, and *hari,* the traditional Japanese term for needle therapy. For some practitioners in Japan, the distinction between *shin* and *hari* is the distinction between acupuncture therapy and needle therapy. *Shin* has an obvious connotation of needle insertion, while *hari* does not have this implication. This is the distinction made by Tōyōhari practitioners in Japan, a traditional school of needling therapy, to distinguish their practice from other *shin*, "acu-*puncture*" practitioners.

The most commonly used needle is the stainless steel *gōshin* or filiform needle. These needles are usually mass-produced by companies that specialize in acupuncture needle manufacture, then either individually packaged and pre-sterilized or packaged in lots of fifty or one-hundred.[6]

The range of somewhat more specialized and therefore less popular needles such as gold and silver needles, copper and zinc needles, the *enshin, teishin, zanshin, chōshin,* and *taishin*, are manufactured by the companies mentioned above, but frequently these needles are made by hand in small workshops, often in the manufacturer's home. Examples of the smaller-scale companies that make hand-produced instruments are the workshops of the late Mr. Hirota Shiono and the Aoki Company.

THE ZANSHIN NEEDLE

The *Ling Shu* describes the *zanshin* as having a large head with a sharp tip that is inserted very shallowly to rid heat-evil at the surface of the skin. The structure of the needle makes it difficult and painful for insertion, thus its use in Japan has tended to follow non-insertion methods. Today, there are a variety of different *zanshin* type needles, many of which are used for the *shōnishin* methods. They are frequently made of brass, copper, or stainless steel.

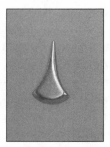

Yoneyama's copper *zanshin* used for *shōnishin*

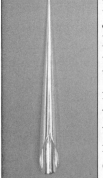

A conical *zanshin*

In some of the traditional schools of practice in Japan, notably the Tōyōhari and Shinkyū Keiraku Kenkyū Kōshin Associations, modified versions of the *zanshin* have been designed. The *zanshin* has been redesigned for more extensive uses that still focus on treatment at the surface of the skin. Silver, copper, and gold *zanshin* have been designed that are conically shaped and used with tapping, rubbing, or pressing methods. For example, we have observed the Arai brothers in Tokyo using the silver variety of this instrument very successfully to improve

---

[6]Some of the better known companies involved in needle production include Seirin, Idō no Nippon, Itō, and Maeda. Of these, Seirin is probably the best known. The quality of their needles is excellent.

circulation in a congested area, such as on the neck, and we use the instruments ourselves for the same purpose.

This particular instrument is hand-made by needle specialists such as Mr. Hirota Shiono of Tokyo whose craftsmanship was well known. It can be applied by tapping with the open end, as a mildly dispersive or draining and moving method. When correctly applied a slightly hollow cupping sound can be heard. This needle can be applied with more direct pressure, using the extended lip of the open end to press points, as a method of circulating qi in congested areas. It can also be used by holding the tapered end to the point for supplementation. This last method is used in the Tōyōhari approach but it requires considerable study to be able to use it successfully.

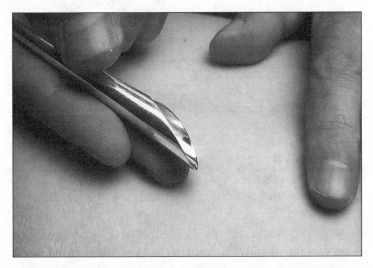

Grasp the conical silver *zanshin* with the thumb and two fingers.

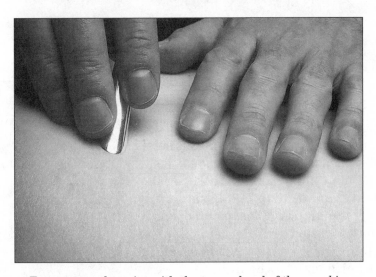

Tap or press the point with the tapered end of the *zanshin*.

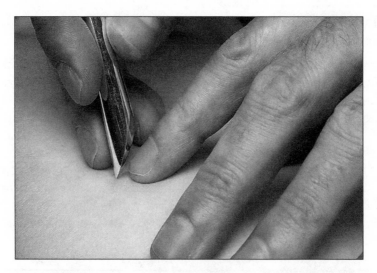

Pressing with the lip of the *zanshin* for qi circulation.

THE ENSHIN NEEDLE

The *enshin* is described in the *Ling Shu* as having a round tip shaped like an egg and is used by rubbing the skin to rid evil qi that is lodged at the flesh level and to improve blood and qi circulation at that level. The implication is that it is useful for promoting qi and blood flow and for ridding evil qi that is a little deeper than that removed by the *zanshin*. This needle is not inserted but used exclusively for rubbing and pressing methods. Typically made of stainless steel, various forms of this instrument exist in the *shōnishin* array of instruments.

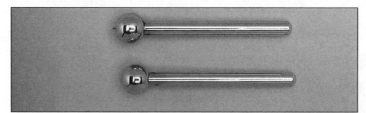

Stainless steel *enshin*

Like the *zanshin*, the *enshin* has also been redesigned for more extensive uses. There are stainless steel *enshin* with completely rounded heads or with rounded heads with a small blunt point. These needles are used to promote qi and blood flow by rubbing techniques. The pointed end is used for congested areas by using tapping-type techniques. Silver versions of the *enshin* also exist which have become favorite tools in a number of the Keiraku

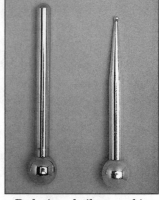

Redesigned silver *enshin*

Chiryō groups. The silver *enshin*, which is relatively popular in the Tōyōhari group, is used primarily on the back regions with long flowing strokes. Silver is by its nature more supplementing than stainless steel. (See discussions of this below.) The use of the silver *enshin* rubbed over a vacuous area is beneficial to increase qi and blood flow in that area. A simple and comfortable method to accomplish this technique for an adult patient is to hold the *enshin* between the thumb and fingers of the right hand. Stroke with long flowing strokes, but not too much pressure, down the bladder channels on the back. After each stroke, follow immediately by a similar stroke of the empty flat left hand. Apply this technique with around five strokes down each line. This improves the bladder channel flow and the tonus of the skin and underlying muscles. On children the techniques are different.

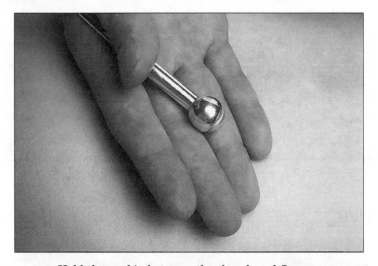

Hold the *enshin* between the thumb and fingers.

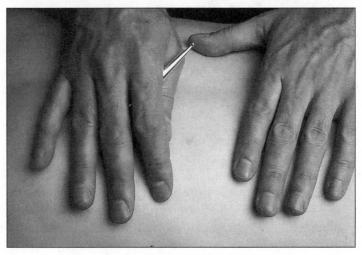

Stroke down the bladder channels,
followed by a similar stroke with the empty hand.

THE TEISHIN NEEDLE

The *teishin* needle is described in the *Ling Shu* as having a round but slightly sharp tip, like a grain of millet. It is not inserted, but is used to press and rub the channel to promote circulation of qi and blood. Care must be taken to not apply excessive pressure, otherwise the *zheng qi* (in Japanese, *sei ki*) will be injured. By using it at the five *shu* points (*jing, ying, shu, jing, he*), it can help promote channel circulation and strengthen and harmonize the blood vessels.

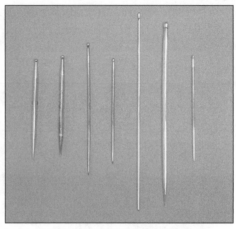

Teishin needles are quite popular in Japan, both in the *shōnishin* methods and in the traditional schools of practice. There are a number of different *teishin* needles. The most common are seen in the photo at right. These *teishin* are made of a variety of different metals, such as stainless steel, copper, brass, silver, gold, platinum, and brass with gold plating.

Various *teishin* needles.

Keiri Inoue invented a form of the *teishin* that gives a larger handle and has the *teishin* itself on a spring-loaded mechanism, so that it is easier to control the pressure applied to points.

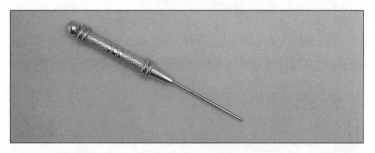

Keiri Inoue's spring-loaded *teishin*.

This particular instrument is useful also as an *enshin*, since, inverting the instrument, a stroking pressure technique can be applied with the rounded end. This instrument is commonly available in stainless steel, but a number of traditionally-oriented practitioners have silver or gold versions. The *teishin* instrument is used primarily for supplementation of qi and/or blood. Different practitioners in Japan have reported over the years that there are occasions where patients get worse with acupuncture, and that this is almost always due to overstimulation. Manaka, among others, thought that very sensitive patients sometimes cannot tolerate inserted needle techniques because they can easily overstimulate. In such cases, many practitioners recommend the use of non-insertion techniques, such as using the *teishin,* in order to stimulate the points more mildly. Manaka reported that in his experience patients who react poorly to treatments using inserted needle techniques almost always manifest vacuity of qi or blood.

Children are almost always more sensitive than adults. Because it is very important to control and regulate the amount of stimulation given when treating children, specialized *shōnishin* methods have evolved. The *teishin* is an important tool in the treatment of children. Non-insertion needle techniques are a specialty of certain groups, such as the Tōyōhari, Tōhō, and Shinkyū Keiraku Kenkyū Kōshin Associations, and are increasingly used in other meridian therapy groups as well. In these associations, the various *teishin* instruments are commonly used.

TECHNIQUES USING THE TEISHIN NEEDLE

We observed a number of different practitioners, including Kōdō Fukushima, Akihiro Takai, Shōzō Takahashi, and Tadashi Takemura, using the basic technique of supplementation with the *teishin.* A simple procedure is as follows:

Step One: Select the appropriate *shu* point for treatment, and locate the "live" point. Press the pads of the index finger and thumb of the left hand lightly together so that their juncture lies exactly over the "live" point. The ring formed by the forefinger and the thumb of the left hand is called the *oshide* (see pp. 65-68 for details.) When you press the pads of the forefinger and thumb, you should be careful not to press them too tightly and be careful not to apply much downward pressure with them.

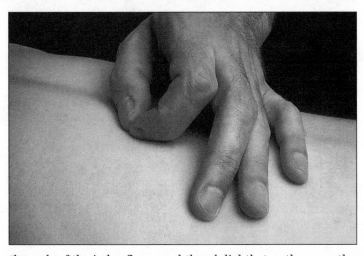

Press the pads of the index finger and thumb lightly together over the point.

Step Two: Next, introduce the rounded end of the *teishin* between the pads of the finger and thumb, slowly advancing it until its tip sits lightly and directly over the "live" point. The *teishin* should now be secured in the *oshide* of the left hand.

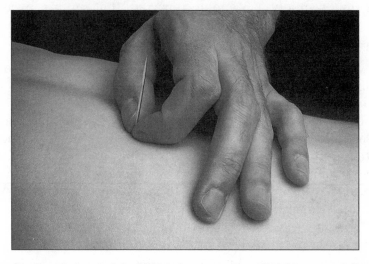

Place the rounded end of the *teishin* between the pads of finger and thumb.

Step Three: Using the right hand, apply very light stroking of the handle of the *teishin* until you feel the qi arrive at the point.

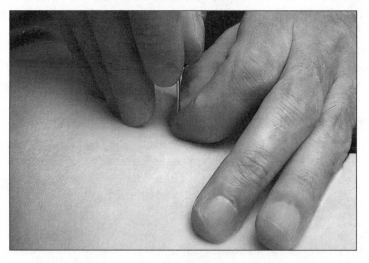

Lightly stroke the handle of the *teishin*.

Step Four: Then remove the *teishin* with the right hand very quickly, simultaneously closing the point with the finger or thumb of the left hand.

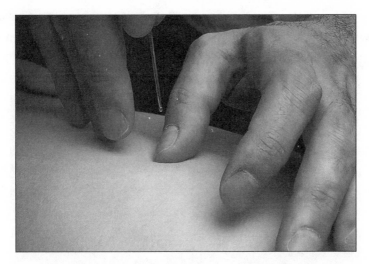

Quickly remove the *teishin* and close the point
with the finger or thumb of the opposite hand.

The removal of the *teishin* and closure of the point should be almost simultaneous; this prevents any leakage of qi. Although this sounds simple, it is actually a very sophisticated and difficult technique requiring many hours of practice to be able to reproduce results repeatedly and reliably. When done correctly, marked improvements in the radial pulses can be noted. This technique is applied in place of regular needles to supplement a vacuous channel diagnosed using yin-yang or five-phase methods. This is one of the techniques used in Tōyōhari.

This method represents the basic supplementation technique using the *teishin*. It is possible to use the *teishin* for draining evil qi, too. The method involves supplementing the qi of the channel so that it becomes strong enough to expel the evil qi. This is a complex technique.[7]

A simpler method, described by Manaka, is that of pressing the acupoint with some degree of pressure so that the *teishin* elicits a slight amount of discomfort and then quickly removing the *teishin* from the point. The left hand does not hold the *teishin*. Rather the right hand quickly presses and releases pressure on the selected point. We observed Mr. Takemura of the Shinkyū Keiraku Kenkyū Kōshin Association using the *teishin* extensively in his practice, both for supplementation and draining techniques. For pain conditions, he applied relatively strong pressure with the *teishin* for somewhat longer periods of time.

There are other *teishin* instruments that only the specialist uses. Mr. Shiono of Tokyo manufactured a dazzling array of *teishin*

[7]For details of this technique, see K. Fukushima, *Meridian Therapy: A Hands-on Text for Traditional Japanese Hari Based on Pulse Diagnosis.*

instruments. Some come with a gold *teishin* at one end of a *zan-shin,* while others are double-ended *teishin,* gold at one end and silver at the other.

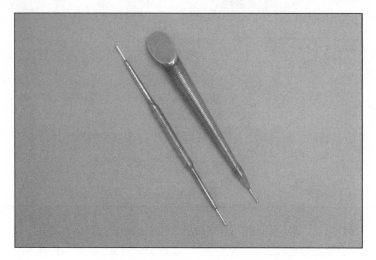

Specialized *teishin* instruments.

A common method of using the *teishin* instrument, usually employing the simpler form seen in the first set of pictures (p. 50) is to use it for locating points exactly. With this method, the exact point locations are determined by looking for distinctive pressure pain. This instrument is very helpful for determining point locations on the auricles and specialized Korean hand points, but this does not constitute treatment.

THE CHŌSHIN NEEDLE

The *chōshin* needle is described in the *Ling Shu* as having a sharp tip, like a halberd, with a long thin body. This needle is inserted to remove chronic *bi* conditions and to treat deeper level diseases. According to Bunkei Ono, it is primarily used to treat deeper level pain conditions or conditions of paralysis or numbness, but it can also be used for supplementation techniques. Pain that is related to a deeper-level evil qi condition likes to be touched and is relieved by pressure. Such pain can respond well to *chōshin* treatment.

The needle is applied horizontally, almost flat to the skin, but it can be applied up to a ninety degree angle. When used with horizontal insertion, the needle is often inserted a considerable length along the needle shaft but because of the angle of insertion, it lies only shallowly in the body. When applied thus, it should be retained usually about one to two minutes (long enough for the qi and blood to arrive). Needles of varying gauges to a length of 5 to 10 *cun* are used. Ono recommends the following treatments as illustrations of the uses of *chōshin* treatment.

ONO'S RECOMMENDED USES FOR CHŌSHIN NEEDLES

Sciatica — GB-30

For sciatica, use a wide gauge (greater than number 10 gauge,) seven *cun* needle. Insert the needle at GB-30 horizontally, threading it down towards the foot. Leave it inserted for some time (longer than 1 or 2 minutes,) before removing.

Paralysis of lower limbs — ST-36 or GB-34

For paralysis of the lower limbs insert a number 10 gauge, 5 *cun* needle at ST-36 or GB-34 horizontally, threading it towards the feet. Leave the needle again for a while before removing it.

Back pain — Bladder channel

For back pain, insert a number 5 gauge, 3 *cun* needle horizontally along the bladder channel, angled down towards the legs. Remove after a couple of minutes.

Ono remarks that this is a specialized method that should not be used often on a patient, and not many needles should be used. After removing the needle, the point of insertion should be rubbed very well.

THE TAISHIN NEEDLE

The *taishin* needle is described in the *Ling Shu* as having a "stick-like" slightly dull tip, used for removing water stagnation at the joints, e.g., water on the knee. The *taishin* tends to be a thick needle, and according to Ono can range in length from 2 to 5 cun. Typically, the longer *taishin* needles are thicker. They can be used for both supplementation or draining methods and are used almost exclusively on the knees or lumbar region. The *taishin* or "large needle" was renamed the *fa zhen* or "fire needle" by later authors, such as Yang Ji-Zhou, author of the *Zhen Jiu Da Cheng* (1601), implying that the *taishin* needle was also being used as a fire needle (probably because it is the most suitable for this purpose given its wide gauge). A fire needle is one that is heated until red hot, and then rapidly inserted and withdrawn from the point. The fire needle technique is used today in China for rheumatic conditions, especially with edemic swellings. Manaka was observed using it on occasion.

Ono describes the supplementation method as appropriate for conditions of severe vacuity. The technique involves rapidly inserting the needle somewhat shallowly to the point, waiting until the qi is gathered, then slowly and very carefully removing the needle, making sure to close the hole. Ono comments that it is important not to cause unnecessary pain with the needle. In order to prevent this, it is important that the practitioner be very centered, breathing deeply from the lower *dantian* area on the abdomen.

The draining *taishin* method is used for significantly replete, stagnated local areas. The needle should be inserted quickly as with the supplementation method, then after the qi arrives, it should be quickly removed in order to release the evil qi.

ONO'S RECOMMENDED USES FOR TAISHIN NEEDLES

Water on the knee, with swollen knees

Use number 9 gauge, 2 *cun* needles. Insert them to two or three pressure pain points on the painful swollen region. The needles should not be inserted too deeply, and the draining method should be employed.

Vacuity and coldness of the lumbar region

Very thick needles, greater than gauge number 10 needles, 3 *cun* long, should be inserted to one or two points in the weakest, most vacuous area in the region. Leave the needles for some time (probably until the areas around the needles are quite reddened). Then remove the needle, slowly, quietly, and carefully in the supplementation method.

Ono comments that with the *taishin* method, it is important to remember that this is a specialized technique, and one not to be used very often. Care must be taken to ensure that the supplementation or draining methods are used appropriately. Usually the posture and breath of the practitioner are quite important.

THE GŌSHIN NEEDLE

In Japan the *gōshin* or filiform needle method is the most commonly used needle technique. This is the same the world around, with most acupuncturists using inserted filiform needle techniques.

What distinguishes the Japanese approach in the use of the filiform needles from approaches used in China and therefore in many other places is that in Japan the needles tend to be thinner, and are almost always inserted using a *shinkan* or insertion tube. Often the needles are only very shallowly inserted, and sometimes are not actually inserted at all, and there is a greater variety in the types of needles available.

While many practitioners around the world now use insertion or guide tubes to aid in the insertion of needles, these tubes were invented in Japan in the late 1600s by the renowned blind acupuncturist, Waichi Sugiyama, who, because of this invention, is often thought of as the father of modern acupuncture in Japan. Almost all Japanese acupuncturists use some form of insertion tube to assist in the insertion of needles. Thus to describe the *gōshin* technique requires that we describe needle sizes and the uses of the insertion tube as well.

Needle Sizes

The most commonly used needle lengths are probably the 1 *cun*, 1.3 *cun* and 1.6 *cun* length needles, with the 0.5 *cun*, 0.8 *cun*, 2 *cun*, 2.5 *cun* and 3 *cun* and longer needles also being used on occasion. Today needle lengths are usually given in millimeters. The 1 *cun* needle is the 30mm needle, the 1.3 *cun* is the 40mm needle, and the 1.6 *cun* is the 50mm needle. The gauges of needles used are seen in the following table:

NUMBER	DIAMETER	Chinese Equivalent
00 gauge	0.12mm	
0 gauge	0.14mm	
1 gauge	0.16mm	
2 gauge	0.18mm	36 gauge
3 gauge	0.20mm	
4 gauge	0.22mm	34 gauge
5 gauge	0.24mm	
6 gauge	0.26mm	32 gauge
7 gauge	0.28mm	
8 gauge	0.30mm	30 gauge
9 gauge	0.32mm	
10 gauge	0.34mm	28 gauge
15 gauge	0.46mm	26 gauge
20 gauge	0.60mm	24 gauge

In Japan, the most commonly used gauges of needles are the number 3 and the number 5 needle. The thinner number 3 needle is the most commonly used. In the root treatment patterns of Manaka, the number 2 or number 3 needle is used in Step One, with the ion-pumping cords, and number 3 needles used for Step Two and most other needling procedures. In the Keiraku Chiryō root treatment patterns, numbers 00, 0, 1, 2, or 3 are used; many practitioners do not use needles thicker than the number 1 gauge needle.

Comparatively, the most commonly used Chinese width of needle is the Chinese number 32 (Japanese gauge number 6) although many practitioners use the number 30 (Japanese number 8.) There is a clear difference in the thickness of needles used.

INSERTION TUBES

The same diversity in size and variety of needles can be found in the variety of insertion tubes available.

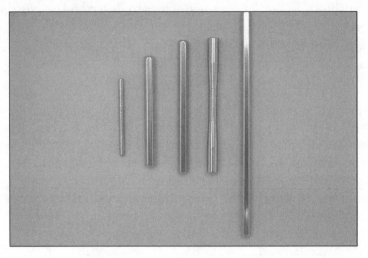

Various metal insertion tubes.

For the insertion tube to be effective, it must be slightly shorter than the needle with which it is used. This difference of length allows a portion of the needle that can be inserted with a tap of the needle handle.

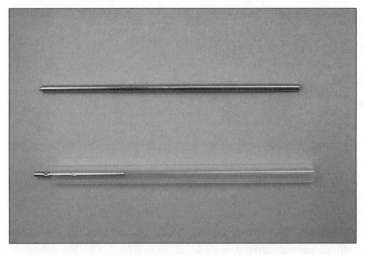

The needle handle extends beyond the length of the insertion tube.

Without a length of the needle protruding beyond the tube, the needle cannot be tapped through the skin to reach the subcutaneous layers. The length of the tube will depend on the length of the needle chosen.

Part of the reason for the Japanese preference for thinner needles has to do with the use of the insertion tube, which provides a mechanical support for the needle and allows for relative ease of insertion. Tapping on the exposed needle handle causes the needle point to pass out of the tube and through the skin in a smooth motion. Without the tube, a thinner needle would bend, rather than pierce the skin.

Another reason for the use of thinner needles lies, of course, in the clinical effects that can be obtained. Using the *gōshin* needling and a thinner needle has allowed for refinements and subtleties in techniques. There are many practitioners who use the filiform needle, but do not actually insert the needle. Instead, they use the insertion tube as a guide in point location.

The following pictures show different needle types with different handles, and different insertion tubes, including the glass and plastic tubes.

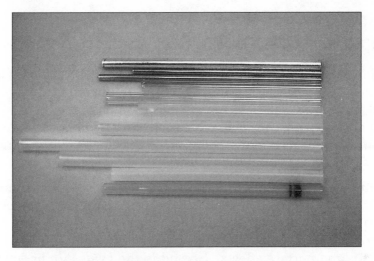

Various metal, glass, and plastic insertion tubes.

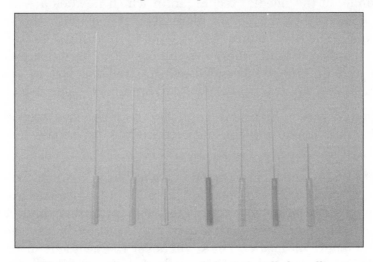

Various lengths and gauges of plastic-handled needles.

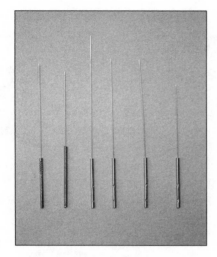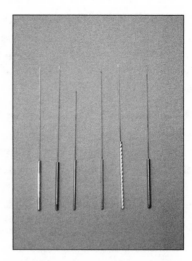

Various metal-handled needles

BASIC PROCEDURES FOR FILIFORM NEEDLING WITH INSERTION TUBE

It is important to emphasize that mastery of the basic uses of the insertion tube and needle must precede the mastery of any more complex technical methods. Learning these uses and techniques is a major emphasis in the education of students in Japanese acupuncture schools; many hours are spent developing certain levels of skill in needle and tube use.

Our essential focus here is on three types of needle techniques. The first is the *chishin* or "leaving" needle technique in which needles are shallowly inserted, not manipulated and not stimulated, and are left in the points for a specified number of minutes in order to obtain appropriate effects. Second is the *kyūtōshin* or "moxa on the handle of the needle" technique in which needles are inserted perpendicularly to the points more deeply than with the *chishin* technique. The needles are then heated by burning a ball of moxa on the handles. Finally there are the basic traditional supplementation and draining techniques, which are essential to the root treatment steps of the Keiraku Chiryō treatment approach.

None of these treatment methods or approaches are possible without first mastering the basic techniques of needle and tube usage.

Usually the needle is inserted to a depth of 1 to 5mm. The average depth of insertion is generally 2 to 3mm. Since the needle is usually inserted at an acute angle to the point, rather than perpendicular to the point, the actual depth of insertion is less than the inserted length of needle. Thus, whenever the needle is inserted at an angle to the point, the actual depth of insertion is almost always very shallow. With perpendicular insertions as used in the *kyūtōshin* approach, the needle is first inserted as far as the tube will allow, and then manipulated and inserted to the appropriate depth.

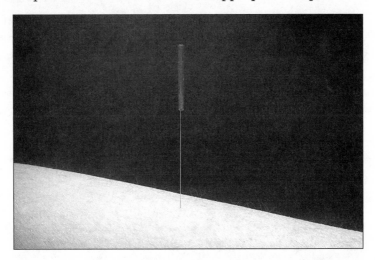

Perpendicular insertion.

When needles are inserted at sensitive points, such as SP-2 or KI-1, it is advisable to insert at a perpendicular angle to the point in order to reduce the sensation of insertion. With these perpendicular insertions the depth of insertion is usually only as far as the initial insertion. These shallow insertions, either at acute or perpendicular angles, leave the needle loosely inserted in the body. Usually the needle will lay flat to the skin or hang loosely at the point.

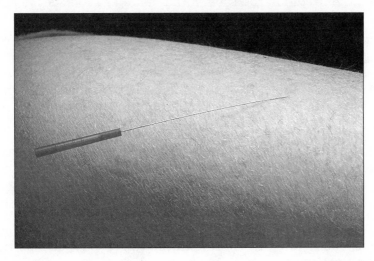

Shallow acute angle insertion causing the needle to lay flat to the skin.

If the needle is standing up on its own at whatever angle it was inserted, it is probably inserted too deeply.

The needle insertion is accomplished by tapping the needle handle lightly so that the needle point is pushed out the other end of the tube. There are a number of techniques and details, which, if carefully attended to, will allow for easy, painless insertions to the required depths.

To use the tube correctly, place the needle in the tube, handle first. Allow the needle to slip down the tube far enough that the point of the needle is just inside the tube and the needle handle is far enough back that it can be held in place by the application of pressure by the forefinger on the needle handle against the tube.

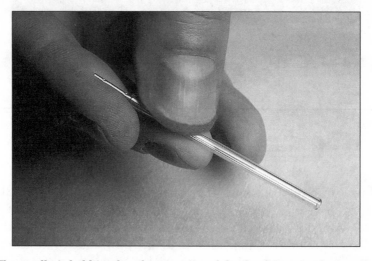

The needle is held in place by pressure of the forefinger on the handle.

The needle and tube are held in one hand, usually the right. Holding the needle in the tube in this manner protects the point of the needle and retains the needle ready for placement on the acupoint. It is important to not place the needle point-first into the tube because of the risk of inflicting self-injury or damaging the point by hitting the tube with the needle's point. This latter issue is a particular problem when using needles made of soft metals such as silver and gold or when using very thin needles (#1 or less gauge).

When you place the tube with the needle inside it on the chosen acupuncture point, it is important that the needle be retracted inside the tube. Were the point to protrude slightly out of the tube, you would involuntarily jab the patient when you place the tube.

In Japan the technique of placing the needle handle first into the tube, and holding the needle in the tube ready for insertion, is accomplished with one hand. This technique is strongly recommended because of the emphasis on palpation for locating reactive points with pressure pain or other unusual sensitivities. One-hand needle placement frees the other hand for palpating, locating, and fixing the acupoint to be treated. The following pictures show the usual method for accomplishing this technique.

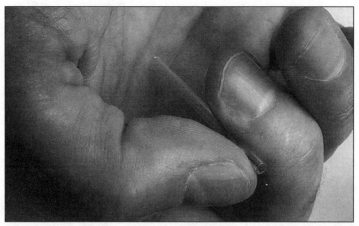

The tube should be held with one end supported in the palm of the hand, the other end free.

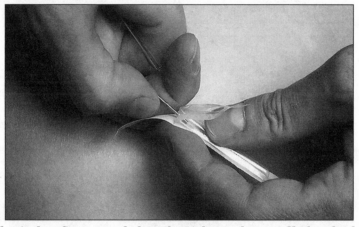

With the index finger and thumb, pick up the needle by the handle, place the tip of the handle at the entrance of the tube and release it, allowing the needle to fall handle first into the tube.

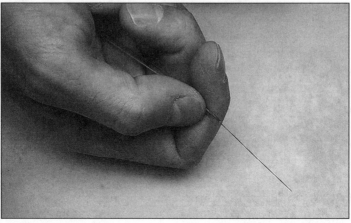

Holding the hand parallel to the ground, turn the tube between the fingers and thumb, so that the end of the tube that was against the palm is now held between the between the index finger and thumb.

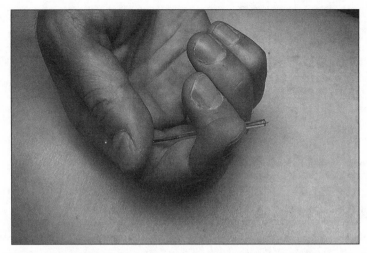

Then tilt the tube back so that the needle handle falls out slightly and can be pressed by the index finger against the tube.

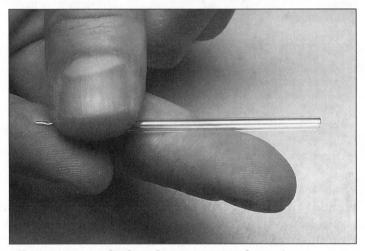

The needle is now ready for placement on the point.

This technique is useful when utilizing needles that come in a package without individual insertion tubes, such as autoclaved needles, single needles in presterilized packages, and silver or gold needles. However, many needles, especially the disposable needles, are already packaged in the insertion tubes, which makes these procedures unnecessary. If the needle you are using is not already placed inside a tube, you may use both hands to place the needle in the insertion tube, though the method described above is preferable.

Whatever technique of placement of the needle in the tube you use, it is important to retain the needle sterility by not touching the body of the needle with your fingers.

While picking up the needle and placing it in the tube, or picking up the already prepared needle and tube, the other hand should be searching for the point indicated. As we have already described, the acupuncture point to be treated almost always shows some kind of palpable response.

Finding and fixing the exact point location takes skill and practice. Often beginners will lose the point once they remove their fingers from it. Because of this, training in Japan emphasizes the importance of the using the fingerpads to locate, then fix or hold the point. Usually the fingers of the right hand hold the needle and tube while the fingers of the left hand locate the point. Whatever your preference, we recommend that you always use the same pattern of holding and locating. If you maintain a standard procedure, each hand will more quickly attain proficiency.

STEPLIST FOR LOCATING THE POINT AND INSERTING THE NEEDLE

1. Using your left hand, locate, fix, and ready the point for needling.

2. Prepare the point thoroughly by wiping it with a moist alcohol swab. (Make sure that the fingers of your left hand which are touching the point and tube—the index finger and thumb—are also thoroughly wiped by an alcohol swab. Correct clean needle techniques must be observed.)

3. Palpate the point to determine the exact location to needle. Usually you will find the point under the pad or tip of the index finger.

4. Make an *oshide* (a ring shape formed by the joining of the pads of the index finger and thumb) over the point. The *oshide* can be circular or semi-circular, either a "full-moon" or "half-moon" shape, whichever is easier and more comfortable for you.

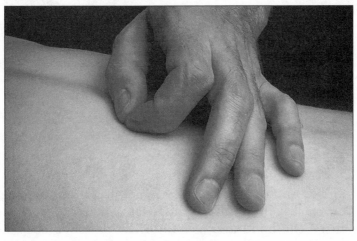

The *oshide.*

The *oshide* serves two basic functions. First, it fixes the precise point location by aligning it exactly below the crevice between the pads of the finger and thumb.

Secondly, the surface between the finger and thumb becomes a guide for the tube and needle, directing them to the point and holding them securely at the point.

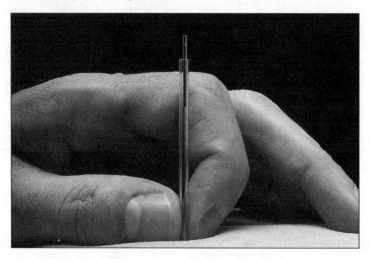

The finger and thumb act as a guide for the tube and needle.

This stabilizing aspect is further enhanced by spreading the remaining three fingers of the left hand upon the patient's skin surface, thereby securing the hand. On the limbs, this will mean lightly grasping that surface body area with those fingers.

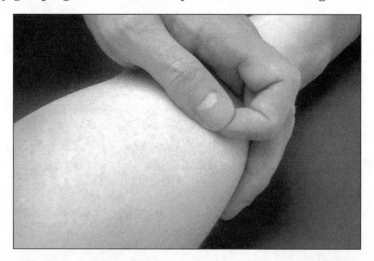

Use the thumb, pointer, and index fingers to stabilize the needle and tube.

It is important that the *oshide* is stable and unmoving. If it moves, the exact point location will be lost. In addition, if you have not stabilized the hand and *oshide* to the patient's body, and the patient moves, either involuntarily because of nervousness or because of poor needle technique startling the patient, then the needle can be inserted in the wrong point, or can jab and irritate the point. In some schools, the *oshide* is an essential structure. In the Tōyōhari school, for example, developing and refining the skill of the *oshide* can take years.

For basic needling techniques with the insertion tube and needle, such levels of development are not necessary. However, there are a few pointers about the *oshide* which can help improve the quality of your practice. Acupuncture is essentially concerned with affecting the qi and channels of your patients so as to restore a more balanced level of functioning. Bunkei Ono stated rather wisely, "The most important aspect of acupuncture is to always remember that everything we do is dealing with qi." Anything you can do to facilitate the movement of qi while needling can be helpful at that point. Allowing your own qi to flow smoothly will usually aid in the transfer and movement of qi in the patient.

Facilitating this requires that you have no tension in your own body while needling. Your *oshide* should be relaxed and not tight; hands, wrists, arms, elbows, shoulders, and neck should be relaxed. The feet should be stable and you should be relaxed in the lower half of your body. To achieve this, center on every point that you are needling so that the point lies directly in front of your abdomen, with your feet slightly apart, knees slightly bent and relaxed, low back straight but not stiff, and breathing focused to the lower abdomen. The *oshide* should be linked to your breath and your lower abdomen.

If this all sounds rather far-fetched and fanciful, or perhaps rather easy, be assured that only careful repetitive practice will allow you to do this appropriately. Surely, the mechanisms of treatment will work without having to pay attention to these details. But these details are the art of the technique; they add extra depth and dimension to the treatment. If every point needled on every patient were done with these techniques in mind, the active engagement of the patient's qi would facilitate much greater clinical results.

To quote the *Nan Jing* (Chapter 78), "Those who know how to apply the needle rely on their left hand; those who do not know how to apply the needle rely on their right hand." The *oshide* is the technical name for the role of the left hand. Aside from locating and securing the point to be treated, the left hand has the role of feeling the "arrival of the qi."

This is very different from modern Chinese acupuncture, where patients are asked if they feel the arrival of the qi (the so-called *deqi*.) We are not looking for this *deqi* sensation, where the patient reports "dull, achy, distended" sensations. Rather, we are looking for something much more subtle–a pulsing, a vitality, or an increased luster that can be detected beneath or in your *oshide*. If you are interested in practicing traditional acupuncture according to the principles described in the *Nan Jing,* detecting this arrival of the qi is a very important aspect of practice. This skill, this art, can be learned, but only over time and only with careful, attentive, repetitive practice. In Japan, we have observed that the Tōyōhari school has mastered and developed techniques for routinely teaching and acquiring this kind of sensitivity and refined technique.

Traditionally, points to be needled should be prepared prior to insertion of the needle. Preparation usually involves the use of some kind of rubbing or pressing techniques, applied by the left hand. This preparation may take a variety of different forms. For instance, for supplementation, Chapter 27 of the *Su Wen* tells us:

> *Rub the point lightly, then harder, then tap or flick the point with your finger to stimulate the point. With your fingernail, press the point slightly, then with finger and thumb, pinch up the skin slightly. This all serves to close the shen. As the patient completes an exhalation, insert the needle.*

For draining techniques, Chapter 76 of the *Nan Jing* tells us:

> *When putting the needle into the ying, using the left hand, rub the point to disperse the qi, then insert the needle.*

There are other descriptions such as these, but all agree that rubbing the point in a variety of ways can be important in preparing the point for insertion. This preparation serves not only to protect the various kinds of qi flowing across the body surface, but it also helps to relax the underlying tissues, thus allowing for greater ease of needle insertion. This is especially important on body areas where the needle is to be inserted into points overlying stiff, tight muscles, particularly if you are using deeper needle insertions, as in the *kyūtōshin* method.

With the correct point chosen, the *oshide* placed, and the needle in the tube poised at the point within the *oshide,* insertion is the next step. The *oshide* should secure and hold the tube and needle on the point.

Pay attention to several important details as you prepare to insert the needle.

•Make sure that the needle is not caught inside the tube and that you insert the point of the needle firmly but painlessly. If the needle is slightly bent, a problem may occur. Sometimes when using the plastic-handled needles, the small bump of plastic where the needle and tube were joined during the manufacturing process can catch inside the tube.

•When you release the needle in the tube (by removing the pressure of your right index finger that is holding the protruding needle handle), the needle should slip into the tube.

•To make sure that the tip of the needle is firmly on the point to be treated, very lightly stroke the needle handle with your right index finger. This helps the needle tip to adhere to the point.

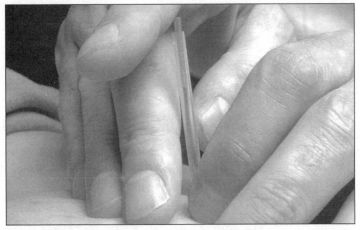

Lightly stroke the needle handle with the index finger.

•When you tap the needle handle, if the needle tip is not touching the treatment point the patient may feel discomfort immediately prior to and during insertion. The needle can jab and on occasion bounce or give increased resistance to the insertion. If the needle tip is already touching the skin, there will be a smooth insertion through the skin when you tap the needle. The insertion is accomplished by several light taps of the right forefinger on the protruding portion of the needle handle.

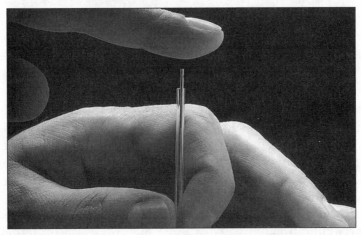

Apply several light taps with the forefinger on the protruding needle handle.

The tapping can be applied with the fingerpad or more proximally along the finger, around the middle joint.

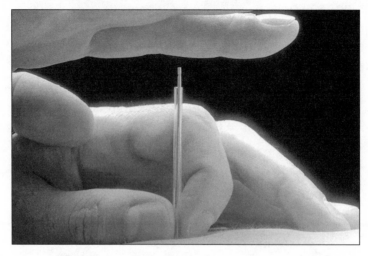

Tapping can be applied more proximally along the finger, around the middle joint.

The force of the tap and therefore the relative depth of insertion decreases as you tap closer to the knuckle, allowing finer and finer control over the initial depth of insertion.

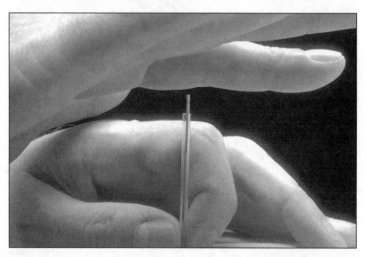

Closer to the knuckle the force of the tapping decreases.

The tube functions to hold the needle on the acupoint, and to keep it straight enough that it will insert without bending. When the needle is tapped, it should insert effortlessly. It is usually better not to tap the needle handle so hard that you tap the tube itself. On some points this can cause unnecessary discomfort. To achieve the best insertions effortlessly and painlessly, remember to keep the left fingers and hand loose and flexible. If you are stiff or tight when inserting a needle, the stiffness tends to transmit to the needle body, and will usually cause some discomfort on insertion.

There are some points, such as KI-1, SI-3, and SP-4, where the thickness of the skin and/or the sensitivity of the points can easily contribute to discomfort when inserting the needle. On such points it is better to tap the needle with a single, firmer blow than to tap with several lighter blows. The difference between the lighter and firmer blows is the degree of control you have over the actual depth of insertion of the needle; lighter taps allow you more control.

Another method of dealing with the more sensitive points is to insert the needle perpendicular to the skin, rather than to insert at acute angles. The general angle of insertion at most acupuncture points tends to be in the direction of the flow of the channels, but for points that are more difficult to needle, or the more sensitive points, it is better to use perpendicular insertions. Points such as GB-20 on the base of the occiput are difficult to needle in a channel-pointing direction; thus perpendicular insertion is generally applied.

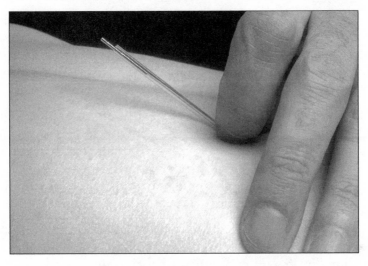

Holding the tube and needle at an angle.

The tube and needle can be held directly perpendicular to the point, or at a variety of different angles. Most of the acute angle needle insertions are done in the 10–20 degree range, that is, almost flat to the skin.

Depending on the point chosen for insertion, the angle of insertion, and the purposes of the insertion, you can adjust the actual depth of insertion with tapping techniques. Generally the needle handle protrudes about 2 to 3mm beyond the end of the insertion tube.

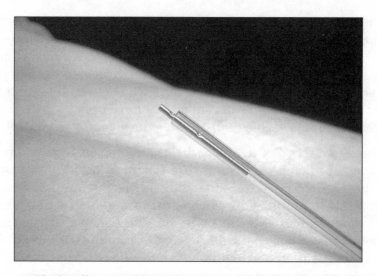

The handle protrudes 2-3mm beyond the end of the tube.

At an ideal depth of insertion, the needle is about half the distance between the end of the needle handle and insertion tube (1 to 1.5mm). This takes the needle deeper than the pain-sensitive layers of the skin but is shallow enough that you can still control the technique.

When inserting the needle at an acute angle to the point, the needle handle may occasionally protrude less than required out of the top of the tube. In such cases you will need to adjust the length of needle handle inserted and thus the depth of insertion so that the needle still enters to around 1.5mm. This might require tapping the needle more than half the length protruding beyond the top of the tube.

Were you to insert deeper on every point, the needle would often be too deeply inserted to administer the appropriate manipulations to the needle. On most points where perpendicular insertions are used (such as some of the more sensitive points or points where deeper insertions are to be used), tap in the needle as far as the tube will allow, but do not tap the tube too hard. In these cases, you will find that the needle tends to be inserted initially to a depth of around 3mm.

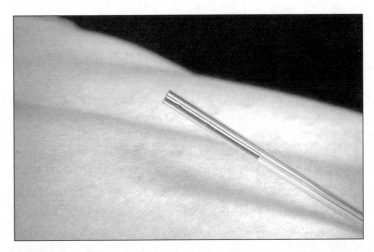

Initial insertion depth of 2-3mm brings the handle level with the tube.

Another technique that can be adjusted to compensate for reactions on the more sensitive points is to vary the amount of downward pressure your *oshide* is applying to the tube prior to and during the insertion of the needle. Usually, the amount of pressure is light, with very little obvious depression of the skin; but with more sensitive points, a firmer downward pressure is helpful because it helps distract the patient from the insertion and stretches the skin more, thereby allowing easier insertion.

Reducing the sensation for the patient can also be accomplished by inserting the needle during the patient's exhalation. For very sensitive patients, instruct them to draw a deep breath and focus on the exhalation; insert the needle during exhalation. The patient's concentration on exhalation helps distract awareness of the sensation of the needle. Inserting a needle on the exhalation is part of the supplementation technique and is usually appropriate.

This whole maneuver is a relatively delicate operation but one easily mastered with practice. It accomplishes needle insertion painlessly and to the appropriate depth. With the light tapping, you have considerable control over the initial depth of insertion. This is important especially in the supplementation and draining techniques.

Always be careful and attentive when inserting a needle to ensure that needle sterility is not lost and to ensure that the correct initial needle depth and angle of insertion are attained. With practice, needle insertion can be accomplished without any discomfort to the patient. Number 3 or number 2 needles are generally used, although on occasion numbers 1 and 2 are used for some techniques or for very sensitive patients. Usually the needles are inserted only enough that they will remain in the point without standing up; they fall or flop over because the insertion is only subcutaneous.

With the exception of techniques such as the *kyūtōshin* method where the needle must be inserted more deeply, or the supplementation and draining techniques, once inserted the needle is manipulated very little if at all.

For most of the insertions required in the approaches described in this text, once the needle has been inserted, the tube should be carefully removed, leaving the needle resting in the point. Certainly for the root treatment methods of Manaka, where needles are inserted and the ion-pumping cords attached, this is all that is necessary.

For the traditional techniques of supplementation and draining, further manipulations are often required. In such cases, insert the needle to the required depth, and remove the tube carefully.

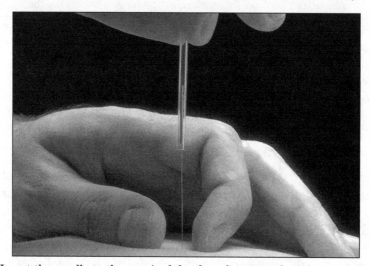

Insert the needle to the required depth and remove the tube carefully.

Then begin to manipulate the needle. Grasp the needle delicately. Support the needle both at the skin and at the handle.

The *oshide* should close over the needle close to the skin, and the needle handle should be held with the index finger and thumb of the right hand in order to administer the appropriate manipulations.

Clean needle technique requires that sterile cotton be used. When holding the needle body near the skin, hold the sterile cotton in the left hand, grasped between the index finger and thumb. With practice, this technique is easily mastered. It is better if the piece of cotton is not too thick because this will hamper your ability to manipulate the needle and feel responses in the *oshide*.

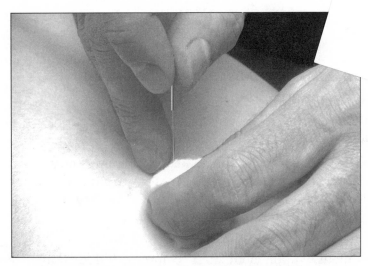

Hold sterile cotton with the index finger and thumb.

Manipulate the needle lightly and delicately with the right hand.

SUPPLEMENTATION AND DRAINING TECHNIQUES[8]

Supplementing techniques from the traditional literature include the following methods:

- Insert the needle at an angle in the direction of flow of the channel treated. (*Ling Shu*, Chapter 1)

- Insert the needle on the exhalation and remove on the inhalation. (*Su Wen*, Chapter 27)

- Insert the needle shallowly first (about 1 to 2mm) obtaining the qi. Then insert a little deeper (to about 3 to 4mm). (*Nan Jing*, Chapter 76)

- Place the finger over the point immediately upon removal of the needle from the point. (*Su Wen*, Chapter 27; *Ling Shu*, Chapter 1)

- Insert the needle so that it is completely painless—literally so that it is like a mosquito bite. (*Ling Shu*, Chapter 1)

- Use silver or gold needles rather than stainless steel needles. (A modern adaptation)

Draining techniques from the traditional literature include the following methods:

- Insert the needle at an angle contrary to the direction of flow of the channel. (*Ling Shu*, Chapter 1)

---

[8]See K. Matsumoto and S. Birch, *Five Elements and Ten Stems*, pp. 160-164, and D. Shūdo, *Japanese Classical Acupuncture: Introduction to Meridian Therapy*, pp. 179-184 for more details.

•Insert the needle on the inhalation and withdraw it on the exhalation. (*Su Wen,* Chapter 27)

•Press the point before inserting in order to protect the more superficial qi. (*Nan Jing,* Chapter 76)

•Insert the needle a little deeper first (to about 3 to 4mm), and obtain the qi. Then withdraw the needle slightly to a shallower depth (about 1 to 2mm.) (*Nan Jing,* Chapter 76)

•Do not close or press the point upon removal of the needle. Sometimes you can stretch the skin around the point in order to reinforce the draining effect. (*Su Wen,* Chapter 27; *Ling Shu,* Chapter 1)

•If draining and supplementing are desired in the same treatment, supplement first before using draining techniques. (*Nan Jing,* Chapter 69)

Stainless steel needles are used in supplementation and draining techniques, but more typically for draining techniques, because of the qualities of stainless steel. However, if properly applied, very thin stainless steel needles can be used successfully for supplementation. Some authors recommend this.[9]

These are basic supplementation and draining techniques, including some techniques for correct needle withdrawal. However, these techniques are infrequently used in general needling of points. They are most important when implementing the root treatment parts of the Keiraku Chiryō treatment style. [10]

For general needling techniques, we recommend using the following methods:

•Wherever possible, insert the needle in the direction of the channel flow at about a 10- to 20-degree angle. On more sensitive points, perpendicular insertion is often preferable.

•Insert the needle on the patient's exhalation; you can also time this procedure with your own exhalation.

•Try to insert the needle painlessly at all points. Ensure that the needle tip is touching the point before tapping the needle handle. Tap the handle with several light blows

---

[9]See, for example, D. Shūdo, *Japanese Classical Acupuncture, Introduction to Meridian Therapy,* p. 187.

[10]For a basic-level of detail necessary to practice this style of needling, see K. Matsumoto and S. Birch, *Five Elements and Ten Stems;* D. Shūdo, *Introduction to Meridian Therapy;* and for more advanced needle descriptions, K. Fukushima, *Meridian Therapy: A Hands-on Text for Traditional Japanese Hari Based on Pulse Diagnosis.*

unless it is on a sensitive point in which case you can use a single heavier blow. Apply a little downward pressure with the insertion tube and a little heavier pressure on more sensitive points. Ensure that you are relaxed and centered on the point before inserting the needle.

•Cover the hole immediately upon removal of the needle from the point. This is best achieved with the use of a dry cotton ball placed over the point as the needle is withdrawn.

•Usually needles can be retained 10 to 20 minutes. However, in the root treatment patterns, the time is dependent on the treatment method and the response of the patient. When using the ion-pumping cords, the needles and cords should be retained no more than twenty minutes, almost always around ten minutes. When applying the Keiraku Chiryō root treatment pattern with supplementation and draining techniques, the needles can be retained until the correct pulse changes occur and there is a decrease in the reactions of the points which were used diagnostically. Sometimes the length of time of manipulation can be very brief— perhaps a matter of seconds up to 1 to 2 minutes; or sometimes a little longer, up to 5 to 10 minutes. The length of manipulation is rarely longer.[11]

CHISHIN *"LEAVING NEEDLE"* TREATMENT SUGGESTIONS

CHISHIN TREATMENTS FROM KANJI SHIMIZU

Kanji Shimizu, the president of the Akabane Association of Japan, wrote an article in which he described the following methods and points for the treatment of common disorders. The list of points represents acupoints that usually show pressure pain in the presence of that disorder. Treatment is applied by using the *chishin* technique on the most reactive pressure pain points. For each disorder, Shimizu recommends the gauge of needle to use, how deep to insert the needles, and whether or not to include some light stimulation techniques. In and of themselves, these suggested treatments do not usually constitute a complete treatment. Shimizu, like many other acupuncturists, has a root treatment method, and uses these treatments as supportive therapy in order to help alleviate the symptoms. He does not specify the length of time that the needles should be retained for the treatment, as this will depend on each patient's condition.

---

[11]Details of these are found in Y. Manaka, K. Itaya, and S. Birch, *Chasing the Dragon's Tail,* and D. Shūdo, *Japanese Classical Acupuncture: Introduction to Meridian Therapy.*

Different authors recommend different lengths of time that the needles should be retained for the *chishin* technique. For instance, while Okabe recommends that they be left up to 15 to 20 minutes maximum, Ono recommends anywhere from 5 to 20 minutes, and Nagahama describes both very short durations of from 20 to 30 seconds and long ones from 20 to 30 minutes. Usually 10 to 20 minutes is the appropriate length of time to retain needles. A good method for determining whether the length of time is appropriate for each patient is to ask the patient if the symptoms feel better. Also, recheck the pressure pain points by repalpating them or monitoring the pulse, following the changes in quality and strength. Shimizu recommends the "vibration needle technique," a gentle manipulation technique where the needle is vibrated up and down in the point along the plane of insertion with an almost imperceptible amplitude of vibration.

Frontal headache

Palpate and needle reactive points from among: GB-14, BL-2, *taiyang*, BL-10, GB-20, TB-15, SI-14, LI-10, CV-17, CV-12, ST-25, CV-4, BL-19, BL-21, ST-36, GB-41. Use number 3 gauge needles inserted about 5mm.

Temporal headache

Palpate and needle reactive points from among: ST-8, GB-5, TB-20, GV-22, BL-10, GB-20, GB-21, SI-14, TB-5, CV-12, LR-14, GB-24, CV-4, BL-18, BL-19, GB-34, GB-41. Use number 3 gauge needles inserted about 5mm.

Occipital headache

Palpate and needle reactive points from among: GV-20, BL-9, BL-10, GB-20, GB-21, SI-14, SI-3, CV-12, CV-3, BL-26, BL-28, BL-60, BL-62. Use number 3 gauge needles inserted about 5mm.

Dizziness

Palpate and needle reactive points from among: GV-20, GB-17, GB-12, BL-10, GB-21, TB-5, LR-14, GB-24, BL-18, BL-14, BL-23, LR-8, GB-34. Use number 3 gauge needles inserted about 5mm.

Insomnia

Palpate and needle reactive points from among: GV-20, GV-22, BL-10, GB-20, GB-21, PC-6, CV-17, CV-12, LR-14, CV-4, BL-15, BL-18, LR-3, GB-34. Use number 3 gauge needles inserted about 5mm.

Trigeminal neuralgia, first branch

Palpate and needle reactive points from among: GB-14, BL-2, BL-10, GB-20, GB-21, CV-12, CV-4, BL-19, BL-23, BL-28, GB-34, BL-62. Use number 3 gauge needles inserted about 5mm.

Trigeminal neuralgia, second branch

Palpate and needle reactive points from among: GB-5, GB-3, ST-3, LI-20, LI-4, CV-12, ST-25, BL-21, BL-25, ST-36 Use number 3 gauge needles inserted about 5mm.

Trigeminal neuralgia, third branch

Palpate and needle reactive points from among: TB-17, ST-7, ST-6, ST-4, TB-5, a reactive point on the chin, CV-12, CV-4, BL-21, BL-22, ST-36. Use number 3 gauge needles inserted about 5mm.

Sciatica

Palpate and needle reactive points from among: SI-3, TB-5, CV-12, ST-25, CV-4, BL-23, BL-25, *josen,* GV-3, BL-26, BL-28, a reactive point on the buttocks, BL-37, BL-54, BL-57, GB-34, ST-36, BL-60. For the lumbar area and lower extremity points, use number 10 gauge needles inserted 10-30mm. For the hand, foot, and abdominal points, use the vibrating needle techniques.

Elbow joint pain

Palpate and needle reactive points from among: TB-10, LI-11, an extra point on the back surface of the elbow joint in the depression between the olecranon process and head of the radius, SI-8, LI-10, TB-9, GB-21, SI-14, BL-13, BL-43, BL-15. For pressure pain points on or near the elbow joint, use number 3 gauge needles inserted about 5mm. For the neck, shoulder, and back points, use a mild vibrating needle technique.

Gastroptosis

Palpate and needle reactive points from among: LI-10, PC-6, CV-12, ST-25, ST-27, ST-29, BL-20, BL-21, BL-22, BL-23, BL-25, ST-36. For the abdominal and back pressure pain points, use number 3 gauge needles inserted about 5mm. For the arm and leg points, use mild vibrating needle techniques.

Cholelithiasis

Palpate and needle reactive points from among: LI-10, PC-6, CV-12, right LR-14, right ST-21, right GB-24, right BL-18, right BL-19, right BL-20, SP-8, GB-34. For the abdominal and back pressure pain points, use number 5 gauge needles inserted 10 to 20mm. For the arm and leg points, use the mild vibrating needle technique.

Inflammation of the maxillary sinus

Palpate and needle reactive points from among: *yintang,* GV-23, LI-20, BL-10, GB-20, GB-21, LI-4, CV-12, CV-4, BL-13, BL-21, BL-25, ST-36. Use number 3 gauge needles on *yintang,* GV-23, LI-20, and LI-4, inserted about 5mm. For the remaining points, use the mild vibrating needle technique.

CHISHIN TREATMENTS FROM BUNKEI ONO

Asthma

Fifteen to twenty needles are applied mainly on reactive points in the upper back region. The needles can be left until the asthma attack subsides. This can take from 30 to 60 minutes.

Tinnitus

TB-21, GB-2, TB-19, TB-18, TB-17.

Difficulty hearing

Same points as tinnitus, but with slightly deeper insertion and leaving the needles for a longer period of time.

Facial paralysis

Select points on the borders of the paralyzed area and on the vacuous areas on the face.

Numbness

Palpate and leave needles in the numb area.

Pain from renal, urinary bladder, or urethral calculus

BL-31, BL-32, BL-33, BL-34, and the area around these.

KYŪTŌSHIN—MOXA ON THE HANDLE OF THE NEEDLE

The *kyūtōshin* method, or literally, "moxa on the handle of the needle" method, is now relatively popular in Japan. According to the research of several authors including Akabane and Tanaka, the *kyūtōshin* method began in Japan around 1930. There is, however, a reference to something that is now understood to be very similar to this method in the *Shang Han Lun* of the late second century. This was called the *onkyu* or "warming" needle method (in Chinese, the *wenjiu* needle method); thus it is likely that the *kyūtōshin* technique or something like it originally began in China. The *kyūtōshin* technique utilizes the burning of balls of moxa on the handle of the needle to apply heat stimulation in addition to the needle stimulation.

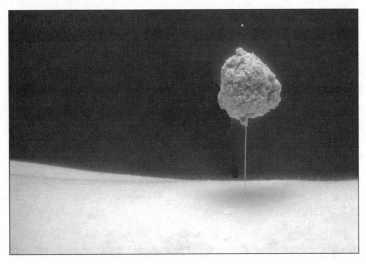

Needles with moxa on the handle—*kyūtōshin.*

This delivers radiant heat to the area around the needle, below the ball of moxa, and a deeper penetration of heat along the needle shaft into the body tissues.

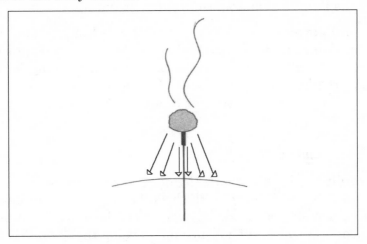

Radiant heat is delivered to the area around the needle shaft.

While there is some debate about the actual depth of penetration of heat along the needle shaft, it is clear that effects are definitely obtained from the radiant heat of the burning moxa. Some authors have suggested, based on research in China, that the application of heat to the needle increases the *hibiki* (nerve stimulation) sensation from the needle. M. Mussat in France has developed an interesting model explaining a possible electrical mechanism of heat application to the needle.[12] Whatever the explanation of the mechanisms and effects of this method, it has definitely proven effective in many cases.

The technique in Japan is different from the modern Chinese *wenjiu* technique in that the degree of heat felt is quite different. In China, the needle and area around it is heated until it becomes quite hot. In Japan, the *kyūtōshin* technique is generally applied so that the heat is felt as a comfortable sensation of warmth. In China practitioners tend to use much thicker needles, often with handles made out of copper, which conduct more heat than the needles used in Japan. Thus a considerably greater degree of heat is conducted along the needle shaft. Further, practitioners in China tend to use a method that places the moxa on the needle so that it sits much closer to the skin. Because the grade of moxa used in China is less pure, thereby burning hotter, a considerably stronger radiant heat is delivered to the surrounding skin than with the Japanese *kyūtōshin* technique.

The *kyūtōshin* technique is briefly described in *Chasing the Dragon's Tail,* where it is one of the more common methods employed to complete Step Two of Manaka's treatment protocol. The *kyūtōshin* technique is thus part of the root treatment method. There are other treatment approaches that employ this technique as part of the root treatment, but most authors describe its uses as part of the local or symptom control treatment approach.

Several Japanese authors describe the techniques and uses of the *kyūtōshin* method. Kobei Akabane published a book devoted to it; Hiroshi Tanaka wrote a series of papers describing it; Yoshio Manaka, Bunkei Ono, and Masāki Imagawa among others wrote about it. The following section is compiled from the works of these authors.[13]

KYŪTŌSHIN TECHNIQUES

According to most authors, the needles used are in the range of the 1 *cun* to 2 *cun* needles, with the 1.3 *cun* and 1.6 *cun* being the most common lengths used. The gauge can be Japanese number 2 to number 5 in width, the most common being the number 3 gauge. With sufficient anatomical knowledge, the technique can be used on

---

[12]M. Mussat, *Physique de l'acupôncture: Hypothèses et Apprôches Expèrimentales,* Paris: Librairie le François, 1972.

[13]Besides acknowledging their work, we would like to thank Hiromasa Okusada and Kazuko Itaya for their kindness and patience in teaching us these techniques.

virtually any area of the body. Some authors describe its uses on
the limbs, back, abdomen, shoulders, neck, face, and even on GV-20.
On areas where only shallower insertions are appropriate, such as
in the interscapular region, the neck, and shoulders, the 1 *cun*
length needle should be used. Use 1.3 *cun* needles on areas on the
back from roughly thoracic seven to the lumbar region. Use 1.6 *cun*
needles on the low lumbar region, buttocks, and hip regions, and the
2 *cun* needles on these regions for more obese patients.

In Japan most stainless steel needles can be used for this technique although special *kyūtōshin* needles are manufactured by companies such as Idō no Nippon. These special needles have handles
with a rough surface which allows the moxa ball to bind well to the
needle handle. Needles with handles that have smooth surfaces are
not a problem for use in this technique although you must be a little more attentive to ensure that the moxa ball is well secured to the
needle handle. Akabane recommends that when using smooth-han-
dled needles, first burn a little moxa on the handle. This will cause
a small deposit of moxa resin to collect on the needle handle, making it stickier and easier for the moxa ball to bind to the handle.
However, this is likely not necessary if you are a little more careful
and follow the guidelines below.

KYŪTŌSHIN MOXA DIMENSIONS

Tanaka advises that the needle be inserted and ball of moxa placed
so that the lower border of the ball of moxa is 2.5 cm from the skin.
Imagawa recommends a distance of from 2 to 3 cm.

Probably the distance you settle on for each needle will depend on
the overall size of the ball of moxa, the area of the body, and the angle
of insertion. Usually, the moxa heat should not be felt too intensely;
rather a comfortable sensation of warmth should be felt. Larger balls
of moxa tend to burn for a longer period of time and thus deliver a
slightly greater intensity of heat than a smaller ball of moxa. Therefore larger balls of moxa should be placed at a greater distance from
the skin than the smaller balls of moxa. Further, the moxa balls
should not be rolled too densely because a more densely packed ball
will burn more slowly and more intensely, thereby delivering more
heat to the skin surface. A more densely packed moxa ball will also
be more difficult to apply securely to the needle handle.

Tanaka recommends that the moxa balls be about 1.8cm in
diameter, and placed so that the needle handle protrudes at least 2
to 3mm below the ball of moxa. This 2mm to 3mm of needle handle
protruding below the bottom of the ball of moxa is important
because it gives you a solid part of the needle to grasp with tweezers either to remove the needle or to pull it back out of the point a
little, if it is too deeply inserted or too hot.

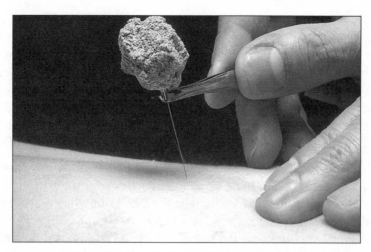

Using tweezers to grasp the needle for removal or insertion depth adjustment.

According to Tanaka, this size of moxa, when rolled to the proper density, will burn and generate smoke for about two minutes and forty seconds. It will stay hot for some time after it stops burning.

The following exercise will help you gain competence with this technique.

•Roll balls of moxa with the goal of consistency in size and density.

•Place the moxa balls on needles inserted into a piece of fruit (such as an apple).

•Time the moxa from ignition until it stops smoking. Set two minutes forty seconds as your time goal from ignition to burnout.

Once you can roll, place, and light balls of moxa that are roughly the same size, which take about two minutes and forty seconds to burn, and which you are able to remove without untoward incident, then your *kyūtōshin* moxa-ball rolling technique is adequate.

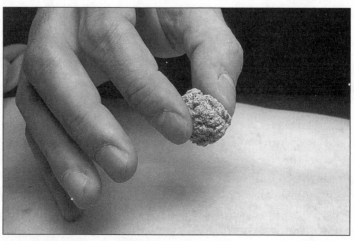

Practice rolling balls of moxa consistent in size and density.

KYŪTŌSHIN AND SEMI-PURE MOXA

For this technique, *wakakusa* "semi-pure" moxa should be used, though if you prefer, the "pure" yellow moxa can be used. We recommend the semi-pure because it burns a little more intensely and delivers the sensation of warmth better than a ball of pure moxa. It is also notably less costly than the pure moxa.

The various grades of Chinese moxa and the dirtier or more impure grades of Japanese moxa are not appropriate for this technique. The semi-pure moxa is yellow-green in color, containing very little particulate matter from the twigs and leaves of the moxa plant. The less pure grades of moxa are greener, with more particulate matter from the moxa plant.

When using this technique, it is important that no ignited particles of plant fall off the ball of moxa onto the skin, and that the ball of moxa itself does not fall off the needle onto the skin. Only the semi-pure and pure grades of Japanese moxa can be used reliably without these mishaps occurring. The Japanese *wakakusa* moxa is produced specifically for this purpose.

KYŪTŌSHIN MOXA ROLLING

The following are guidelines for rolling moxa properly. First pick up a piece of moxa roughly the following size:

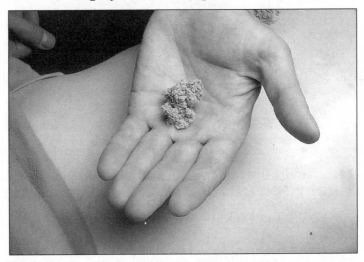

Pick up about this much of the loose *wakakusa* moxa.

Holding it in the palm of the hand, tap it with the side of the palm of the other hand. This helps dislodge and settle out small particles of plant fiber left in the moxa.

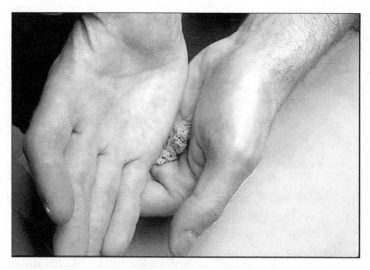

Tap the palm of one hand with the side of the other hand.

Holding the piece of moxa in the palm, place the other palm over it. Using a gentle rotation motion, roll the piece into a ball shape.

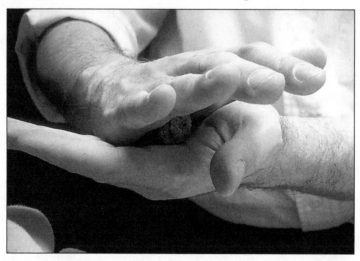

Lightly roll the moxa into a ball, cupping the palms of each hand slightly.

Hold the hands at a slight angle to the floor so as to allow any remaining particles of plant fiber left in the moxa to fall out.

Once the ball of moxa is rolled, it is ready for placement on the needle handle.

There are several different approaches for placing the moxa ball. You can gently split the ball in half, then holding each half in the fingers of each hand, position the two halves at the correct height to either side of the handle of the needle. Firmly, but without further compressing the moxa, press the two halves of the moxa ball back together, so that they bind securely.

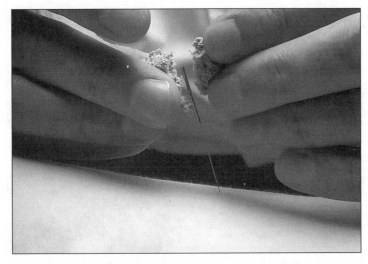

Position the two halves and press them back together securely.

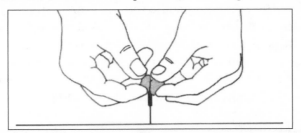

Another method is to split the moxa ball partially, leaving the upper surface of the ball still joined, then hold it over the handle of the needle and press the two halves together so that they bind.

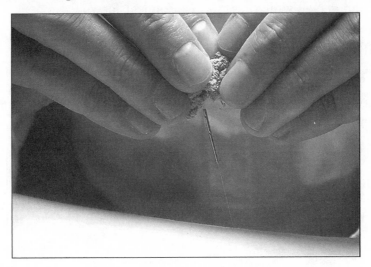

The upper surface of the moxa ball is still joined as it is positioned and secured.

A third method is to press the ball of moxa down over the handle of the needle with one hand, while holding the needle securely so that it is not pushed further into the body.

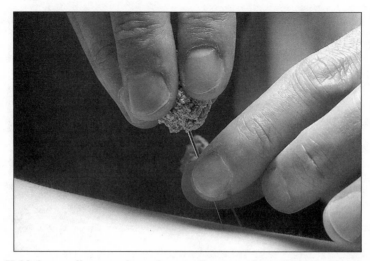

Hold the needle securely and press the moxa down over the handle.

A final method using a needle handle kept aside for this purpose is to press the handle of the needle into each ball before application. Leave a small hole the width of the needle handle in the moxa ball. The application then becomes rather easy. It merely requires the gentle placement of the ball of moxa onto the needle handle, by slipping the handle of the inserted needle into the hole.

KYŪTŌSHIN PRECAUTIONS

For beginners, we recommend the first, second, and fourth methods over the third because with the third, the possibility of pressing the needle further into the point is greater than with the others. Try each and decide which method works best for you.

Whichever technique you use for the moxa placement, be careful when placing the moxa ball on the handle of the needle. There is often a tendency, especially for beginners, to apply a slight downward pressure, inserting the needle a little deeper. If this passes unnoticed, when the moxa is ignited, it can become too hot for the patient and possibly become a problem.

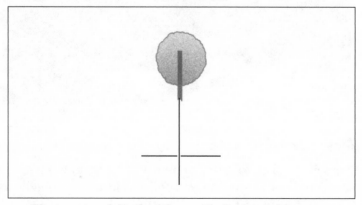

Placement and depth of the needle for *kyūtōshin* moxa.

When applying the moxa ball to the needle handle, make sure that a portion of the moxa ball always sits firmly over the top of the needle handle so that the handle top cannot be seen. To ensure that this happens, be certain to press the halves of the moxa ball firmly together over the top of the needle handle and then along the needle handle. Keep in mind that the top of the needle handle should *not* be visible; the bottom of the needle handle *should* be visible.

Once the ball is placed on the handle of the needle, check to make sure that it is properly centered in the moxa ball. A ball that is not centered on the needle handle can burn in such a way as to pull itself off the needle handle and fall off. This might cause an accident for the patient. Close visual inspection is important, as is a gentle but firm tapping of the moxa ball.

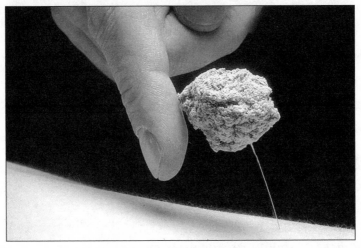

Gently but firmly tap the moxa ball.

If the ball is correctly applied, you should not be able to see any portion of the needle handle through the moxa ball, except the portion below the ball.

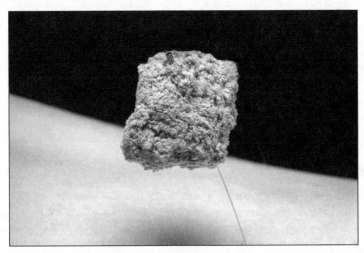

An incorrectly placed moxa ball allows the top of the needle handle to show.

When tapping it, the ball and needle will sway back and forth, but the ball will not slip or move on the needle handle. If inadequately attached, the moxa ball will slip down the needle to the skin or just fall off to the side. It is much better to find this out before igniting it!

After placing the ball on the needle, inspect the surface of the ball, especially the lower surface, looking for small particulate matter that might be hanging. Remove such pieces of matter before igniting the moxa. On occasion, these pieces can fall off onto the patient, giving them an unexpected and unwanted minor burn.

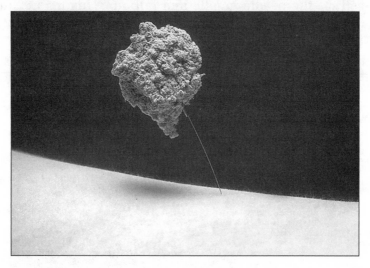

Remove hanging particulate matter.

The needle should be inserted perpendicularly to almost all points. For this technique (unlike all others recommended in this text), the needle is regularly inserted more than a few millimeters. The depth of insertion will vary depending on the body area, but it is usually about 1.5 centimeters or deeper.

When applying this technique, we are not looking for a *hibiki* or nerve stimulation sensation. In fact, some authors specifically recommend that if a *hibiki* or nerve stimulation sensation is obtained, the needle should be withdrawn and reinserted close by. The needle should be carefully inserted to a depth sufficient to support the weight of the ball of the moxa, without bending over too much. Because the needle is inserted to these depths, the technique is almost never used on bony areas of the body, or on areas where there is very little underlying flesh.

Typically, the technique is used on points where pressure pain and muscular knots can be palpated. For example, when using the technique on related back-*shu* points, the needles are inserted into the pressure-sensitive tight muscle bundles on either side of the spine rather than the normal point location which might lie to the side of the muscle bundles. Because needles are placed into pressure-sensitive tight points on the body, it is better to palpate, find, and then mark all the points to be treated before inserting any needles. Sometimes, palpating one point while a needle is already in another can be uncomfortable for patients and make it difficult for them to distinguish the reactive point.

Before lighting the moxa, be sure that you have a metal tray or bowl, tweezers, and some small shields ready and immediately available—all the necessary equipment for carrying out the procedure and dealing with any mishaps on hand. The metal tray or bowl is important if the moxa gets too hot, requiring that the needle and moxa be removed and put down, or if the moxa ball falls off the needle, requiring rapid pick-up and disposal. The tweezers are necessary to pull the needle back out of the point, if the moxa is still burning. If the moxa heat becomes too intense because of the proximity of the moxa to the skin, or if, for some reason, the needle is too deeply inserted into the point, it must be removed quickly. The small shields are important because, if the heat becomes too intense, rather than have the patient feel too much heat, it is better to block or shield the excess heat with the shields, then remove them after the moxa ball has passed its peak of heat. These shields can be made of a variety of materials. We recommend using folded aluminum foil because it creates a good reflective surface, providing a protective effect for the skin.

We strongly recommend that the practitioner remain with the patient while doing this technique.

IGNITING THE MOXA

Once the needles are inserted, and the moxa balls are placed and checked to ensure that they are secure, recheck your preparedness to deal with possible mishaps, then light the moxa. Usually it is better to light all the balls at once, rather than one or two at a time. This latter approach takes much more time while authors such as Ono and Manaka consider the former approach to give a greater synergistic effect. If, for example, you were to apply this technique to BL-23 and BL-25, as you might do as part of Step Two in Manaka's treatment approach, you would light all four moxa balls at the same time.

The method of lighting the balls will depend on your preferences and the patient. Usually a lighter or match will do.

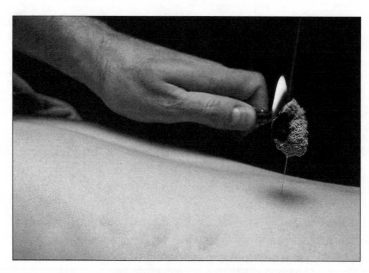

Lighting the moxa ball.

The problems with using a lighter are that it must be held at an angle, which allows the end to get quite hot, which might, on occasion, cause a self-inflicted burn. Also, the whooshing sound of a lighter flame and the sudden sensation of heat that usually accompanies it can make a nervous patient even more nervous and jumpy. On the low back, this is not such a problem, but if working up around the shoulders or neck, lighters may make patients nervous.

When using a match, always strike the match away from the patient. Wait for the flame to settle down, and then light the moxa. One disadvantage of matches is that occasionally they burn down before igniting all the balls of moxa, requiring that another match be lit. A match, when burned down, can also burn you slightly.

A third method which is less desirable is to ignite the moxa balls with the lighted end of an incense stick. Overall this method is safer than the two mentioned above (though they are minimally dangerous), but the moxa burns much more slowly with this technique, and it is thus much more time-consuming.

It is usually preferable to light the moxa ball on its bottom surface. The advantage of lighting the moxa like this is that as the moxa burns, it burns upward and binds to the lower portion of the needle handle because burning moxa contracts slightly and gives out a resin which helps bind it. Thus lighting the moxa on the bottom surface helps the moxa ball adhere to the needle handle more firmly.

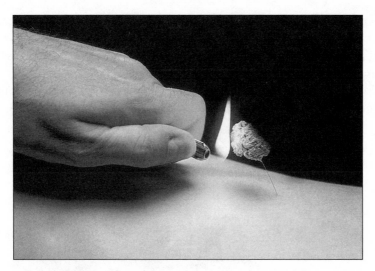

Lighting the moxa ball on the bottom surface.

On occasion, we have observed that lighting a moxa ball on one side can cause the moxa ball to become unsecured. As the moxa burns, it contracts to that side, tending to loosen its hold on the other side. If the needle handle is somewhat off center and sitting on the unlit side of the moxa ball, it can cause the ball to lose its hold on the needle handle and fall off.

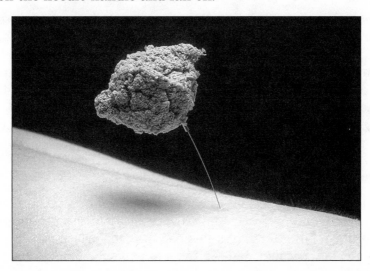

An off-center needle handle on the unlit side can cause the moxa to fall off.

There are occasions when the needle tends to lean over to the side, either before the moxa ball is fastened to it, or after it is fastened. There are several causes for this leaning. After the insertion of the needle to the point, the underlying muscle tissues begin to relax, which might pull the needle over to one side. If patients are somewhat thin and weak-muscled, deeper needle insertions can create a greater degree of muscular changes and the muscles may become unable to support the needle (especially with the moxa on its handle). Another cause occurs when the body area tends to incline the needle over to one side slightly, as, for instance, with the sacral *liao* points. Also, if the needle is not inserted deeply enough to firmly support the weight of the moxa, and if the ball of moxa is too big, or relatively too big for that body area on that patient, the needle may lean.

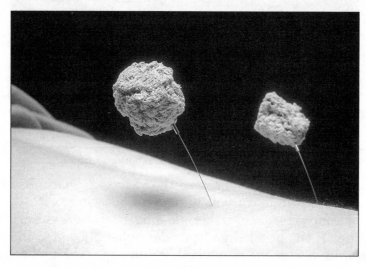

If the ball of moxa is too big, the needle may lean.

Kyūtōshin can still be applied in any of these cases, but the situation is a little more difficult, requiring more attention and work on your part. If the piece of moxa is too big, remove the moxa before igniting it, and make it smaller so that the angle is improved towards the perpendicular. For a needle that is too shallowly inserted, remove the moxa ball, and reinsert the needle a little more deeply, until you feel a slight grip of the needle. This should be done with great care on areas where needles cannot be inserted deeply to begin with. Also remember that we are not looking for a *hibiki* (nerve stimulation) sensation.

For the other cases, or whenever the needle is inclined to one side, light the moxa on the top surface, close to the needle handle, so that it can bind to the handle near the top surface. As the moxa burns, the ball becomes lighter and you will observe that frequently the needle slowly straightens up towards the perpendicular. In cases where this is not occurring sufficiently, place your fingers on the other side of the needle and pull the skin slowly and gently away from the needle, until the needle rises up to the perpendicular. Hold it there. This technique will help with a needle that is keeled over to the side or in cases where the point is getting a little too hot.

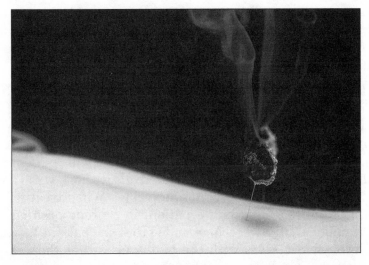

As the moxa burns, an inclined needle moves more to perpendicular.

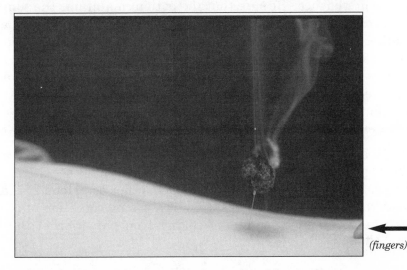

(fingers)

Gently pull the skin away from the needle with your fingers.

When using a lighter or a match to light the ball of moxa, be very careful not to let the flame touch the needle body below the handle of the needle. On one occasion, one of the authors was lighting a moxa ball with a window open. A draught blew the flame lower than intended. It struck the needle body only very briefly, but long enough that the needle rapidly became red hot, and, with the weight of the moxa ball, bent over to ninety degrees. This left the lighted moxa ball burning very precariously on the needle handle which gave the author quite a surprise. The needle was safely removed without alerting the patient at all to the problem.

Should a problem occur with the *kyūtōshin* technique, it is best to stay alert and handle it as expeditiously as possible, so as not to disturb the patient or make the patient anxious. If a moxa ball slips off a needle when lit, quickly and confidently pick up the moxa ball, being careful not to drop it onto the patient, and place it on the metal tray or into water. Usually, when a ball slips, it tends to roll, and most of the time manages to roll off the body and onto the table, allowing ample time to deal with it.

Patients who are disturbed or anxious will be uncomfortable and will often move around abruptly. This movement is not desirable. Usually it is a good idea to instruct patients to settle into a comfortable posture and not move while the technique is being applied. It is also a good idea not to talk much with patients when utilizing this technique. An animated discussion, with hand or head movements, is definitely not desirable. When treating points on the posterior surface, with a patient in a prone position on the table, Manaka and Itaya recommended that the patient lie with the arms down by the sides with the palms up rather than raised to support the head. However, if this posture is too awkward, comfort takes precedence. Be sure that the patient maintains the same posture during *kyūtōshin* treatment. On one occasion one of the authors observed a patient decide to move his arm while *kyūtōshin* was being applied up around BL-18. The needle keeled over from a ninety degree angle to a very acute angle, and the moxa ball almost touched the skin. Always check to assure that that the patient is comfortable before locating and treating the points.

One to five moxa balls can be burned on each needle. In Manaka's approach, usually two are burned. This is probably a good average for each needle. If the patient is extremely sensitive, it may be preferable to use only one moxa. On other occasions, it is a good idea to use three or perhaps more if a strong condition of coldness can be determined by feeling coldness on palpation of the lower abdomen.

KYŪTŌSHIN MOXA BALL REPLACEMENT

To remove a burned moxa ball and replace it with a fresh one, it is important to not pick up a ball which is still burning or smoldering. After the moxa ball has stopped smoking, it remains red-hot for some time. Wait for the heat to dissipate completely before removing the ball. We recommend using your fingers rather than trying to remove the ball with a tray or some kind of instrument. First, hold the palm of the hand over the moxa ball. When no heat is felt and no red embers are visible in the ball, it is ready for removal. Place all fingers below the ball, closing them so as to make contact with the bottom surface of the ball. Then draw the fingers up, thus lifting the ball. Carry the ball to the tray and drop the ashes onto the tray. Remember not to touch the needle handle because it often remains quite hot.

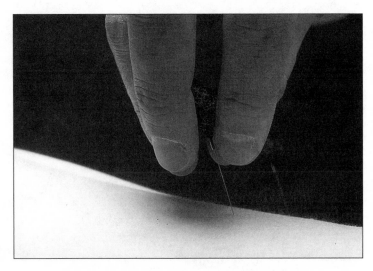

Place the fingers below the ball to lift it off safely.

When properly done, little or no spent ashes are dropped onto the skin of the patient, and no burning ashes are dropped. If you make a mistake and pick up a ball that is still burning, try not to respond reflexively and drop it on the patient. Instead, carry the ashes swiftly over to the tray and set them there. Check carefully that there is no heat left in the ball before picking it up.

A special moxa ball removal spoon has been created in Japan. The slit in the spoon allows you to place the spoon underneath the moxa ball and to then remove it.

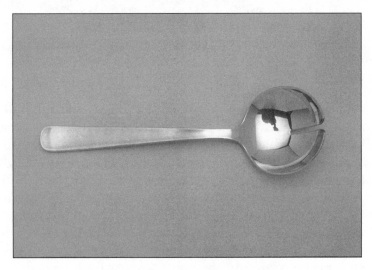

Special moxa ball removal spoon.

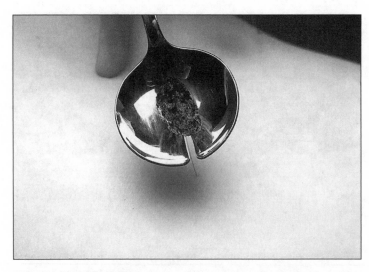

Slide the special moxa ball removal spoon under the spent moxa.

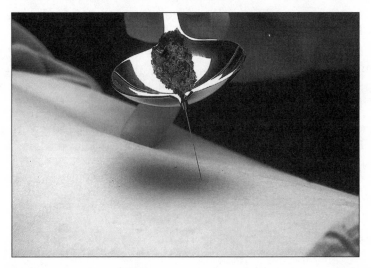

Lift the spent moxa off the needle with the special moxa ball removal spoon.

If the needle must be removed while the ball is still hot, use the tweezers. Grasp the needle carefully and gently by the bottom portion of the handle which protrudes below the ball of moxa, and withdraw it and place it in the tray. This situation may arise if the patient becomes anxious for some reason, or if the heat builds up too intensely, or if some portion of the moxa falls and strikes the patient's skin. Usually, if the heat sensation is too intense, withdrawing the needle a few millimeters is sufficient to deal with the situation; if not, then use the heat shield. One of the authors has observed a needle sink into the point, almost to the needle handle, while a moxa ball was still burning on it. This created very intense heat and discomfort for the patient and required immediate withdrawal of the needle. This particular problem occurred because of an attempt to save time by looking for pressure pain points on the auricle while the *kyūtōshin* technique was being applied. As the pressure pain point was found, the patient involuntarily tensed up and the resulting muscle spasm pulled the needle down into the point. The moral of this story is that you should not do anything else while the moxa is burning!

SMOKE VENTILATION

With practice this is a simple, easy, and relatively quick technique to apply. As beginners, the moxa looks very precarious and unsafe, and there is a tendency either not to want to do it, or to use some other technique for heating the needle. Also, the production of smoke in such quantities can be a problem both for patient and practitioner, particularly if it there is not an adequate ventilation system in place.

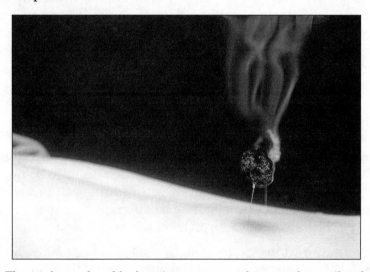

The smoke produced by burning moxa must be properly ventilated.

If you are inclined to try using a moxa pole held near the handle of the needle, instead of placing moxa directly over the needle handle, the smokeless moxa pole can be used. While this cuts down on smoke production and certainly to the inexperienced is easier and seemingly safer, the disadvantage is that it becomes harder to judge the correct dosage of heat delivered to the point and area around it. Often much more heat is delivered than with the *kyūtōshin* technique. Further, you must stand holding the pole close to the needle handles, and can heat only one needle at a time, thereby losing some of the synergistic effects that come from heating several needles at once. However, if you work where smoke is not permitted, or cannot be adequately ventilated, there may be no alternative but to use the smokeless moxa pole. If you are using the pole because the other technique seems unsafe, then concentrate on accelerating your technique practice, so that you can improve enough to apply it in the clinic.

You may want to consider installing a ventilator system with metal ducts into each treatment room that can be connected to a fan on the roof. In our clinics we have used flexible piping (laundry dryer piping will do) inside each treatment room that is attached to a movable and extendible arm which can be placed over the burning moxa. This system works quite well. With this system we have had no further problems with moxa smoke since it is ventilated as soon as it is produced.

Another method that has been developed in Japan to try to improve on the safety aspects of this technique is to use a small metal cap in which the ball of moxa is placed, and which is then placed over and onto the needle handle. While this technique definitely improves on the safety factors by almost eliminating the risk of the moxa overheating the point or area around it, and the risk of dropping small burning particles onto the skin, it certainly has its problems. First, because of the extra weight of the metal cap, either the needle has to be inserted more deeply, which often is impossible, or thicker-gauge needles have to be used. Neither of these alternatives are options we prefer, primarily because our general approach is "less is better" and because a thicker needle will deliver much more heat to the point. Also, almost all the radiant heat effects are lost because the cap shields the skin from the radiant heat. Some authors have speculated that more clinical effects in the *kyūtōshin* technique come from the radiant heat, rather than from heat conduction down the needle handle. If you use this cap technique, be aware that the effects obtained may be different that those achieved by placing the ball of moxa directly on the needle handle.

If you are working in an environment where burning any substance is not permitted, you can consider using a heat lamp. If you use an infrared heat lamp you can leave it over the needles for at least 10 minutes. Make sure it is not too hot for the patient.

The *kyūtōshin* technique described above is safe, effective, and easily mastered. When you practice the technique at home on fruit or other objects, make sure that you can roll the same sizes and densities of moxa routinely, and place them onto the needles routinely without having them fall off, slip down, or cause some other problem while burning. Then you are ready to try the technique on real patients.

It is often said that if the patient feels a comfortable sensation of warmth penetrating into and through the body, the treatment is very effective. If, when treating the lower back of a patient with any of a number of symptoms, but with accompanying coldness of the lower abdomen and/or back, while burning the moxa, the patient describes a sensation of warmth spreading through to the abdomen, this is a very good sign.

PRECAUTIONS AND CONTRAINDICATIONS

It is essential with this technique that the patient be comfortable at all times. A distressed patient will not respond well to the treatment and may complicate the circumstances by unexpected movements. To this end it is important to pay special attention so as to avoid letting the heat build up too intensely. What constitutes excessive heat for each patient will differ. For some, only a slight amount is too much; for others, a large amount just feels good. Usually you want to deliver heat between these extremes. Ono recommends not letting the area around the needle become very red because this is a sign of too much heat. If the area starts turning red, ask the patient if they feel comfortable. If they are comfortable, then nothing needs to be done; if they are uncomfortable, then apply a little shielding with your finger to cut down on the amount of heat delivered to the skin.

When placing the moxa balls, pay careful attention to the actual depth of insertion and the angle of the needle. If the needle inclines heavily to one side, then you will need to be careful in lighting the moxa and may need to pull the needle to an upright position by gently pulling on the skin, as described above. Generally this technique is not used on areas where there is little bulk of underlying muscles.

Do not talk much with the patient during this procedure because an animated discussion can cause the needles to move. Always make sure that patient is comfortable before lighting the moxa balls, and instruct them not to move.

In some acute conditions, it is better not to apply this technique in the affected areas; distal points are better. For example, in cases of acute lumbar pain with local inflammation of the spine, joints, or muscles and with strong local pressure pain, treat distant points on the legs rather than on the back itself. When the condition is chronic, with less local pressure pain and inflammation, the technique is very appropriate.

CLINICAL USES ACCORDING TO MANAKA'S STEP TWO TREATMENT

In *Chasing the Dragon's Tail* we gave indications and a number of case histories showing how the *kyūtōshin* technique is used on the *back-shu* and other acupoints as Step Two in Manaka's treatment protocol. What follows are a number of strategies that can be used as part of Step Two treatment in this protocol, or that can be used simply to relieve symptoms. Ono recommends the following techniques as part of overall treatment:

Hemorrhoids

Use 3 to 4 needles in the area around the anus.

Lower abdominal dull pain

BL-30 or BL-28.

Cold lumbar area

BL-52 or BL-25.

Sciatica

GB-30, and selected appropriate points along the pathway of the pain.

Paralysis of the lower limbs

BL-40 or BL-60.

50-year shoulder (chronic painful shoulder with difficulty moving)

LI-15.

Stiff shoulder

GB-21 with shallow insertion (use 1 *cun* needles).

CLINICAL USES ACCORDING TO TANAKA'S METHODS

Tanaka gives a very different logic for the uses of this technique as the whole treatment for the "50-year shoulder" and rheumatism of the knee. His point selections are based primarily upon the underlying musculature and the effects that the technique has on those muscles.

50-year shoulder

With the patient lying prone (abdomen toward the treatment table), palpate and treat the following points: BL-22 and BL-18 *(latissimus dorsi)*, BL-43 and SI-14 *(rhomboideus and levator scapula)*, TB-15 *(trapezius)*, SI-11 *(infraspinatus)*. With the patient lying on the untroubled shoulder side, rotate and slightly abduct the painful shoulder; treat in the two depressions formed on the acromion, LI-15 *(deltoid)*, and TB-14 *(infraspinatus)*, also LI-14 *(deltoid)*, TB-13 *(deltoid)*, LI-16 *(supraspinatus)*. Then have the patient change to the supine position (back toward the treatment table) and treat LU-1 and an extra point 2 *cun* medial to the end of the clavicle on the posterior ridge of the clavicle.

Rheumatism of the knee

This technique should not be used if the knee is in the first stages of inflammation, with redness, heat in the knee, and fever in the body. If the knee is swollen, but without the fever and redness, then the technique is indicated. With the patient lying supine, place a small pillow under the knee and palpate and treat ST-32 *(rectus femoris),* SP-10 *(vastus medialis),* GB-33 *(vastus lateralis),* LR-8 (crevice of the joint), SP-9 and GB-34 (muscles of lower leg). If the knee is clearly swollen, add the eyes of the knee. If the medial side of the knee is sore, add an extra point on the upper ridge of the medial condyle of the femur. If the lateral side of the knee is painful, add GB-33. Then have the patient lie in a prone position, placing a small pillow under the foot in order to give slight flexion. Palpate and treat KI-10, BL-39 (crevice of the joint), and an extra point 2 finger-widths medial to BL-55 *(triceps surae),* an extra point posterior to GB-34 *(triceps surae),* an extra point a few *cun* above KI-10 *(semitendinosus and semimembranosus),* and an extra point a few *cun* above BL-38 *(biceps femoris).*

If the popliteal crease is clearly swollen, use KI-10, BL-55, BL-39, and a point above the popliteal crease directly above BL-40 to make a rectangle, plus BL-40. Do not do BL-40 at the same time as the others because the knee will get too hot. It is also important to check and treat the lumbosacral region, especially if the region is cold for the patient or cold to the touch. Palpate and treat BL-23, BL-25, BL-32.

Tanaka's treatments are interesting, but require that many points be treated with *kyūtōshin.* If you have a hard time with the smoke of the moxa, or if you have a hard time ventilating the smoke out of the room, this kind of approach is probably not for you. In general, we almost always recommend performing a root or general treatment first, followed by a few simple procedures for the symptom-control portion of treatment. With such an approach, you would generally not need so many points. However, if you have a patient with one of these symptoms who has been unresponsive to treatment, this very symptom-oriented approach might prove helpful.

CLINICAL APPLICATIONS OF AKABANE'S TECHNIQUES

In his book, *Kyūtōshin Ho,* Akabane describes the work of a Mr. Sato, who used the *kyūtōshin* technique exclusively on all of his patients. While these treatments are interesting, they are not very practical since they usually employ more moxa burning than even those of Tanaka's. The amount of smoke generated is enormous, and without an extremely efficient method of smoke removal, it will be inappropriate for use in most Western acupuncture clinics. Akabane himself, though, recommends the *kyūtōshin* method for a wide variety of different disorders. The following are some of these:

Heavy-headedness, headache

After lightly stimulating the painful area with the *sanshin* or touching-needle technique, or the intradermal needle methods, use *kyūtōshin* on points such as BL-10, GB-20 on the affected side(s). If only one side is affected, Akabane recommends using this technique on that side 2 to 3 times and then his draining needle technique on the other side.

Facial paralysis

Many patients are not comfortable having the *kyūtōshin* technique used on the face, because it makes them very nervous. If the patient will allow you to use it, have the patient lie on their side, and after finding and selecting the pressure pain points on the paralyzed area, use 1 *cun* needles with 1 to 2 moxa balls on each. Next, lightly stimulate the area further with needles such as the intradermals. Then use the draining needle technique on the healthy side.

Stiff shoulders

Find pressure pain points on the shoulders, and if the reaction spreads to the neck or upper back, use on those areas, too. Apply the technique to those points. Usually shoulder stiffness is a result of internal problems, and thus treatment must also be directed at those problems (i.e., root treatment).

Whiplash injury

Kyūtōshin is effective for the treatment of whiplash injuries, and is very useful if applied to the pressure pain and tight muscular points on the upper back, which are typically on or near the upper thoracic vertebrae or on the bladder lines in the interscapular region. In this case, use the 1 *cun* needles and shallower insertion. Some practitioners prefer not to use this technique in this region because of the possibility of needling too deeply and puncturing the lungs. Probably it is better for beginners to avoid this area, but provided appropriately shallow needling is used, it is not a problem.

With the patient lying face down, find and treat these reactive points. Akabane adds that the addition of an intradermal needle (See Chapter 6) to a distinctive pressure pain point on one of the midaxillary lines can reinforce the effects of treatment.

50-year shoulder

Check the patient's range of motion, and mark distinctly painful pressure pain points. Try treating 2 or 3 of these first with *kyūtōshin* and then check the range of motion again. If there is no change, choose 2 to 3 other points and repeat the procedure. Usually it is much better not to overstimulate the patient. Instead, repeat the procedure on future visits, rather than try to treat all pressure pain points at one sitting. After using the *kyūtōshin* technique on the affected side, use the draining needle technique on the healthy shoulder and then place an intradermal on the midaxillary line on the affected side.

Gastroenteric disorders

Mild disorders can be treated by *kyūtōshin* on ST-36, and pressure pain points on the back are useful. For serious cases of ulcer or cancer of the stomach, it is better not to treat. For milder stomach ulcer symptoms, *kyūtōshin* should be avoided on the abdomen and is best applied to the back and on the neck around BL-10. In addition, add an intradermal needle to the midaxillary line pressure pain point. For a simple case of stomachache or hyperacidic stomach, treat pressure pain points on the abdomen and back.

Diarrhea

In either acute or chronic cases, *kyūtōshin* on pressure pain points on the abdomen, around CV-10 to CV-12, ST-36, CV-14 or left ST-26 and on the back can be very effective.

Gastroptosis, Atony of the stomach

Select pressure pain points from within a radius of 12 to 15 cm from the navel and pressure pain points on the lumbar region, and ST-36.

Lumbago

First palpate and treat reactive points on the abdomen, especially a point in the lower left quadrant of the abdomen. Typical points on which pressure pain is found on the lumbar region and to which the technique can be applied from 3 to 5 times are: BL-25, GV-3, BL-23, BL-52, BL-18.

Sciatica

Palpate and select pressure pain points on and around Lumbar 2 to Lumbar 5, both on the spine and just to the sides, and on the posterior superior iliac spine, lateral to the lumbar eye points. Also, on the affected limb side, treat the pressure pain point on the buttock. If the pain is only down the back of the leg, BL-38 is useful; if to a wider area, such as down the gallbladder channel, GB-31, GB-33, or BL-40 will be useful. Do not use the technique more than three times on any point.

Gynecological disorders

The main treatment points for symptoms such as lower abdominal discomfort, leukorrhea, heavy-headedness, stiff shoulder, anxiety, insomnia, and so forth, are on the lumbar and abdominal regions. Points such as BL-23, BL-52, BL-25, GV-3, *jōsen,* and to the sides of and below the navel are useful.

High blood pressure

Most patients with an elevated blood pressure have stiffness of the neck and shoulders, often with a feeling of heavy-headedness. It is important to loosen up these areas. With the patient sitting, palpate and treat from among BL-10, GB-20, GB-21. Treat on the upper back if pressure pain and stiff points are found. Also, with the patient lying prone, palpate and treat pressure pain points on the lumbar region. Treating ST-36 can also be useful.

Poor appetite

Palpate and treat reactive points to the sides of the navel, CV-12, on the right subcostal region, around BL-20, and GV-9.

Many options exist for the uses of the *kyūtōshin* method. The treatments cited above are illustrative only. For any symptom with accompanying vacuity signs and cold or cool areas, for conditions of deep cold and vacuity, and for general supplementation, the *kyūtōshin* method is an excellent technique to use.

Chapter 5
Kyū—Moxibustion

A Brief History

Though most moxa therapy was practiced by acupuncturists and moxibustionists, much of the long history of moxibustion practice in Japan included folk medicine, where family members treated other family members, or where moxibustion therapy was practiced by monks or nuns in various Zen temples. Although moxibustion is primarily practiced as a clinical specialization in Japan today, it is still a common—though less popular—practice to have patients apply some form of moxibustion technique on themselves or some family member as a form of home therapy.

Today, separate licenses for acupuncture and moxibustion allow for a high degree of specialization in the use of moxa and for an extension of its uses into areas where it has either not been widely used before or is currently not used by most acupuncturists outside Japan.

While there have been a number of specialized classical moxibustion books from China, such as the *Zu Pi Shi Yi Mai Jiu Jing (Eleven Vessel Moxa Text)*, the *Yin Yang Shi Yi Mai Jiu Jing (Yin Yang Eleven Vessel Moxa Text)*,[1] the twelfth century *Huang Di Ming Tang Jiu Jing (Yellow Emperor's Ming Tang Moxa Text)*, and the nineteenth century *Shen Jiu Jing Lun (Miraculous Moxibustion Classic)*, highly specialized use of moxibustion is now found primarily in Japan.

Some relatively modern Japanese moxibustion specialists, such as Isaburo Fukaya, who practiced for over 60 years, Takeshi Sawada, who inspired a whole generation of practitioners with his uniquely brilliant and powerful treatments, and Seiji Irie, the leading proponent of Fukaya's style, studied the Chinese classical literature extensively. In fact, many of the techniques derived from their

---

[1]Both were found in the Mawang Dui graves, dating from the second century B.C.

studies of the classics. One of Fukaya's favorite texts was the *Huang Di Ming Tang Jiu Jing (Yellow Emperor's Ming Tang Moxa Text)*.

Though Sawada wrote no books, his student, Bunshi Shirota, wrote both about Sawada's work and his own. Much of the material found in Shirota's books comes from Sawada. While Sawada used moxa almost exclusively, only occasionally using gold needles, Shirota practiced acupuncture as well as moxibustion, and wrote more than eight volumes about both therapeutic modalities. Toward the end of his sixty years of practice, Fukaya wrote more than ten volumes almost exclusively concerning the use of moxibustion, and little, if any, mention of the practice of acupuncture. Irie wrote a moxa text about the treatment methods of Fukaya, the *Fukaya Kyū Hō (Moxa Methods of Fukaya),* which remains quite popular. He continues to write articles about moxibustion practice. A number of other non-moxibustionist specialists wrote extensively about the practice of moxibustion. For instance, the late Yoshio Manaka, an internationally renowned practitioner and researcher, wrote a moxibustion text for the layperson,[2] and has extensive references to moxibustion therapy in his other texts.[3]

TECHNIQUES OF CURRENT MOXA USE IN JAPAN

In this chapter we will focus on clinical details by describing some of the more commonly used moxibustion techniques. We will cover the following general areas:

• Types of moxibustion currently in use in Japan.

• Techniques of *okyū* or direct moxibustion, including recommended applications and prohibitions; numbers, size, placement, and lighting of moxa, and precautions and contraindications.

• The general treatment ideas of Sawada.

• A list of points used for specific diseases from Shirota.

• Indirect moxa techniques such as *ibuki* moxa that can be used at home as substitutes for *okyū* moxa.

• Techniques of *chinetsukyū* or cone moxa, including numbers of applications, precautions, general treatment strategies, and recommended techniques and prohibitions.

---

[2] Y. Manaka, *Okyū no Kenkyū (Moxibustion Studies)*.

[3] See Y. Manaka, K. Itaya, and S. Birch, *Chasing the Dragon's Tail*, pp 206-217, for a list of moxibustion treatments from Manaka and Shirota. This book also contains an essay by Kazuko Itaya on the history and nature of moxibustion therapy, a compilation by her of Japanese research on the physiological effects of moxibustion, and a further compilation of classical references to the points contraindicated for the use of moxibustion (cf. pp. 348-361). A useful series of essays on moxa therapy authored by Junji Mizutani can be found in the special Spring 1998 issue of the *North American Journal of Oriental Medicine*.

The practice of moxibustion can be divided into two general categories. These are traditionally called the *yukonkyū* (scarring) and the *mukonkyū* (non-scarring) moxibustion techniques. Techniques that have moxa burnt directly on or down to the skin are scarring or "direct" moxibustion techniques. Traditionally, direct moxibustion resulted in scarring, though today this technique does not have to form scars. The non-scarring techniques utilize moxa applied indirectly on the skin. In these techniques moxa is either placed on the skin, but not burned down to the skin, or burned through another substance which shields the skin. Some practitioners utilize a wide variety of techniques that apply heat to the skin, where the heat source is not necessarily burning moxa.

SCARRING TECHNIQUES

The three scarring or direct moxibustion techniques are the *tōnetsukyū, shōshakukyū,* and *danokyū* methods. The *tōnetsukyū* technique is the most commonly used. Also called *okyū,* it refers to the placing of small pieces of moxa punk directly on the skin which are then ignited by incense, and allowed to burn down to the skin in order to stimulate the selected acupoint. This technique was the most commonly used by Fukaya, Irie, and Manaka, and is the major focus of this section.

The *shōshakukyū* technique is used specifically for cauterizing warts, corns, and the wounds of poisonous insects or snakes. It is less commonly used and thus not a focus of this book.

The *danokyū* method applies large moxa cones to cauterize the skin at the acupoint and is followed up by the application of an irritating herb paste, which causes the formation of a small ulcer with a purulent exudate. After the exudate production slows down, a second herb paste is applied to heal the wound. This method is used to cleanse the blood, to treat blood stasis, and to improve liver function. As with *shōshakukyū,* this method is not used very commonly and thus is not a focus of this book.

NON-SCARRING TECHNIQUES

There are many forms of non-scarring or indirect moxibustion. In some, the moxa is placed on top of a paste or substance so that the heat intensity is reduced and more diffuse. Examples of this are bean paste moxa, where the moxa is placed on a small amount of miso; garlic moxa or ginger moxa, where the moxa is placed on top of a slice of garlic or ginger; and salt moxa, where the moxa is placed on top of a mound of salt. These are techniques used widely in China.

The *onkyū* moxa method is commonly used in Japan by lay practitioners. Moxa placed inside a bamboo tube or a ceramic or unglazed bowl is ignited. As soon as heat is felt on the bottom surface of the tube or bowl, these are pressed to the points or areas to be treated.

Other applications utilize moxa placed on a small platform so that the heat of the moxa irradiates the point but the moxa makes no direct contact with the skin. Examples of this kind of technique are the *ibuki* moxa methods and the moxa-box method (commonly used in China).

The *ibuki* method can easily be substituted for the *okyū* method and is suitable for home therapy because there a lower risk of patients burning themselves. Fukaya, Sawada, Shirota, Irie, and Manaka normally used direct moxa and would teach their patients to use moxa techniques at home. We also recommend use of the *ibuki* moxa for home therapy because there is less chance of a self-inflicted burn or scarring. However, if patients appear able to use the direct moxa techniques without burning and scarring themselves, or if they have a family member or partner to do it for them, you may be able to teach the patient, family member, or partner to use direct moxa.

Indirect application can also be done using moxa rolled up into a pole shaped like a cigar, which is then ignited and held over the acupoint, area, or needle being treated. There are a variety of kinds of moxa poles available, and their use is often part of a Chinese-style practice.

A moxibustion method commonly used by Keiraku Chiryō practitioners in Japan is the *chinetsukyū* method. Relatively large cones of moxa are rolled and placed at the acupoint, and can be removed as soon as the patient begins to feel a little heat, or after the heat is felt a little more intensely. This places moxa directly on the skin, but is considered a non-scarring or indirect method because the moxa is removed long before it burns down to the skin, thereby giving only mild heat stimulation.

The *kyūtōshin* method, discussed in the last chapter relative to the type of needle used, involves placing a ball of moxa on the handle of the needle and igniting it to give heat stimulation to the needle, points, and surrounding areas.

Additionally, there are readily available devices or tools used to apply heat to acupoints without actually burning moxa, such as self-heating hot packs that stay warm for a number of hours and apply a relatively constant heat to the point or area stimulated, and electrical heating instruments designed to apply heat either to a small point or to a larger area.

Of these diverse methods of direct and indirect moxa treatment, the *okyū,* the *ibuki,* and the *chinetsukyū* methods will be described in some detail below.

MOXA PUNK "GRADES"

Many grades of moxa are available in Japan. There are several grades of "pure" moxa, "semi-pure" moxa, and finally "crude" moxa. The crude moxa is used in moxa poles and with various instruments, none of which are discussed here. The semi-pure moxa is used specifically for the *kyūtōshin* and *chinetsukyū* techniques.

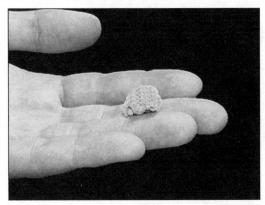
Pure moxa.

The pure moxa is used in *okyū* applications, and is processed specifically for use in this method. Thus, when applying the direct *okyū* moxa methods, always use pure moxa, and never the semi-pure or crude moxa. The pure moxa is processed so that only the moxa "wool" remains, with most of the plant fiber and particles either sieved or washed out. This allows for a very soft, malleable moxa-wool that can be easily molded to shape. It burns with less intensity, thereby allowing for greater control over the amount of heat applied to the acupoints. With appropriate techniques, this allows the practitioner to control the degree of heat applied and not burn or scar the point. The semi-pure moxa has more fiber and particles left mixed in with the moxa-wool; the crude moxa has much more fiber and many more particles left in it. The greater the amounts of fiber and particles in the moxa, the harder it is to roll the moxa to the desired shape and size, and the hotter it burns. This makes it more difficult to control the amount of heat delivered to the point by the moxa punk.

OKYŪ—DIRECT MOXIBUSTION

Rolling moxa to the right shape, size, and consistency is a skill attained only with hours of careful practice. In Japan, students in acupuncture school spend many hours learning and perfecting their moxa rolling, placing, and burning techniques, so that they can pass the rather difficult practical parts of the curriculum of the various schools and national licensing exams. In the West, this level of repetitive diligence is less common, though still very important, as a general level of skill must be attained so that moxa can be used effectively and repeatedly without burning and scarring the patient. To this end, the following points should be observed:

•Roll the moxa correctly, both with respect to a consistent size and a consistent degree of compression.

•Generally the moxa should be felt as slightly hot to the patient, but not uncomfortable and not to the point of burning the skin.

•If the moxa is rolled too large or is compressed too tightly, it tends to burn hotter and deliver a more intense heat to the point, which if not properly controlled can blister and scar the skin.

•To ensure the delivery of the correct degree of heat to a point, make sure that the moxa cones are rolled to the same size with the same consistency. Once able to do this, you can ensure that the same dose of heat is delivered to the point with every cone, thus giving you much greater control over the total dosage delivered.

•When correctly applied, the heat of the moxa is generally like a brief pinprick. Sometimes it even elicits the same stimulation sensation obtained normally with needles.

•Perfecting delivery technique requires constant practice in moxa rolling. You might set tasks for yourself, such as rolling and placing twenty moxa in a row that are all the same size and consistency.

•The moxa cone or punk sizes are usually very small, ranging from thread size, to sesame size to half-rice grain size—usually the biggest used. The piece of moxa should be shaped either in a thin rod shape, or like a grain of rice. What is important is to ensure that when the piece of moxa is placed on the skin, it stands up with only minimal contact with the skin. A piece of moxa that has a wide base is not desirable because it will burn hotter as it burns down towards the skin. The following pictures show the shapes and sizes of moxa relative to a U.S. 10-cent coin (1.7cm diameter):

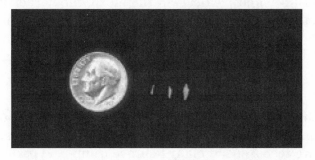

Sizes of moxa relative to a U.S. 10-cent coin.

The moxa should not be densely packed or rolled tightly. When rolling the moxa, mold the moxa to shape and size without compressing it. The rolling is usually done between the pads of the thumb and forefinger of whichever hand is the easier to use. Ideally, the piece of moxa should be rolled without the finger and thumb touching. This assures the most correct pressure because it molds but does not compress the moxa. When correctly rolled, the moxa should be loose but well formed.

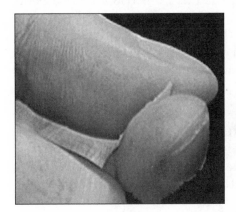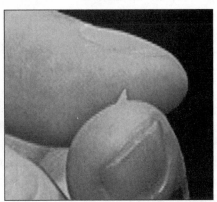

Rolling moxa.

There is a Korean form of pre-rolled moxa that can be used as direct moxa, called *sook*. This is made of a combination of mugwort (moxa), wormwood, and sagebrush. This burns differently from pure moxa, delivering a hotter pinch of heat. It also burns very slowly, and can thus increase the time of a treatment. While this may be a useful technique for some, especially the absolute beginner who has not yet achieved good technique, we cannot overemphasize the importance of using hand-rolled pure moxa. Achieving consistency comes with regular and steady practice, and once skill is gained, you will have much more control over the intensity and duration of heat delivered to the point.

PLACING THE MOXA PUNK

Moxibustion is applied to a palpably reactive point. Chapter 3, Palpation, describes common reactions to seek which for *okyū* are usually points with knots or indurations and pressure pain. After determining what points to check, that is, those indicated for the symptoms, palpation is used to determine exact point locations. Moxa therapists usually palpate more points and areas of the body than most acupuncturists. There are two reasons for this. First, the point treated is usually very small, and because the piece of moxa is also very small, it is easy to miss the point, if even by a few millimeters. When one misses the point, the success of the treatment may be seriously compromised. Second, moxibustion practice is very pragmatic; it strongly de-emphasizes theory. Because theoretical methods, including patterns of diagnosis and so forth, are not part of mainstream moxibustion practice, the method of selecting points has to shift away from a theoretically selected point and is determined empirically by palpating points.

Palpation is the tool that moxibustionists use to find the exact point to be treated. In fact, in their relatively frequent study groups, moxibustionists in Japan, such as Seiji Irie, practice point location, even after many years of clinical experience. They recognize, as should any practitioner, that point selection and location must be extremely precise when using moxa. After finding the point, mark its location with a pencil or pen.

Once you have selected a point on which to apply moxibustion, the next step is to place the moxa so that it stands upright, directly on the point. For some, this is often the hardest step and requires considerable practice. It can be a little difficult because the actual size of the moxa punk can be very small, and if your fingers are big, or if your hands tend to sweat a little, you will find doing this takes much practice to master.

In order to place the moxa punk on the point you must first hold the moxa correctly. Probably the simplest approach is to hold the small moxa punk lightly between the finger and thumb, so that it protrudes slightly. To facilitate placement of the punk, position it point-down, without squashing it, standing it up at an angle, or having it fall over on its side.

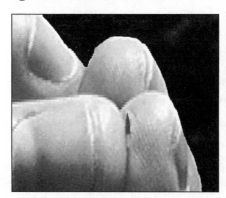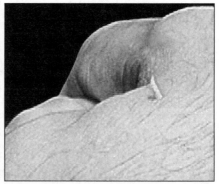

With the moxa protruding slightly between thumb and finger,
gently but firmly position it point-down.

You can help achieve placement of the punk, so that it stands up and does not fall off the point, by moistening either the point or bottom surface of the punk with a little water. Some recommend using a very thin film of wax- or oil-based balm on the point. We recommend using water, as once balm is on your finger tips, it is difficult to manipulate and place the moxa punks. Moistening the point or bottom surface of the punk with a tiny amount of water works well without precipitating further rolling and placement difficulties. If you moisten the point with water, you should be careful not to put too much water on the point. Too much water would interfere with the moxa burning down all the way, and the treatment might end up ineffective.

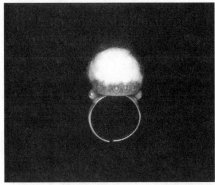

A ring with a wide clasp holds the cotton ball.

Traditionally, the point was moistened with a very thin application of saliva, or the bottom of the piece of moxa was touched to the tongue. This particular practice is now, for obvious reasons, almost obsolete. Instead, a number of new approaches have been adopted. Perhaps the best is the use of a small ring constructed with a wide clasp so that it can hold a cotton ball in it.

The cotton ball is dipped in water so that it becomes moist, without dripping. When moisture is needed, the point can be moistened by wiping the pad of the little finger across the cotton ball and then across the point.

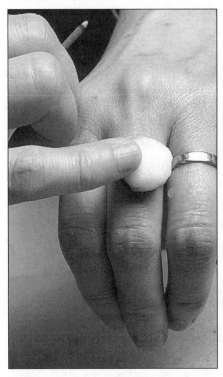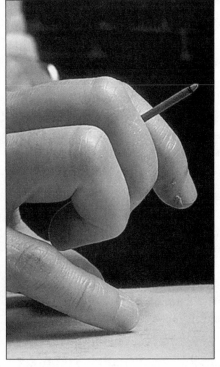

Wipe the pad of the little finger across the cotton ball, then across the point.

Or, you may lightly touch the bottom surface of the moxa punk to the cotton ball and then place it on the point. If you cannot locate one of these rings, which are readily available in Japan, you can place a few drops of water on the back of the hand, or place a moist cotton ball on a nearby tray, and either wipe the little finger or touch the bottom surface of the piece of moxa there.

If the tips of the index finger and thumb holding the piece of moxa become too moist, the moxa often sticks to the finger and thumb and is difficult to place at the point. Thus care must be taken not to get too much moisture on the finger and thumb. This whole procedure is really quite easy, but it does require practice.

Westerners tend to have more body hair than do Japanese. This poses particular problems when applying moxibustion to points. On the head, the best method of dealing with the presence of hair is to use hair clips that firmly secure the hair, splaying it out from the point. When done professionally, the patient will lose no more than a few hairs with the burning of moxa on a scalp point. On the body, hairy areas are a little trickier because pins or clips can't be used to move the the the hair aside. Taping the hair down is ill advised because removal of the tape can be painful. Instead, the recommended technique is either to trim off the hair immediately at the point, or to remove it with the lighted end of an incense stick. Trimming any hair with scissors may be disturbing to patients, but if the patient agrees, it is also a suitable solution.

The use of the lighted incense stick is good, because the patient accepts it as part of the therapy. To accomplish this technique, hold the incense close to the lighted end between the index finger and thumb. Then placing the tips of the finger and thumb on the skin, apply a sweeping motion over the point. The patient will feel a slight sensation of warmth as the unnecessary hair is removed from the area immediately around the point.

The moxa punks are really quite small and take a certain amount of practice to be placed consistently. Practicing the technique of rolling and placing moxa is helpful. As a simple exercise, try to roll and place twenty moxa punk of equal size and consistency on a surface. Make sure that they are all roughly the same size, shape, and consistency and are all standing up. Try this with thread-, sesame-, and half-rice sizes. Once you have mastered this, and can quickly, reliably, and efficiently roll and place the moxa, then you are ready to proceed.

A Japanese company makes so-called *kyūtenshi* or "skin shields," which allow you to fix the exact point location and ensure that the moxa stimulates only the point you wish to stimulate. The shields are made of foil on an adhesive base, with a small hole at the center of the foil. These shields may be useful for nervous beginners or very nervous patients, but they are likely unnecessary once you have mastered good moxa techniques.

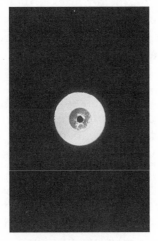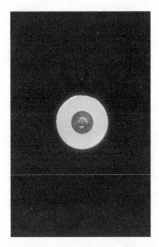

Kyūtenshi moxa shield.   *Kyūtenshi* with moxa on it.

IGNITING THE MOXA

Lighting the moxa is also a skill that becomes easier with consistent and patient practice.

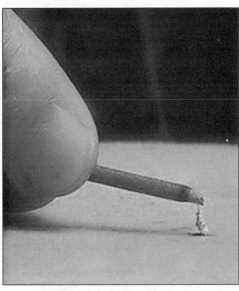

Lighting the moxa with incense.

Because the piece of moxa is very small, the moxa must be lit with burning incense. However, the incense will often lift the moxa off the point when you try to light the moxa with it. To prevent this from happening, give the incense a very slight rotation as you touch the moxa. This helps the incense roll off the moxa thereby leaving it in place. Again, though this is a relatively easy procedure, you need to practice it before any consistency can be achieved.

It is useful to regularly remove the ash from the lighted end of the incense stick. Accumulations of ash on the end of the incense stick commonly cause the moxa punk to lift off the point. If your hands tend to get a little moist while doing this procedure, it is a good idea to draw your index finger and thumb along the incense stick and over the lit end very quickly, in order to remove the ash.

The ashes can then be rubbed lightly onto the end of the finger and thumb, tending to give them a drier surface, which will be better for rolling and placing the moxa. It is generally better to use a thicker stick of incense to light the moxa. A thicker stick will burn more slowly, giving you more usage. Since it burns more slowly, there will be a slower buildup of ash on the lighted end of the incense. In Japan, companies makes special incense for moxibustion use.

NUMBERS OF MOXA APPLICATIONS

With direct moxa techniques, cones are usually burned an odd number of times. We can speculate that this is because tradition teaches that odd numbers are yang in nature and even numbers are yin. Moxa therapy, being somewhat yang in nature, would thus be applied an odd number of times. Whatever the reasons, the moxa is typically applied three, five, or seven times. There are, of course, exceptions to this which are usually specified in the literature. Guidelines for the number of moxa applications are, perhaps, a little different from what you would imagine. Most moxibustionists in Japan state that the moxa heat should be *felt* three, five, or seven times.

Often when an appropriate point is selected, the patient does not feel heat at the point, even when the moxa burns all the way down to the skin. In such cases, the recommendation of burning three moxa at the point is understood to mean that moxa is burnt at the point until the patient has *felt* it three times. On some points this might take over one hundred moxa! For example, in an acute gastrointestinal upset with diarrhea and vomiting, the point *uranaitei* on the plantar surface of the foot is usually indicated. Often either the left or the right point is reasonably sensitive to the burning moxa, and the patient feels heat after only a few applications. But often the other side takes many moxa punks before the heat is felt. In such a case, you might find that as soon as the heat starts being felt at the point (for example, after 50 or so moxa applications) the symptoms start to improve, and you should continue to moxa until the patient has felt the heat a total of three, five, or seven times.

When you find a reactive point that is insensitive to the moxa, it usually indicates that that is a good point to treat. The greater the insensitivity, the more severe the problem reflected at that point. Though it takes time to apply, it is the best way to treat the patient with moxa and is a good opportunity to improve your moxa application skills. In such cases, it is not the best solution to keep increasing the size of the moxa until the patient feels the heat. Keeping the moxa pieces the same size will help you gauge the degree of severity of the patient's condition and helps assess the likely length of treatment, thus assisting your prognosis.

CONTROLLING THE AMOUNT OF HEAT: PREVENTING BURNS AND SCARS

The sizes of moxa we have described here, the thread-, sesame-, and half rice-sizes, can deliver quite a sharp pinch of heat to a point. The smaller pieces tend to deliver a quicker, less sustained pinch of heat, while the larger pieces tend to deliver a more intense, more sustained pinch of heat. The heat sensation can penetrate into the body and is often felt as though a needle were inserted. Patients also describe feeling travelling sensations, just as they often do with needling.

In general, though, it is a good idea to be able to control the degree of heat delivered to a point and to be able to control the rate at which the heat is delivered to a point. An excessive degree of heat, delivered very rapidly to a point, might have good clinical effects, but can be very uncomfortable for the patient, and may disturb the treatment. There are also some people who are extremely sensitive at any treatment point selected: any degree of moxa feels too hot. In such cases it is essential to ensure that a minimal degree of heat is delivered to the point, and that you control the rate at which it is delivered.

For your moxa rolling techniques to be proficient, you must be able to roll consistently and place and ignite small, thin sizes of moxa. In particular, repeated use of the thread-size moxa, when professionally applied, will usually neither burn nor scar the point. In order to distract the patient from the small but sharp pinch of heat that such moxa delivers, Fukaya recommended the use of pressure around the point. This technique does not reduce the intensity of the heat itself. Rather than just pressing around the point with the fingers, Fukaya preferred to use a bamboo tube pressed firmly to the skin around the point. Now glass tubes are available for the same purpose.

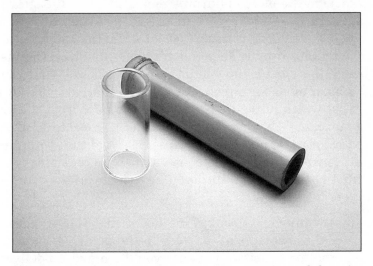

Glass and bamboo tubes used to create pressure around the point.

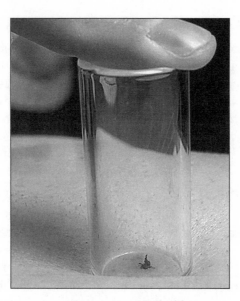

A glass tube is applied to reduce sensitivity to moxa heat.

If your techniques are not so refined, or if you want to reduce the risk of burning and scarring the point completely, you need to reduce the degree of heat that is delivered to the point by the moxa. There are three simple techniques that can be employed to reduce the degree of heat delivered to the point and/or the rate at which it is delivered. The first is simply to extinguish the moxa at the same time that the patient begins to feel the heat. This can be done by simply tapping the moxa cone and compressing it to the skin. Done correctly, this extinguishes the moxa immediately without burning you or the patient because the moxa punk is so small it will snuff out as soon as you tap it.

In order to use this technique well you must understand exactly at what level in the piece of burning moxa the patient begins to feel the heat. Waiting for the patient to say it is hot, or asking the patient when it is hot, is often too late. The moxa punk usually burns down quite rapidly so you don't have time to extinguish the moxa before there is too much stimulation. It is best that you have practiced burning enough pieces of moxa so that you already know the depth at which patients usually feel the heat from the piece of burning moxa, and that you keep the finger you use to snuff out the moxa ready for rapid deployment. It is essential that your pieces of moxa are consistently the same size and same consistency or texture. Practice on yourself until you have a good idea of when the sensation of heat is felt.

One disadvantage of the *okyū* method is that you have not much control over the rate of heat delivery to the point. Another disadvantage is that on sensitive patients you often end up delivering a sharper, more intense heat to the point than was intended. To help offset this last problem, it is generally a good idea to make sure that the initial pieces of moxa are snuffed out sooner than normal. Then, if you ascertain that no or very little heat was felt, you can let the pieces burn down a little further before snuffing them out. It is important that a firm enough tap is applied to the moxa to snuff it out. If your tap is too light, either the moxa will continue to burn, delivering too much heat to the point, or it will lift off on the end of your finger and burn you.

A second method of decreasing the heat intensity of the burning moxa is to leave the ashes of previous moxa on the point and place new pieces of moxa upon those ashes. This tends to reduce the amount of heat delivered to the point, as the skin is being shielded by a thin layer of ashes.

However, when applying this technique, if the moxa of previous pieces has not completely burnt, and remains on the point, the next piece of moxa can reignite those remains, thus generating a more intense heat than a normal piece of moxa would deliver. To prevent this, make sure that the moxa cones are snuffed out before this can happen. Sometimes placing a new moxa cone on the ashes can be more difficult than placing one on the skin itself, because you cannot moisten the ashes, you can only moisten the bottom surface of the new piece of moxa.

The third and perhaps best technique for controlling the amount of heat delivered to the point, and one that also gives you more control over the rate of delivery is as follows. After placing the moxa punk at the point and igniting it, place the index finger and thumb of your free hand to the side of the piece of moxa, with a cone-shaped gap between the finger and thumb.

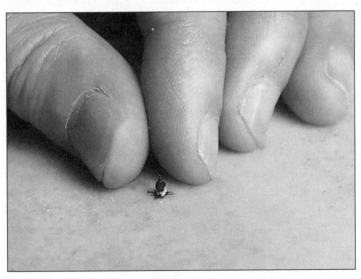

Position the index finger and thumb around the moxa as shown.

As it begins to burn down, slowly roll the finger and thumb over the piece of moxa, so that the cone-shaped space sits directly over the piece of moxa. This slows down the rate of flow of air to the piece of moxa, depriving it of oxygen and thus slowing down the rate at which the piece of moxa burns.

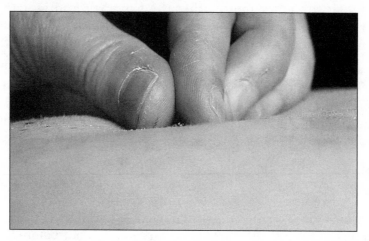

Roll the finger and thumb over the moxa to slow the rate of burning.

When done correctly, the heat is no longer felt as a distinct pinch of heat, but rather as a milder, more drawn-out sensation of heat. If the finger and thumb are too widely spaced, insufficient control of air flow will occur, and the moxa will burn hotter than intended. If the finger and thumb are not sufficiently spaced, the air flow will be cut off and the moxa will snuff out before heat is felt. Usually, your index finger and thumb will not feel much heat as the moxa burns, but if you do it incorrectly, you can feel too much heat and possibly cause yourself a little irritation. Done correctly, you will never burn yourself, and the technique is completely safe and effective. Learning this technique well takes repetition. First practice doing this on a flat surface, then on yourself.

Finally, you can gain more control over the degree of heat delivered to a point by combining the first and second methods, or by combining the second and third methods. Practice and experience will help you judge what is appropriate for you and for each patient.

The techniques of controlling the degree of heat delivered to the point are important from a traditional point of view as well. Usually a milder degree of heat delivery is seen as being more supplementing, because the less the patient feels the heat, the more supplementing the treatment, and conversely, the stronger the heat delivery, the more draining the treatment. This principle is articulated in *Ling Shu* Chapter 51, where it says, "To disperse with moxa, blow on it gently," which makes it burn hotter.[4]

[4]See K. Matsumoto and S. Birch, *Five Elements and Ten Stems*, p. 166.

PRECAUTIONS AND CONTRAINDICATIONS

The following are a few contraindications and precautions for the use of direct moxa:

•When treating children, generally the moxa is not allowed to burn down to the skin.

•When treating inflamed areas or inflamed joints, do not burn moxa on points in the inflamed area; rather, select and treat local points that are proximal and distal to the inflammation.

•Burning moxa on the face is generally not recommended because of the risk of scarring.

•Avoid applying moxa when the patient is very hungry or has just eaten a big meal.

•Avoid the use of moxa in very serious cases, such as the last stage of cancer, a very high fever, or extreme fatigue.

•It is ill-advised to use moxa on the lower abdomen of a pregnant or possibly pregnant woman.

•Avoid moxa application for an hour before or after taking a very hot bath or sauna.

•Avoid treating with moxa if the patient has recently consumed alcoholic drinks.

•Avoid using moxibustion over large blood vessels.

•Avoid the use of direct moxibustion over areas of dermatological diseases.

•There are contradictions in the traditional and modern literature as to which points are contraindicated for use with moxa. Nevertheless, it is good idea to become familiar with these contraindications and follow them.[5]

•Care should be taken when using moxa on diabetic or allergic patients because the site of moxibustion therapy can more easily become irritated or infected than on non-diabetic or non-allergic patients.

•Usually, when applying moxa on a diabetic patient, only points on the torso are selected.

•When applying moxa, it is always a good idea to locate and treat the points while the patient remains in one treatment position.

[5]See Y. Manaka, K. Itaya, and S. Birch, *Chasing the Dragon's Tail* pp. 355-361 for details.

Though direct moxa is prohibited for an inflamed area such as an arthritic joint, or for a seriously ill patient with high fever, contraindications for the use of moxa in patients with euphemistically termed "hot" conditions are not recognized and do not apply. Traditionally moxibustion therapy has been used successfully on patients with all kinds of health problems, whether or not they have so-called "hot" conditions.

SAWADA'S TAIKYOKU MOXA THERAPY

Mr. Sawada had an interesting treatment method which he termed *taikyoku* (in Chinese, *taiji*, the great ultimate), the "root" or balance treatment. Unlike Manaka's approach, where the root treatment typically uses ion-pumping cords, or the Keiraku Chiryō schools, where supplementation and draining techniques are used to balance the channels, Sawada used moxa on a specific set of points for all patients, regardless of symptoms or conditions, to produce general balancing effects. After using this general set of points, he would select other points specific to the patient's symptoms and conditions. The selection of this second set of points was based on empirical knowledge of the points and their palpatory responses. The general points he felt were good for overall body balance.

From this combination of root and symptom control therapies, Mr. Sawada obtained extremely good results. His case records hold numerous examples of successful treatment of advanced cases of diseases such as tuberculosis, where he had an extremely high success rate long before penicillin or antibiotics were available. Many practitioners in Japan still use Sawada's general treatment method; some, like Manaka, have devised alternate combinations of points having the same general balancing effects.[6]

Sawada considered disease an imbalance of the blood circulation. He viewed circulation as part of the body's self healing mechanisms. He believed that stimulating and improving the circulation using the *taikyoku* treatment to improve the body's self-healing powers could potentially treat anything, and was particularly good for chronic diseases.

To get the most benefit from Shirota/Sawada treatments, moxa the following points from the *taikyoku* treatment and then select and treat a few points indicated for the patient's specific problem. Select those points that seem most appropriate and treat them as a set. You can moxa each point three, five, or seven times depending on the sensitivity of the patient, the number of points chosen, the severity of the patient's condition, and the ease and rapidity of your moxa rolling techniques.

---

[6]See Y. Manaka, K. Itaya, and S. Birch, *Chasing the Dragon's Tail* pp. 177-179 for details.

An introduction to Sawada's *taikyoku* treatment, the points, and some guidelines for their selection are outlined below.[7]

Point	Application	Usage
GV-12	most patients	helps regulate the nervous system
BL-18	most patients	specific for the liver
BL-20	most patients	specific for the spleen and stomach
BL-22	important, but not commonly used	specific for the triple burner
BL-23	almost all patients	specific for the kidneys
Sawada's GB-25[*1]	commonly used	specific for the kidney
BL-32	most patients	regulates the bladder
CV-12	most patients (less with children)	good for the spleen and stomach
TB-4	most patients especially on the left side	
LI-11	most patients	regulates large intestine and skin problems
ST-36	virtually all patients except gastric hyperacidic patients	good for digestion
Sawada's KI-3[*2]	most patients	good for the kidney
BL-15	not so commonly used	
LI-10	not so commonly used	
LU-6[*3]	not so commonly used	
LI-2	often used on children especially combined with GV-12	
SI-10	not so commonly used	
GV-8	not so commonly used	can be good for liver problems
TB-15	used on many patients	
BL-13	not so commonly used	
GB-34	not so commonly used	
Sawada's BL-43[*4]	not so commonly used	
an extra point, 1 *cun* above BL-18, 1 *cun* lateral to the spine	not commonly used	

[*1] Location: BL-52.
[*2] Location: near KI-6.
[*3] Location: $1/3$ distance from LU-5 to LU-9, $3/10$ that distance.
[*4] Location: BL-44, lateral to BL-15.

[7]This introduction is based on Bunshi Shirota's works, *Shinkyū Shinzui (Basics of Acupuncture and Moxibustion)*, pp. 8-16 *passim; Kyūryō Zatsuwa (Miscellaneous Lectures on Moxa Therapy)*, pp. 207-209, and *Shinkyū Chiryō Kisogaku (Fundamentals of Acupuncture and Moxibustion Therapy)*, pp 423-424.

This basic set of points presented above can be useful for chronic and stubborn problems, especially those that have been unresponsive to other treatment methods. They can be treated each time the patient visits the clinic. For some patients it is useful to have a relative or partner at home treat the point set daily. Recently we had a patient present with an advanced case of cystic fibrosis who was awaiting a lung transplant operation. This *taikyoku* moxa treatment, applied daily by the patient's partner, was the primary treatment and proved extremely helpful for the patient.

In the next section, there is a list of moxa treatments from Shirota's *Kyūryō Zatsuwa*. Combining the *taikyoku* treatment with the appropriate symptom control points can be very effective. Using the points mentioned for a specific disease can be helpful after any of Manaka's root treatment methods and/or the Keiraku Chiryō approaches outlined in Chapter 2.

MOXIBUSTION TREATMENTS FROM BUNSHI SHIROTA

The following is a list of highly recommended moxibustion treatments for over fifty common disorders. These treatments are recommended especially for acute problems. Taken from Bunshi Shirota's book *Kyūryō Zatsuwa* (pp. 210-213), they form a kind of emergency therapeutic repertoire. Points are selected as usual by palpation. Care should be taken to mark the most reactive points and to treat only the more reactive points. On occasion, though, if the symptoms persist, the rest of the points can be used.

Headache
GV-20, GV-16, GV-12, BL-10 (or above BL-10), LI-10.

Migraine headache
BL-10, TB-15, GB-17, BL-7, GV-20.

Earache
TB-17, GB-2, KI-3, HT-3, TB-9, LI-10.

Stomatitis
BL-14, LI-11, LI-15.

Toothache
Upper jaw: BL-14, ST-44, TB-10, LI-10.

Lower jaw: LI-7 (Sawada's location),[8] BL-13, LI-4.

---

[8]Sawada's LI-7 is located as follows: when the index fingers and thumbs of both hands are interlaced so that the index finger of one hand is placed on the styloid process of the other hand, the point is in the depression between the muscles right under the tip of the index finger. This is likely the same point named LU-7 in modern Chinese practice (TCM).

Gingivitis

LI-11, LI-10, BL-14.

Nasal congestion

GV-22, BL-10, LI-10, HT-3.

Epistaxis

GV-16, GV-23, GV-14.

Cerebral hemorrhage

GV-20, BL-20, LI-10, ST-36, LI-40.

Cerebral anemia

PC-4,[9] LI-10, ST-36, HT-7, SI-1, GV-22.

Eye pain

TB-22, LI-11, BL-23 *huato* point,[10] Sawada's LI-4.[11]

Throat pain

KI-3, LU-5, GV-12, BL-11 *huato* point, LU-7,[12] TB-17.

Chest pain

SI-11, BL-43. For pain that runs vertically, add KI-3;
for pain that runs horizontally, add LR-14,[13]
for pain in the whole region of the chest, add PC-4.

Heart pain

PC-4, SI-11, HT-7, GV-10, CV-17, CV-14.

Breast pain

CV-17, SI-11.

Spasm of the stomach

ST-34, BL-50, LR-13.

[9]PC-4 is located approximately 1/3 the distance from PC-3 to PC-7, 3/10 of that distance.

[10]The BL-23 *huato* point is 0.5 *cun* lateral to the midline of the spine, at the level of BL-23 (lateral to the intervertebral space between Lumbar 2 and 3).

[11]Sawada's LI-4 is just distal to the junction of the first and second metacarpals where a pulse can be felt.

[12]LU-7 is located on the lung channel, on the line between LU-9 and LU-5, 1 ½ *cun* proximal to LU-9, just proximal to the styloid process of the radius.

[13]LR-14 is located in the subcostal region, at the tip of the 9th costal cartilage, slightly medial to the mammary line, level with CV-13.

Stomachache from hunger

GV-9, BL-17, CV-16, CV-14.

Gallstone colic

CV-12, right ST-21, BL-50, GB-36 (or GB-40), above right LR-14, above right ST-19, right BL-19 *huato* point.

Pain in the cecum area

CV-6 (moxa 30x), ST-34, LR-8, one thumb width lateral to right BL-25.

Abdominal pain

LR-13, GB-25, CV-9, CV-12, ST-34 (whole abdomen).

Colic

KI-16, CV-12, CV-6, BL-50, Sawada's GB-33 (3 *cun* below GB-32).

Bladder pain

CV-3, CV-4, ST-28, CV-6, LR-8, BL-32.

Urethral pain

LR-8, CV-2, CV-3, KI-12.

Hemorrhoid pain

LU-6, BL-33, GV-2.

Hemorrhoidal hemorrhage

LU-6, BL-32, BL-33, BL-27, *josen,* BL-23, GV-3.

Anal prolapse

BL-32, BL-33, GV-20.

Hemorrhaging of internal organs

Stomach or duodenal ulcer: GB-34.
Intestinal hemorrhaging: BL-27, GB-34.

Uterine bleeding

GB-34, BL-27.

Hemoptysis

PC-4, TB-8, KI-3.

Pleurisy

PC-4, GB-35, GB-21, LR-14, BL-17.

Peritonitis

LR-13, CV-9, LR-8.

Palpitations

PC-4, HT-7.

Intermittent fever

SI-2, SI-3.

Pneumonia, influenza

SI-3, BL-11 *huato* point, GV-12, Sawada's GB-33.[14]

Catching cold (wind evil)

BL-12, GV-12 (moxa 21x).

Food poisoning

ST-44, *uranaitei*[15] (moxa 15-20x).

Diarrhea

Watery diarrhea: ST-34, BL-33.

Explosive diarrhea: BL-60.

Constipation

Sawada's HT-7,[16] left SP-14.

Difficult labor

BL-67, tip of the little toe.

Morning sickness

TB-4, CV-12, CV-14.

Carbuncle (including boils)

LI-11, LI-10, LI-4, SI-6.

Urticaria

LI-15, BL-12, LI-11.

Skin diseases (e.g. eczema, miliaria)

LI-15, LI-11, GV-12, BL-12.

[14]Sawada's GB-33 is located(3 *cun* below GB-32.

[15]*Uranaitei* is located on the plantar surface of the foot posterior to the phalanges-metatarsal joint of the second toe. Place a dot of ink in the center of the pad of the second toe, fold the toe down towards the plantar surface of the foot, where the ink dot touches the foot is the point *uranaitei*.

[16]Sawada's HT-7 is located in the depression on the wrist crease between the heart and small intestine channels.

Blepharitis

LI-11, TB-22.

Tinnitus

HT-3, TB-17.

Dizziness

GB-43, GB-12.

Hypomenorrhea

SP-6, SP-10.

Menorrhagia

GB-34.

Detoxification (including intoxication)

KI-9.

Pain of the heel bone

BL-61.

Speech disturbance

GV-15.

Edema

KI-3, KI-1, ST-44, GV-20.

Erysipelas

Extra point one *cun* proximal to PC-3.

IBUKI MOXA

Instructions for home therapy using the ibuki moxa technique can be given to the patient, as it is relatively risk-free and easy, and permits moxibustion therapy to be practiced safely at home.

There are several forms of *ibuki* moxa. The most common has only moxa inside it, while the others have various herbal substances admixed. Some Korean moxa products, such as the JSA moxa, use the same approach as the *ibuki* moxa. Another Korean product, the KMI moxa, uses a combination of moxa, wormwood, and sagebrush, which tends to leave a yellow resin deposit. We would recommend in particular Japanese *ibuki* moxa and the Korean JSA moxa products.

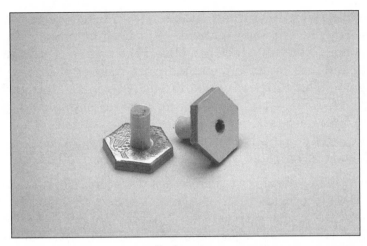

Ibuki moxa.

They both share a common mode of application: a little piece of moxa is placed on one end of a platform having a sticky surface on the other end. This method allows for moxa to be placed on the point without the moxa actually touching the skin. Thus it is safer than the *okyū* method for patients to use at home, as patients without good skills in *okyū* might easily burn themselves. The sticky base prevents the moxa from shifting position and allows easier handling of the hot moxa as it can be picked up off the skin by grasping and lifting the base.

To apply the *ibuki* moxa, hold the base firmly, peel off the wax paper that protects the sticky base, and position the base firmly over the point, making sure that the hole in the middle of the hexagonally shaped base sits over the point to be stimulated. Ignite it like a piece of incense and then place it on the point to be treated, or light it once positioned on the skin, using either incense, a match, or a lighter.

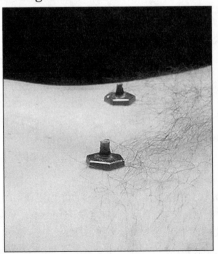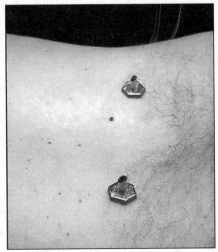

Ibuki moxa positioned on the back.

Usually the heat of the moxa is felt as being mild, not at all uncomfortable. On some patients, the heat becomes a little too intense, and, if left untended can blister the point slightly. To offset burning and discomfort and eliminate the risks of blistering, follow these guidelines: as the *ibuki* moxa burns down far enough for the patient to feel the heat, lift the platform off the skin; then replace it on the point, lift again, replace again, and so forth; continue doing this until the moxa has burned out. This way the heat does not become too concentrated and intense and will not blister the point.

When using *ibuki* moxa, there are occasions when the patient hardly feels the heat. In such cases continue applying the *ibuki* moxa (as above with direct moxa) until the patient feels the heat. Usually burning or blistering occurs only when the patient feels the heat, and leaving the *ibuki* on the point will not create a problem. Depending on the severity of the case, you can apply one to five or more *ibuki* moxa to a point, but usually one to three is enough, and is likely the best recommendation you can give to the patient for home therapy. If working with a pair of points, such as left and right SP-6, the *ibuki* moxa cone can be moved from point to point as soon as the heat is felt at each point. Thus it might be placed on left SP-6 to begin with, and as soon as the heat is felt there, it should be lifted off and placed on right SP-6. When heat is felt there, lift it off and place it on left SP-6 again, and so forth. Moving the moxa platform back and forth like this is not only economical, but it lessens the amount of stimulation given to each point and reduces the total volume of smoke produced.

The *ibuki* moxa can be used as a substitute for any of the moxa treatments discussed above. If a patient suffers from a particular complaint, palpate the appropriate points, marking those that are reactive. After applying treatment in the clinic, give the patient *ibuki* moxa, along with instructions on how and where to apply it to stimulate the selected points while at home. Used in this fashion, the *ibuki* moxa can be an invaluable aid in the treatment of difficult and chronic problems.

An even more general use of the *ibuki* moxa is as a method of warming areas that are typically cold, or cold to the touch. Often the lower abdomen is cold or cool to the touch. This is seen in patients with weakness of the lower burner, problems of the bladder, problems of the intestines, and gynecological or menstrual problems.

Have the patient apply the *ibuki* moxa at the coldest points on the lower abdomen, or focus on general tonic points such as CV-6 and CV-4. This treatment can be helpful for the overall condition as well as the patient's symptoms. Another general use of the *ibuki* moxa is as a gentle stimulus to release muscle tension in the neck and shoulder regions. All the yang channels and some of the yin channels pass through the neck and shoulder regions, which can cause a bottleneck effect, where channels are frequently obstructed, along with the accompanying muscle tightness and stiffness. Often a little gentle heat in this region applied to the tightest, stiffest points or muscles is helpful for releasing this tension. If you decide to have patients try this at home, make sure to instruct them to not let the moxa become too hot, by moving the platform around a little more frequently than at other points or body areas.

CHINETSUKYU—CONE MOXA[17]

The advantage of using *chinetsukyū* (cone moxa) is the superlative control of heat applied to the point, which allows for a very precise as well as general supplementation effect. Because the moxa cones burn much more slowly than the regular direct moxa cones or punks, you have much more time to remove the moxa at the appropriate moment. This technique is suitable for a range of uses including general supplementation of qi, movement of qi in obstructed channels, mild supplementation effects as a complement to techniques such as bloodletting, and fixing wrong or improper treatments.

The moxa cone can range in sizes, depending on the practitioner. What is important is to determine the size you prefer to use and to use it consistently. Typical sizes of these moxa cones are seen relative to a U.S. 10-cent piece in the following picture:

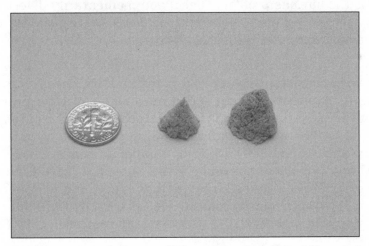

Cone moxa size relative to a U.S. ten-cent piece (1.7cm diameter)

As is apparent, these moxa cones are considerably larger than the direct moxa cones or punks.

---

[17]For this section we are particularly indebted to Masahiro Kurita and Kōei Kuahara for their excellent instruction.

We recommend the use of the "semi-pure" moxa that was used also for the *kyūtōshin* (moxa on the handle of the needle) technique. Using a flat surface, take a piece of moxa and compress it between the thumb, forefinger, and middle finger of one hand, simultaneously pressing or rubbing it against the flat surface so as to apply pressure from that surface and give the cone a smooth bottom surface.

To make the cone come out in the right shape, apply a twirling motion with the thumb and fingers. This twirling motion should stem from the wrist rather than the fingers and thumb. When rolling the moxa cone, compression is essentially applied by the force of the fingers from the sides, from the force of the fingers pressing down and rubbing on the flat surface, and from the rotation force of the fingers and thumb. The reason it is important to apply pressure from all sides like this is to produce an evenly compressed moxa cone.

An unevenly compressed moxa cone will burn unevenly. For example, it might burn down very quickly through the center of the cone, where you cannot see it, while appearing to burn slowly on its edges. This will cause the cone to get hot very quickly. When the cone gets hot with surprising speed, you must move quickly to remove it, thereby increasing the chances of dropping the cone and burning the patient. Furthermore, if too much heat is delivered to the point, the effect is more draining. If you were trying to supplement a point, too much heat would be counterproductive. Also, there is the obvious problem that if you momentarily divert attention to something else, you might be too slow responding to the intense heat and burn or blister the point.

To avoid all these problems, you should be able to roll the moxa cones with consistent compression and uniform size. Mastering this skill requires spending a certain amount of time practicing rolling the moxa before applying the technique on a patient. To this end, we recommend practice rolling the cones until you can quickly and without effort roll a number of cones which, when placed side by side, are of roughly the same size, have flat bottom surfaces, and when squeezed lightly have the same relatively firm consistency. Don't roll the cones too loosely, as they will burn more quickly, giving you less time to judge precisely when to remove them.

Once you have mastered the cone-rolling techniques, you must learn the application techniques. The cones are ignited using a burning incense stick and are typically burnt only about halfway down.

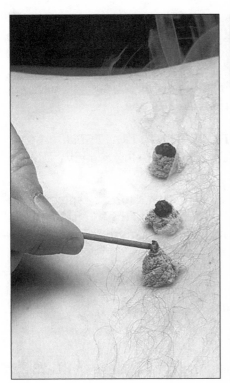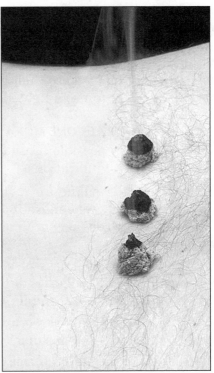

Chinetsukyū moxa.

To let them burn much further usually delivers too much heat to the point. Thus when you remove the cone, the wider half of the cone will still be burning. Rather than let it keep burning, and thus unnecessarily smoke up the treatment room, we recommend keeping some water handy in a metal bowl. As the patient begins to feel the heat (which is felt more as a sensation of warmth) pick up the cone by its base and drop it, point down, in the water in the bowl. This extinguishes the lighted moxa cone immediately.

It is also important to remember that moxa, by its dry nature, will not stick to the skin very well. To prevent the moxa cone from rolling around while lighted (a disturbing experience for both practitioner and patient), we advise moistening the bottom surface of the cone before applying it to the point. Float the moxa cone, bottom surface down, on the surface of the water in the bowl for a few seconds. This will ensure that a certain amount of water will remain on the bottom surface of the cone. Next, carefully remove the cone and place it on the back of your hand before applying it to the point. This maneuver serves two purposes. First, it assures that the bottom surface of the cone is sufficiently moist to stick to the skin. Second, it allows removal of any excess water and warming of the water before applying the cone to the desired treatment point.

Having gained sufficient mastery of these techniques, you will be able to moisten and place half a dozen cones at the same time, without any worry of burning the patient. But, as with all other techniques, only practice makes perfect! We also recommend starting out applying no more than three moxas at a time. To light the cone, it is better to use a lighted incense stick.

GENERAL CONE MOXA TREATMENT STRATEGIES

There are many possible uses of cone moxa; below we give a few of the most general indications.

•For overall weakness of qi, typically with a lung or spleen vacuity pattern, apply cone moxa to GV-14, and a point to either side of GV-14. Use one cone on each point, ensuring only light heat sensations.

•For overall weakness of qi, especially if reading and distinguishing the radial pulses is difficult, try applying cone moxa to left and right ST-25, CV-12, and CV-6 or CV-4.

•For overall weakness of qi, especially with weakness of the lower burner, use cone moxa on CV-6.

•For lower burner problems in general, cone moxa to BL-23 and GV-3 can be helpful.

•For any chronic problem, cone moxa to *pi gen* can be helpful.

•For any problem in the upper half of the body, with soft, vacuous-feeling skin and/or muscle tightness in the supraclavicular region, apply cone moxa to reactive points.

•To correct a mistaken treatment, where too much stimulation was given, or the wrong diagnosis was made, try applying cone moxa repeatedly to GV-14 until the patient feels better or the radial pulse improves. This may require the use of many cone moxa. The same technique can be used on CV-6 in the same manner for the same purposes. The signs of a mistaken treatment are a radial pulse that is worse than before the treatment began (e.g., faster, weaker, and more floating), or if the patient complains of a strange or unusual feeling or fatigue.

•To correct an overdose of bloodletting (i.e., letting of too much blood), cone moxa may be burned at GV-14 or CV-6 or at the site of the bloodletting. An overdose of bloodletting usually only occurs after excess amounts of blood are let when bloodletting and cupping are used together. (See Chapter 10 for more detailed discussions).

•For a patient with fever, apply cone moxa[18] repeatedly to GV-14, and let the moxa be felt a little hotter.

[18]Though contrary to the recommendations of many modern Chinese texts, where moxibustion is contraindicated in the presence of heat, efficacious use of moxa for fever is confirmed by more recent Chinese studies (e.g., Tian & Wang, 1987, and Wang, Tian, and Li, 1987).

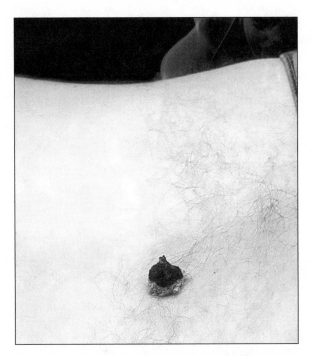

For a fever, the cone moxa is burnt further down and is therefore hotter.

•For diarrhea, apply cone moxa to four points immediately above, below, and to the two sides of the navel; let the heat be felt a little stronger. For stiff neck, headache, or stiff shoulders, apply cone moxa to BL-10, GB-20, or GB-21.

•For dermatological problems, such as a rash, insect bite, or itching, apply the cone moxa directly on the problem area and let it be felt a little hotter.

•For contusions, palpate around the edges of the contusion, and apply cone moxa to encourage qi and blood flow to the injured area.

Chapter 6
Hinaishin—Intradermal Needles

Hinaishin (literally, "skin-inside-needle") or intradermal needles–sometimes called subcutaneous needles are an extremely useful treatment modality. There are different types of intradermal needles made of silver, gold, or stainless steel that are manufactured in different sizes or gauges (3mm, 4mm, 5mm, 6mm, 7mm, 8mm) and equipped with solid handles or coiled wire handles. The following show a number of different types at their actual sizes:

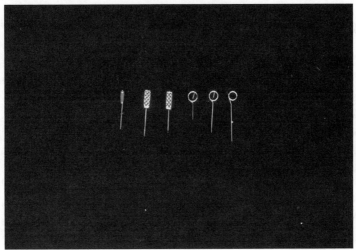

Varieties of the most commonly used *hinaishin*.

The most commonly used, and covering perhaps the broadest range of applications, are the 3mm and 6mm stainless steel needles. We recommend using the Japanese intradermals, which are individually packaged and presterilized and tooled to the correct thickness for safe, painless use.[1]

---

[1]The Chinese have been using intradermal needles and describing the use of intradermal needles for a number of years now. They now manufacture their own needles. However, the Chinese intradermal needles are much thicker, longer, and are inserted more deeply inserted. Because of this difference in size, they are unsuitable for many of the uses described here.

INTRADERMAL POPULARITY

Intradermals are used by almost all acupuncturists in Japan today. Since their invention they have helped spark a resurgence of interest in acupuncture, especially in the study and practice of Keiraku Chiryo or channel therapy. Because they are inserted so shallowly, with no stimulation or sensation, they adhere to the principles of the Keiraku Chiryō groups.

Intradermals were invented in the early 1950s by Kōbei Akabane of Japan. He originally designed them for use in his famous "Akabane channel-balancing" treatments of the left and right branches of the channels. Today they are used not so much with the intention of balancing the channels, but more for the gentle and continuous treatment of specific points for the relief of specific conditions.

The main difference in use between these needles and regular needles is that intradermal needles are inserted very shallowly into the points. Then they are taped and left in place for up to one week to provide gentle and continuous treatment while they are in place.

INSERTING INTRADERMAL NEEDLES AT THE ACUPOINTS

MARKING THE POINT

As with almost all the techniques described in this volume, points are selected on the basis of known or empirical effects—uses of the points and the presence of some palpable reaction, such as pressure pain, tension, tightness, a muscle knot, and so forth. Once a point has been selected for treatment, mark it so that it cannot be lost. This can be done either by pressing the point with a blunt probe such as a *teishin* in order to leave a small dent, or by marking either side of the point with a pen. (Avoid needling into an inkspot!) With practice, this marking will become unnecessary as you become more sensitive to what you feel when palpating and as you become accustomed to palpating with one hand and holding the prepared needle with the other.

DETERMINING THE ANGLE OF INSERTION

After selecting and marking a point, ascertain the natural crease or fold of the skin at that point. A skin crease is a clearly visible line in the skin, and common on the wrists, knees, elbows, and other joints. A skin fold is one that only becomes visible with movement or is that plane along which the skin folds with movement. On the abdomen the skin fold is usually horizontal, that is, running from left to right or right to left. On the low back, the skin folds also run horizontally. On the upper back between the shoulder blades, the fold is more vertical. Knowing the natural crease or skin fold is important because the needle should follow the crease in order to reduce the risk of irritation. While not all authors agree on the optimal angle of insertion for intradermal needles, the following illustrations show the angle of insertion for each body area that we have found safe, effective, and useful.

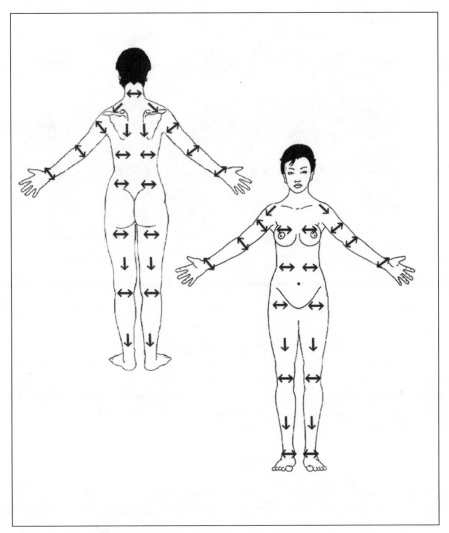

Angle of *hinaishin* insertion for body areas.

When not needling near a joint on the limbs (e.g., GB-31), you can angle in the direction of channel flow. If needling near a joint (e.g., SP-10), it is better to insert at an angle perpendicular to the channel. On the torso, the angle of insertion should always be parallel to the floor, i.e., perpendicular to the channels, excepting needle placement in the interscapular region. Here, you should angle either with or against the channel flow. On the spine, the intradermals are typically inserted in the intervertebral spaces, perpendicular to the spine, and parallel to the floor.

Before inserting the needle, use an alcohol swipe to sterilize the skin surface. The needle should be picked up using fine tweezers. To do this correctly, the tweezers should not grasp the needle by the handle. It is better to grasp along the body of the needle, near the handle.

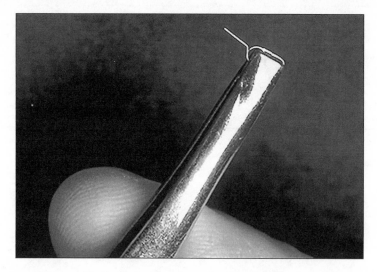

Grasp with the tweezers along the handle of the needle.

The weakest part of an intradermal needle is where the body and the handle join. To protect this weak spot, care should be taken to avoid bending the needle when inserting it. Unless your technique is inadequate, this should not be difficult to avoid, particularly when using the stainless steel needles described in this section. Sometimes intradermals made of silver or gold, which are softer metals, will test your mastery of insertion skills.

USING TWEEZERS TO INSERT THE INTRADERMAL NEEDLE

Tweezers with a grasping surface that does not extend along the whole surface, serrated edge tweezers with edges thicker than the thickness of the needles, or pointed tweezers that taper to a point, all hamper efficient handling of intradermals because of their small size. Tweezers that have a clear, wide grasping surface are much better. The best tweezers to use when handling intradermal needles are those with non-serrated, flat grasping surfaces where smooth contact can be made along the length of both surfaces. In our experience, inexpensive and readily available eyebrow tweezers have worked best for handling intradermal needles.

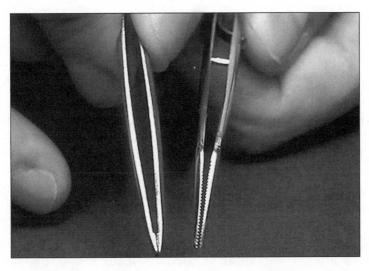

The flat-edged tweezers (on left) are better for intradermal use.

DROPPED OR BENT INTRADERMAL NEEDLES

Unfortunately, because the intradermal needles are so small, it is not uncommon for practitioners to drop and lose them. This may happen because the tweezers are ill-suited to handle the needles. Sometimes, the needle falls out of the package as it is opened or as the needle is grasped. Sometimes holding the needle in the tweezers with one hand while trying to do to other things distracts the practitioner from keeping pressure on the tweezers, thereby allowing the needle to fall out. If the needle should fall on a work surface such as the treatment bed, and especially if it should fall on the patient, it is important that you do your utmost to find it. Any dropped needles are, of course, disposed of by normal means. To help prevent such mishaps, work carefully and methodically, and avoid doing too many things at the same time.

If a needle bends while being inserted, it should be replaced, as bent needles run the risk of inadvertent deeper insertion which might cause irritation.

INTRADERMAL NEEDLE INSERTION DEPTH

Though intradermal needles are used by different practitioners in many different ways, the literature we have researched and the practitioners we have observed recommend insertion of intradermal needles to no more than half, and usually less, the length of the needle body. It is incorrect to insert intradermal needles to the hilt. This means that the needles are inserted from 1mm to 3mm only. On the 3mm intradermals, the typical insertion is about 1 to 1.5mm. On the 6mm intradermals, the typical insertion is 2 to 3mm. Some groups of practitioners prefer even shallower insertion.

INTRADERMAL NEEDLE SIZE

The size of intradermal needle used will depend largely on the body area treated, and to a lesser extent on the size, build, and other factors of the individual patient. In general, when working on the limbs, especially when near any of the joints (knees, ankles, elbows, and wrists), you should use the 3mm length needles. It is possible on large framed people to use the 6mm needles for the mid-points of the thigh and upper arm. When working on the torso, the 6mm needles can be used on virtually all points on the posterior of the body, including the upper, middle, and lower back, the spine, the shoulders, and the hips. On the spine, when working from T8 down, the 6mm needles can be used, but in the interscapular region, that is, T7 and up, it is better to use the 3mm intradermal needles. When working on the anterior portions of the torso, it is generally better to use the 3mm intradermals, especially if working on the abdominal region. Any points on the hands or feet should be treated with the 3mm needles. Points in the auricles should always be treated with the 3mm needles. Points on the neck are usually better treated with 3mm needles, but, depending on the patient's build and the exact point being treated, the 6mm can be used. On the face, the 3mm are usually better, but if working closer to the ears, as for example, ST-7 for TMJ type problems or teeth problems, the 6mm needles can be used.

Guidelines for placement of 3mm needles

•The limbs, especially when near any of the joints (knees, ankles, elbows, and wrists)

•Anterior of the torso, e.g. chest, abdomen

•On the spine from T7 up

•Points on the hands and feet

•Points on the auricles

•Points on the neck (average or smaller build)

•Points on the face

•Reflex or microsystem areas of the body, such as the auricles and Korean hand reflex areas and points

Guidelines for placement of 6mm needles

•Midpoints of thigh and upper arm on large-framed patients

•All points on the posterior of the torso, e.g., upper, middle, and lower back, the spine, the shoulders, the hips

•On the spine from T8 down

•Points on the neck (larger build)

•Points on the face for TMJ or teeth problems

INTRADERMAL NEEDLE INSERTION

There are two techniques used for the actual insertion of the needle. Neither method involves forcing the needle into the point, as forceful insertion can be painful and often may bend the needles, especially if they are silver or gold. The first method involves displacing the skin away from the needle point, holding the needle point over the acupoint to be treated and slowly allowing the skin to slide back over the needle, so that the needle inserts by the return spring or elasticity of the skin and not by a push of the needle itself. The following are the steps to use for this method:

1. Locate the point and wipe it with an alcohol swab, then hold the needle with tweezers and place the needle over the acupoint so that the point of the needle lies directly over the acupoint.

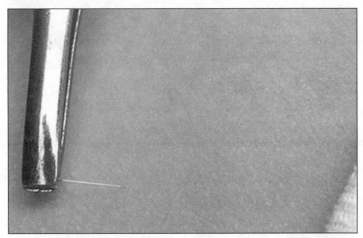

Hold the point of the needle directly over the acupoint.

2. With the finger of the other hand, move the skin away from the point of the needle.

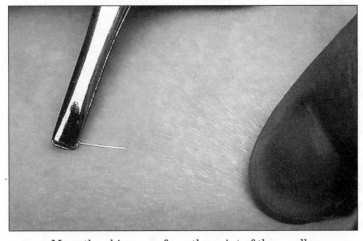

Move the skin away from the point of the needle.

3. Adjust the position of the tip of the needle point to ensure that it lies directly over the marked acupoint in order to allow the needle to insert into exactly the right location.

4. Angle the needle very slightly into the skin.

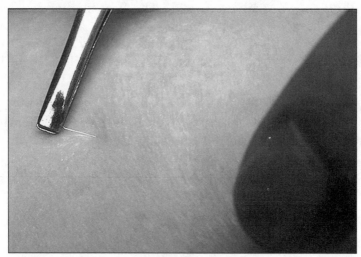

Angle the needle into the skin.

5. Gently and slowly release the skin, allowing the immobile needle to contact and penetrate the skin as it moves back into its normal position. This should be done smoothly and without effort, thereby allowing the needle to be inserted with minimum pressure.

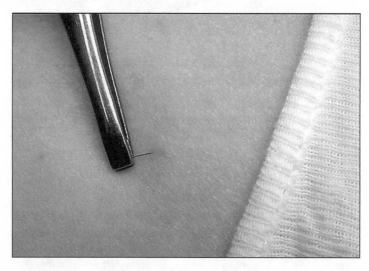

Gently release the skin.

6. Depending on how deeply the needle penetrates, you may need to use the tweezers, while still grasping the needle, to slightly increase or decrease the depth.

The second method is usually easier when using stainless steel needles and when treating a patient with flaccid skin, such as an elderly patient. The needle point is held with tweezers at the acupoint; with the fingers of the other hand, the skin behind the needle is pulled, so that the skin is slowly drawn over the immobile needle to achieve insertion. This method can also be seen as a series of steps:

1. Locate the point and wipe it with an alcohol swab.

2. Hold the needle with tweezers and place its tip so that it lies directly over the desired acupoint, angled slightly into the skin.

3. Touch the point of the needle to the skin.

4. With the free hand, slowly and smoothly pull the skin from behind the needle so that the skin is drawn up over the needle which must be held steady throughout the procedure.

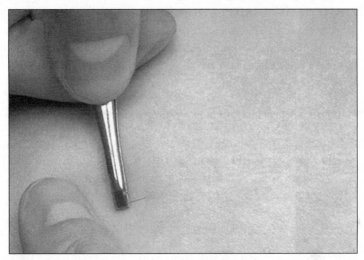

Angle the needle into the skin and pull the skin gently from behind.

5. After the needle is inserted, adjust the needle so that it lies at the correct depth.

When the needle is inserted properly using this technique, patients should not feel the needle insertion at all. Frequently they will ask if the needle is in yet.

The method of insertion of intradermal needles to reflex or microsystem areas of the body, such as the auricles and Korean hand reflex areas and points, is the same as that previously mentioned, except that 3mm intradermals are always used on these areas. The insertion is best achieved by holding the tip of the needle exactly at the desired point while holding the auricle or hand firmly and securely. The needle is then inserted about 1mm using smoothly applied pressure from the hand holding the tweezers and needle. It is hard to displace the skin in the auricles or on the hands, and points are much smaller on both these surfaces. Thus it is better to push the needle through the skin which seems to be the simplest and most painless insertion method.

On the auricles, it is unnecessary to insert intradermal needles so that their points enter into the underlying cartilage. Inserting the needle to a depth so that the inserted portion of the needle lies between the skin and cartilage of the ear, which is easily observable, is optimal. Needles that are left inserted into the underlying cartilage tend to give much more stimulation and patients complain much more about them. Taping needles in the auricles should be done in the same manner as on regular body points, but it is more difficult because the auricles are so small and have so many folds and uneven surfaces.

It takes practice to attain skill at intradermal insertion. Before using intradermals in the clinic, practice the techniques on yourself. When the insertions are routinely painless, you will be ready to use intradermal needles on your patients. Careful and attentive practice is paramount when using these tiny needles. You should not hurry, as haste is likely to be the cause of bent needles, dropped needles, or missed points.

We recommend practicing with the stainless steel intradermal needles rather than the softer silver or gold needles, because they are less likely to bend. When you have mastered the method using stainless steel needles, you will be ready to practice with silver and gold intradermals, though they are not used as often.

DEPTH OF INTRADERMAL NEEDLE INSERTION

Once you have inserted the intradermal following one of the above methods, it should lie in the skin between the superficial fascia and the deep fascia. It is important that intradermals be inserted this deep and no deeper because they are usually left in place for a number of days. If they are inserted too deeply so that they enter to underlying muscular tissues, then whenever those tissues contract and move, the intradermal needle will move as well, possibly causing unnecessary discomfort and increasing the risk of irritating the patient's condition or the point being treated.

To ensure that the needles are inserted to the correct depth, apply a simple test. Apply gentle pressure to the handle of the needle. If you observe the inserted part of the needle easily raising the skin, this is the correct needle depth. If you cannot see this, pull the needle back out slightly and apply gentle pressure again. If the skin still does not raise with this test, then pull the needle back out further and angle the needle so that it is more shallowly placed. If this still doesn't work, remove the needle altogether and reinsert it.

On the hands, it is important to not insert the needle too deeply because the hands are used and move so much throughout the day. Once the point is located, insert the needle to a maximum insertion of about 1mm. Be very careful when taping the needle to make sure that it is secure. Unfortunately, needles on the hands seem very easy to lose because they are easily rubbed off.

ASSESSING CORRECT APPLICATION

Problems with the use of intradermal needles are rare. Because of the protective and anti-infective properties of the superficial fascia, and because the needles are carefully taped in place, the risk of infection from the use of intradermal needles is almost insignificant. Providing the instructions are correctly observed, selection and placement are double checked, and the patient is given clear instructions concerning care and removal of the needles, there is usually no problem. There are cases, discussed later in the text, where they would not be selected or where they would be used with great care.

When the intradermal is doing its job correctly, the reaction at the point treated—the pressure pain, tension, knot—will decrease. To assess this, use the finger pad to reapply pressure to the point about one to two minutes after inserting the needle, making sure to apply the pressure directly on the needle. Because the needle is flat with the skin, the needle itself will not bend or cause irritation with this pressure. In order to ensure that the needle is working and the reaction has decreased, it is important to apply at least the same or more pressure as applied in diagnosing the point. If the patient reports that the reaction is substantially decreased or gone, the needle can be taped in place.

When the goal of treatment is an easily assessable problem such as conditions of pain, restricted ranges of motion, and so forth, you will usually see an immediate improvement in the patient's symptoms as well as a reduction in the pressure pain or knot at the point treated. It is always a good idea to have patients demonstrate the amount of pain and/or restricted motion that they have prior to beginning treatment. Immediately after insertion of the intradermal needle, have them repeat the motions or activities that cause the pain and restricted motion. With a good point selection and location, these symptoms will have improved immediately.

However, if the reaction at the point shows no change or is only a little better, and if the patient shows no signs of improvement in pain levels or degrees of mobility, leave the needle a little while longer and then check the point again. If the reaction is substantially decreased or gone, and/or the patient shows improvement in the pain or range of mobility, tape the point.

In almost all cases, provided the point selection and location is good, sufficient results can be obtained using stainless steel intradermals. If the changes are slight or if there are no changes, you must reconsider the appropriateness of the point location, the accuracy of the point location, and the adequacy of a single point. If these factors are ruled out, inappropriate needle type should be considered. Sometimes such a determination is easy, but often it is difficult to decide.

If there is no clear improvement in the symptoms or reaction at the point using a stainless steel needle with good point selection and location, it is usually a sign to leave the needle as it is. Tape it and look for another point, or a point to reinforce the first point. Repalpate around the point or affected area, being careful to try to identify what is clearly the most reactive point. If you find another point which seems more reactive than the one needled, remove the needle from the first point and insert a new one at the new point.

If there is really no change in the reaction and symptoms, this could be due to incorrect selection or incorrect needle type. If you have used every means to reverify point selection and location, and you can determine that the point treated is clearly the more reactive point, but there are no signs of vacuity or weakness, remove the needle and look to different body parts or areas to treat. If, however, there are signs of weakness and vacuity in the point or area treated, you may want to consider using a silver intradermal needle. If these signs are evident, try removing the stainless steel needle and inserting a silver one.

Repeat the above procedures to assess efficacy. Remember, if the first point you have treated was clearly the most reactive, but there are no signs of vacuity or weakness, remove the needle and look to different body parts or areas to treat. In general, the most common finding is that another intradermal needle in another point is necessary. The next most common finding is that the point location is inaccurate. Much less common is the determination that a different type of needle is required.

TAPING AN INTRADERMAL NEEDLE

Usually two or three pieces of tape are sufficient to ensure correct taping of an intradermal needle.

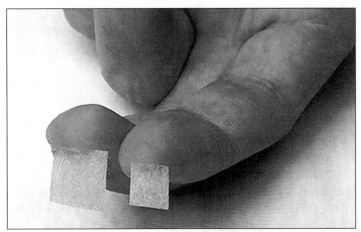

Two pieces of tape secure the intradermal properly.

The first piece should be a smaller piece that is placed underneath the handle of the needle. This acts as a pillow which prevents the handle of the needle from stimulating any other points.

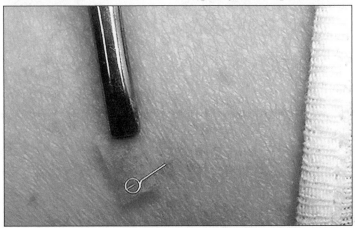

The first smaller piece acts as a pillow.

The second piece of tape should be placed over the needle and the first piece of tape, to cover both like a blanket.

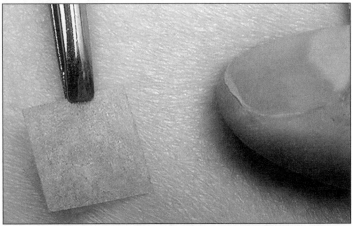

The second larger piece acts as a blanket.

The second piece of tape must be larger than the entire length of the needle. When applying the second piece of tape, it is essential to stretch the skin surrounding the needle and then place the tape. This is important because when the patient moves around after therapy, the skin will be stretched. If the tape had not been applied to stretched skin, it will likely come loose as the skin stretches. It is also a good idea to place the second piece of tape so that it makes contact first with the skin at the point end of the needle and is then applied upward along the body of the needle, covering the handle of the needle last. This is important because applying the tape from the handle end first can push the needle in more deeply or cause the needle to jab the patient once it is taped up, and thereby requiring that it be retaped.

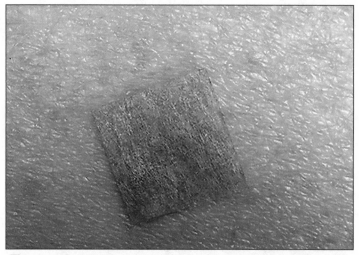

The second piece of tape completely covers the inserted needle.

Sometimes a third piece of tape is applied in the same manner as the second in order to ensure that the needle is secure. Whether or not to use this third piece of tape depends on the point treated, the patient, and the preferences of the practitioner.

If a good-quality tape has been used to secure the intradermal, it is usually safe for the patient to shower, bathe, or swim. Patients should be cautioned not to rub or scratch the taped area, and not to dry the area too vigorously. They should also be advised to check the tape and needle occasionally to make sure that everything is in place. If the tape comes loose soon after the treatment and before it is time to remove the needle, the patient should tape over the original tape in order to secure the needle and tape.

We recommend the use of the half-inch MICROPORE™ tape for taping the intradermals. Precut pieces of tape in white or beige tone are now available which may be peeled off and applied. The precut tape comes in various sizes appropriate for the "pillow" and "blanket" pieces.

After taping the needle it is always a good idea to palpate the needle lightly to check for signs of discomfort. If the patient reports that the needle causes some discomfort, ask if the discomfort is like a needle stabbing or pinching or if it is like a dull aching. If it is like a needle stabbing or pinching, the needle **must** be retaped. Frequently this involves removing the needle altogether and reinserting and taping again. If the sensation is a dull achiness, which occurs mostly in auricle points, it is usually no problem. If the patient shows discomfort from the sensation, it is better to retape it.

If at the end of treatment or when dressing the patient reports that the needle is causing discomfort, there are usually two probable causes. Either the needle is jabbing, in which case it **must** be removed and reapplied, or the point treated is on a hairy area, and some hair has been caught by the tape.

If some hair has been caught by the tape, most patients will confuse the sensation of pulled hair with the sensation of an uncomfortable needle, and will, once out of the clinic, remove the needle and nullify any benefits of its placement. It is a good idea to carefully trim away any hair that might be caught by the tape, though clearly it is better if this has been done prior to the initial taping.

REMOVAL OF INTRADERMAL NEEDLES

Not all practitioners agree on the best angle for removing the tape and needle. The following is what we have found to be simple, safe, and effective. It can be done at the patient's next visit, or instructions can be given to the patient for removal at home. Peel back the tape slightly, grasp the tape at the pointed end of the needle, and pull the tape towards the handle of the needle. As you remove the tape, the needle will also be pulled out, since the handle of the needle is usually caught between the underlying small "pillow" of tape and the larger overlying "blanket" of tape. Remember to "close" the hole using the needle removal technique.

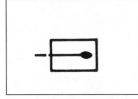 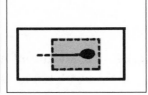 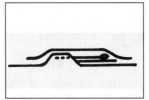

The needle rests on the pillow tape. Needle and pillow are completely covered.

Removing the tape and needle at other angles runs the risk of causing a very slight skin tear on the point as the needle is pulled out; however, the risks are usually minimal. The angle of removal recommended here represents what we consider to be the optimal method.

Usually intradermal needles are left in place only for a few days. The practitioner should always instruct the patient on how to remove the needle for two reasons. First, the patient's subsequent visit may not allow the practitioner to remove the intradermals in a timely fashion. Second, sometimes needles cause irritation to the patient. If this happens, the needle should be removed right away.

After removal of the tape, check to make sure that the needle has been caught in the tape and removed. On odd occasions, the needle will be left in the skin, and will need to be removed. On even rarer occasions, if the tape has become loose, the needle may not be found when the tape is removed. We suspect that in these cases the needle may have washed out from under the tape and down the drain of the shower.

Sometimes needles will fall out of their own accord as the tape becomes loose or gets caught by something. Usually this results in no mishap. The patient may be disappointed by this because there may be a slight increase or return of symptoms, but even more often the patient feels that they have lost a part of their treatment.

Intradermal needles can be left inserted for up to a week. If you are treating the patient on a weekly schedule, you can remove the intradermals during the next office visit. If the patient comes more often for treatment, for instance, two or three times a week, it is still a good idea to remove the needles at the beginning of each treatment. If the climate is very hot and humid, or if the patient naturally sweats a great deal, the needle should be removed after an even shorter period of time, as in such conditions the tape will frequently become loose and dirty. Optimal removal is after three to four days. Sometimes the second day is better, but this judgement will depend on the patient and environment.

Often when patients remove the intradermal at home, they forget the best method for removing the needle. So far this has not caused any problems.

PATIENT CONCERNS

Occasionally an extremely sensitive patient may feel irritation from the needle after a relatively short time. For such patients, where the amount of stimulation must be carefully regulated and controlled (we have seen this in patients with multiple sclerosis, multiple allergies, extreme fatigue, stress, and so forth), it is better to instruct the patient to remove the needle the next day at the latest or whenever they feel any sort of discomfort or unease with the stimulus from the intradermal. In such cases, more monitoring of the patient is required because this extreme sensitivity can also predispose the patient to periods of greater discomfort or aggravated symptoms.

Sometimes the removal of the tape and needle will reveal a slightly red and inflamed looking point. Such cases are signs that the needle was slightly irritating to the patient, but not enough to take notice and remove it. We have not seen any persistent problems from this. However, patients should be made aware of this possibility and its probable resolution within a few days. Assuring them that it is relatively normal and nothing to worry about is helpful.

With some patients there may also be skin irritation where the tape has been. Usually the hypoallergenic tapes will not cause such reactions, but there are some patients who are so reactive that this type of skin irritation will nevertheless occur. If this seems to be a persistent phenomenon with a particular patient, it may be that intradermals are an unwise selection for that patient because there is no suitable tape. Before giving up, it is a good idea to try different tapes; also try having the patient leave the needle in place for only a few hours, at most for a day. Often patients will have some idea that they are likely to be allergic to the tape.

While it is very rare for the needles to cause discomfort or concern, if at any time a patient becomes disturbed about the presence or sensation of an intradermal, they should be reassured that you are always available to discuss their concerns help them resolve any difficulties. As the practitioner, you know what the needle is doing there, and a doctor unfamiliar with the use of intradermal needles will not; thus it is clearly to your advantage to keep on top of the situation by taking the necessary precautionary measures.

INTRADERMAL NEEDLE CONTRAINDICATIONS

If you want to use an intradermal needle on a child of fifteen years or younger, always instruct the parents or the responsible person who brings them for treatment about what has been done. If the child is younger, for instance, ten years or less, you should be aware that they are usually more sensitive and the needle should not be left for more than a couple of days. If you have used a needle on a much younger child, for example, one five years old or younger, take further precautions by instructing the parent to remove the needle within hours or, at the latest, by the next day in order to prevent overdose. For infants, intradermal needles are not normally used because they give too much stimulation.

If you are treating a patient who suffers from circulatory disorders or who is predisposed to circulatory disorders, take particular care when using intradermal needles. For a patient who is diabetic, use intradermals only on the torso, not on the limbs. However, if the diabetic patient suffers from peripheral neuropathy, judge according to the severity and extent of the condition of the patient whether intradermals should be used at all. If the needle were placed in such a way as to allow bacteria to enter the needle wound and cause an infection, the patient would have less resistance to combat the bacteria because of the diabetes and neuropathy. This could lead to a very serious situation for the patient. Use of intradermals on diabetic patients should be restricted or prohibited according to the extent and nature of any complications they might have.

Treatment of patients with compromised immune systems also falls under the same restrictions, and for the same reasons. For example, the risk of inadvertent bacterial infection from an infected needle wound in a patient who has tested HIV-positive would be highly undesirable.[2]

Treatment of patients having other immuno-suppressant complications with intradermals should also be considered carefully. This is especially the case if a patient manifests tendencies to develop skin lesions from small cuts and so forth. Individual assessment must guide the practitioner as to whether or not the intradermal needles can be used or should be avoided. Patients who might have chronic fatigue syndrome, for example, or patients with systemic candida yeast infection, have been treated with intradermals without any apparent problems. We can add, however, that patients who are immune-compromised are often quite run down and fatigued, which tends to predispose them to greater sensitivity. If intradermal needles are used at all, they should be removed earlier in order to prevent problems that can follow prolonged application.

Intradermals can be used on patients who are carriers of or are actively infected by diseases such as hepatitis. However, great care must be taken when removing and handling the needles of these patients to avoid the risk of disease transmission from patient to practitioner. Always handle the removed needles of all patients with tweezers, holding the tape rather than the needle itself.

Besides the above precautions and restrictions which were garnered from discussions we have had in the classroom, we know of no other restrictions. None of these precautions and restrictions were found in the Japanese literature.

---

[2]Some practitioners think that so long as no major diseases have developed, or that the patient has not actually developed AIDS, limited and careful use of intradermal needles is acceptable. In the case of patients who have more advanced problems and have developed AIDS, even greater care need be taken. Depending on the case, it may be completely contraindicated. At the very least, the use of intradermals on HIV-infected patients should be performed with great caution; thorough monitoring and clear instructions to the patient are required.

POINT SELECTION GUIDELINES FOR INTRADERMAL NEEDLES

You should be careful not to use too many intradermals during one treatment. Recall the adage, "less is better": it is better to pick fewer points rather than try to use too many. There are some general rules that help narrow point selection.

1. It is usually better not to use two intradermals on the same channel trajectory or stream. Some practitioners do this, but within the framework we have been suggesting, where intradermals are used as the last step in a series of steps for a single treatment, we think it is better to use only one needle per stream. If you place an intradermal on right BL-23, it is better not to place another intradermal anywhere else on the right bladder channel. However, it is fine to place one on the left bladder channel, depending on the point and the nature of the dynamic set up between the points used. This is good advice for the other eleven channels and the *du mai* and *ren mai,* too.

2. Do not use intradermals of different metals in one session. The reason for this is that taping a silver needle to one point and a stainless steel or gold needle to another sets up a small but continuous current between these two which will flow as long as both needles are retained. Usually this provides too much stimulation. There are possible exceptions to this rule, but generally you should use needles made of the same metal. In most cases, this entails the use of stainless steel needles.

3. Usually when selecting points referenced for the treatment of particular conditions to alleviate a patient's symptoms, such as a painful shoulder, you may palpate all around the shoulder to find and select one or two of the most reactive sore or tense points. Place intradermals to those. This can be very helpful for relieving the local pain. If you select this particular type of therapy, it is better not to use any other recommended points.

4. Within the treatment approaches described herein, intradermal needles are frequently used in Manaka's overall treatment procedures. He especially liked to use them on auricular points, where he would use many. Using auricular points drastically reduces the possible overdose to a channel because there is no direct stimulation on the channel. In such cases, treatment involves insertion of needles in the auricles until clearly observable changes in the condition occur, such as reduced pain or increased range of motion.[3]

Usually, if this approach is used to relieve symptoms, one or more intradermal needles are left in the auricles. To keep the overall numbers down and to avoid giving too much stimulation, it

---

[3]See Y. Manaka, K. Itaya and S. Birch, *Chasing the Dragon's Tail,* pp. 217-232.

is better to use few or no intradermal needles on body points when auricle points are selected. If you use three or four needles in the auricles, then use one or no needles on the body. If there are already two needles on the body and you want to supplement the effects with auricle points, use only one or two intradermal needles. Remember that less is better than more.

Manaka had a favorite combination for the treatment of pain. He would use his three-point isophasal combination with intradermals. If a patient complained of shoulder pain, he would palpate on the shoulder to find the worst and most affected channel and point to place an intradermal there. Then he would palpate in the auricle on the same side of the body in the auricular shoulder region looking for the sorest point, and would place an intradermal there. Finally, he would palpate the hands in the shoulder reflex area based on the Korean hand acupuncture scheme to find the most painful point and leave an intradermal there. This made a total of three needles. The effects of this three-point isophasal combination were quite remarkable.

GENERAL THERAPEUTIC VALUE OF INTRADERMAL NEEDLES

As we have just suggested, treatment of local problems with intradermal needles can be very effective. When the correct point is selected, as the pressure pain or other reaction in the point decreases, so do the symptoms. This is particularly the case with immediately assessable conditions such as pain, stiffness, or decreased range of motion. For instance, placing an intradermal on a sore or reactive *jōsen* to address lower back problems can be amazingly effective for relieving the problems.

Intradermal needles can be used as the primary mode of therapy or they can be used as an adjunct to other therapies, such as five-phase, extraordinary vessel, moxa, and so forth. Their real value lies in the fact that they provide safe, gentle, and powerful continuous effects. They can be extremely valuable when used as a local pain control or symptom control aid in order to supplement a more complex clinical practice. Sometimes they provide surprising therapeutic effects.

Another way they can be used is for supplementing the clinical treatment of chronic problems such as problems of vacuity. For instance, using intradermal needles on the sore or reactive back-*shu* points which correspond to the vacuous organ/channel can be a helpful supplemental technique because of the continuous stimulation the intradermals provide. They can be extremely effective in the treatment of underlying vacuity.

Some members of the Toyohari Association use intradermals in the following way. They recognize four basic diagnostic patterns: lung vacuity, spleen vacuity, liver vacuity, and kidney vacuity. Following the dictum from the *Nan Jing* (p. 69), "For vacuous conditions, supplement the mother," they use both the corresponding back-*shu* point and the corresponding back-*shu* point of the mother channel. Since not more than one intradermal should be placed on the same channel stream, one back-*shu* point is treated on one side and the other on the other side. The primary channel back-*shu* point is treated on the right side on women (the yin side) and the left side on men (the yang side). This gives the following general treatment patterns:

VACUOUS CHANNEL	MALES	FEMALES
lung	left BL-13	right BL-13
	right BL-20	left BL-20
spleen	left BL-20	right BL-20
	right BL-15	left BL-15
liver	left BL-18	right BL-18
	right BL-23	left BL-23
kidney	left BL-23	right BL-23
	right BL-13	left BL-13

In this treatment method, the intradermal needles are actually inserted less deeply than we have described above. Often they only pierce the skin, sometimes only 1/2mm to 1mm.

The following is a list of treatments from Akabane's *Hinaishin Hō (The Method of Hinaishin),* pp. 132-137, which suggests some uses of intradermal needles. For each condition, palpate the points indicated and treat those that show clear reaction.

Frostbite

TB-4, ST-41. These points are also useful for numbness or pain of the tips of the fingers or toes. They may also be used for pain in the wrists or ankles and numbness of the hands and feet. In the latter cases, adding a small amount of bloodletting at the *jing* points will help reinforce the treatment.

Dysmenorrhea

Jōsen, SP-6, SP-10. The needles are best inserted just before or at the onset of menstruation and left in place for five days. Repeating this for several consecutive periods is often very helpful.

Gynecological diseases

Check the whole lower back region, especially *jōsen*; below L2 (GV-4 area), and to the sides of L2, usually from 3 to 5 cm from the spine; below L4 (GV-3 area) on the upper region of the sacrum. Check on the abdomen, especially inferior and lateral to the navel and slightly above the *pubis symphysis.* Also compare right and left SP-6 and SP-10.

This category includes associated lumbar pain, discomfort in the lower abdomen, heaviness of the head, headache, stiff shoulder, leukorrhea, and heaviness of the legs. Select the more reactive points.

Labor

Jōsen and nearby sensitive points, and the sensitive point on the midaxillary line. (Compare left and right sides, treat the more sensitive side.)

To aid with labor, and to help reduce the pain, place intradermals at *jōsen* and nearby sensitive points, on the midaxillary line, on the more sensitive side. (Caution: see high blood pressure category, p. 161.) Insert two intradermals, one at *jōsen* and the other on the most reactive point on the midaxillary line, either on the scheduled day of delivery or a few days before. If this gives some feeling of relief within five minutes of insertion, it usually means that these two needles will be effective.

Postpartum contraction pains

SP-6.

For postpartum contraction pains, insert intradermals at SP-6. When the patient is discharged from the hospital, remove all the needles.

Hemorrhoids

Jōsen; BL-28 or BL-31 (not for very chronic conditions nor anal fistula).

Pressure pain is found near *jōsen* and either near BL-28 or BL-31. Place intradermals on two points, usually *jōsen* and one of the right- or left-sided reactive points. If prolapse accompanies the condition, insert intradermal needles to *jōsen* and the right and left reactive points (3 needles), and then moxa GV-20.

Asthma

LU-1, KI-25, KI-26, GB-21, back-*shu* points, midaxillary line.

Look for pressure pain points on the chest around LU-1, KI-25, KI-26, on the midaxillary line, on the more sensitive side, on the back in the interscapular region, and on the shoulders, roughly around GB-21. These points can temporarily stop the asthma attack, but it is necessary to treat appropriate back-*shu* points, too. It is often difficult to cure asthma, so it is necessary to treat for relatively long periods of time. If using intradermal needles, it is usually necessary to treat every 7 to 10 days.

Pulmonary tuberculosis, pleurisy

Chest, shoulder and upper back regions, back-*shu* points, pressure pain points on forearms.

Pressure pain points appear, as in asthma, on the chest, shoulder, and upper back regions. Intradermals will help with the pain and cough associated with these conditions. Choose the more reactive points which are usually easy to find because the patient will often feel strong discomfort on palpation in those regions. It is also good to treat appropriate back-*shu* points, and pressure pain points that appear on the forearms. If the patient is particularly weakened and fatigued, *do not* use intradermal needles because they can overstimulate these patients, which is contraindicated. Often poor appetite will accompany these diseases. In such cases, place intradermals on the midline in the epigastric region and around ST-36. An intradermal can be placed on the reactive midaxillary line point to enhance effectiveness.

High blood pressure

Midaxillary line.

Compare pressure pain responses of left and right sides of the midaxillary line, and leave an intradermal at the sorer of the two. Also bloodlet SP-1 on the side that is less sensitive to heat.

Mumps in children

Around TB-17.

Treat the most reactive point around TB-17. For very young children, it is better to use the metallic grains or press-spheres.

Tonsillitis

Tonsil region below the mandible.

Palpate on the right and left sides of the tonsil region below the mandible, and mark the more painful one. Use the contralateral draining technique on the opposite side withdrawing after a pressured sensation is felt. Then place an intradermal needle at the reactive point. For children, the metallic grain or press-sphere is better.

Toothache

Area of ST-5 and ST-7.

Palpate and treat sore points above the areas of ST-5 and ST-7. Usually placing an intradermal on the diseased side and then using the contralateral draining technique on the same point on the other side works well. In children, the press-sphere is better than the intradermal.

Digestive diseases

Abdominal or back regions; around SP-8; SP-1.

If there is referred or associated pain on the abdominal or back regions, look for pressure-sensitive points on both surfaces and place intradermals at them. Also look for pressure pain around SP-8 for most acute cases and place an intradermal there. Bloodlet SP-1 on the side less sensitive to heat.

Diarrhea or constipation

Area around ST-27.

Palpate around left and right ST-27 for diarrhea or constipation and place intradermals at the reactive points.

Hepatic diseases

BL-18, BL-19; sore point on right shoulder, sore point over the liver; LR-8; SP-1.

Compare right and left BL-18 and BL-19; place intradermals at the more sensitive points. Palpate and treat the sore point on the right shoulder, and a sore point over the liver on the ribs. Also palpate and treat on the knee around LR-8. Bloodletting SP-1 can also be helpful.

Neck and shoulder pain

Sensitive local points.

Have the patient move their head in all directions to determine where pain is felt. After fixing the location of the pain, palpate, looking for pressure-sensitive points, and place intradermals on these. Do not use too many.

Pain of the shoulder joint

Sensitive local points.

Have the patient move the arms to find the location of the pain. After determining the location, palpate to find pressure-sensitive points and treat these with intradermals. Do not use too many.

Intercostal neuralgia

Sensitive local points.

After determining which rib space levels are affected, palpate close to the spine on that side in those intercostal spaces. After finding pressure-sensitive points, leave intradermals at those, and then palpate in the intercostal spaces on the chest and leave intradermals at the sore points there. Typically, the reactive points on the chest are found under the breast.

Lumbar pain

Sensitive local points.

Have the patient bend and move the lower back to determine the sore area. Then palpate in that area to find pressure-sensitive points. After finding these, treat them with intradermal needles; *jōsen* is often helpful for a variety of low-back pain disorders.

Sciatica

Sensitive points on lower lumbar and sacral areas; below BL-36.

If not a result of spinal injury, sciatica can respond well to the use of intradermals. Have the patient lie prone with pillows as extra support. Palpate for pressure-sensitive points on the lower lumbar and sacral areas and leave intradermal needles at the sorest of these. Also palpate on the upper leg, somewhere below BL-36, and treat the reactive point, if one is found, with an intradermal needle.

Foot pain

Along the line joining the malleoli.

Palpate along the line joining the two malleoli and leave intradermals at one or two sore points.

Knee pain

Around the head of the greater trochanter; around and above the knee (SP-10 or ST-34).

For pain in the medial portions of the knee, palpate around the head of the greater trochanter and place an intradermal needle at the reactive point. Then have the patient kneel or bend the knees, (if possible) and palpate around and above the knee looking for pressure-sensitive points. Treat these. They will often be found around SP-10 or ST-34.

Contusions

Sensitive local points.

Place intradermals to reactive points around the region of the contusion. Then use the contralateral draining technique on the opposite side.

Periostitis

Sensitive local points.

Treat reactive points in the affected area with intradermals, even if inflammation (a sensation of warmth) can be felt.

Broken bones

Sensitive local points.

To help reduce the pain of the broken bone, palpate around the break and place intradermals at the most reactive points.

Scrofula

Sensitive local points.

Leave an intradermal at a reactive point on or to the side of the raised area. This is better repeated again and again so that a needle is in place almost continuously.

INTRADERMAL RECOMMENDATIONS FROM BUNKEI ONO

Bunkei Ono recommends the use of the intradermal needle for several conditions as follows:[4]

Lumbar pain: Use five to six needles on the pressure-sensitive points in the lumbar area.

Shoulder pain: Use two to three needles on the pressure pain points in the painful area.

Migraine: GB-40.

Sciatica: Seven to eight needles on pressure pain points in the painful area.

---

[4]B. Ono, *Keiraku Chiryō: Shinkyū Rinshō Nyūmon (Meridian Therapy, an Introduction to Classical Acupuncture)*, pp. 254-256.

Chapter 7
Empishin—Press-Tack Needles

The *empishin,* like the intradermal, is a kind of needle left inserted in the acupoint on the body surface in order to provide a gentle, continuous effect. What distinguishes it from the intradermal needle is that the shaft of the needle comes out perpendicular to the needle handle, like a small thumb tack.

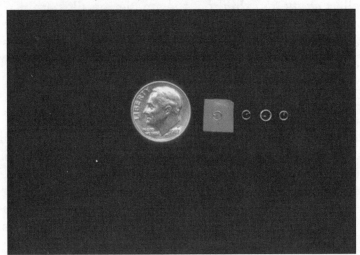

Different types of *empishin,* relative in size to a U.S. 10-cent piece (1.7cm).

Thus when used, the empishin needle is inserted slightly deeper than the intradermal needle because the needle is applied perpendicularly to the skin surface, whereas the intradermal is applied at a very small angle, so that it is parallel to the skin surface.

The *empishin* needle was invented in China a few decades ago. Like the intradermal needle, it is used mostly to supplement the general treatment by providing symptom relief. Many restrict its application exclusively to points on the auricles which is where its use seems to have originated. Several practitioners in Japan have reported good results using it on points on the body as well.

In this section we will focus on its use on body points and only briefly discuss its use on auricular points. Following the guidelines we outlined in Chapter 2, we try not to give strong stimulation in treatment. The use of *empishin* in the auricles is relatively strong stimulation because the needle point inserts into the cartilage of the auricle. We prefer to use intradermals in the auricles because the needle point lies between the skin and cartilage thus giving milder stimulation. This treatment is also more comfortable for the patient, with less risk of infection. (See Chapter 6.)

TYPES OF EMPISHIN

Like intradermal needles, there are several types of *empishin*. They are usually made of stainless steel, with needle shafts of 2mm, 2.6mm, or 3.2mm, and handle widths from 3mm to 5mm. (See the pictures on page 165.) Based on our clinical experience, we recommend the PYONEX needles. They are presterilized and come preattached to adhesive tape for easy application.

Empishin are constructed of a single strand of wire, wrapped to the correct shape. For adults, the slightly larger needles are used, for smaller adults and children, the smaller needles are used. The maximum depth of insertion is usually a little less than 2mm to about 3mm, which for almost all body areas, especially those with underlying muscular tissues, is safe and effective. A variation of the stainless steel *empishin* are the tin-plated and gold-plated *empishin*. These are commercially available, but not commonly used.

It is thought that the *empishin* needles can be useful for conditions that are chronic and stubborn because they give a mild and continuous stimulation to the point, but one that is a little different than the intradermal because the amount of stimulation is stronger. The *empishin* tends to be used more for pain whereas the *hinaishin* has a wider range of applications. They can also be used for acute disorders. Kobayashi and Chō[1], discussing their uses primarily in the auricles, list the following conditions that respond well to their use: rheumatoid pain, neuritis, traumatic pain, chronic bronchial asthma, ulcerative disorders, epilepsy, spermatorrhea, enuresis, and impotence.

Other authors give a broader range of uses for acute disorders which include a wide range of musculoskeletal and joint disorders, digestive disorders, and nasal problems.[2] (See p. 171 for a list of suggested uses.)

---

[1]Y. Kobayashi and K. Chō, *Zusetsu Jishingaku (Illustrated Ear Acupuncture Study Guide)*.

[2]F Shiozawa, "Treatment Effects of the *Empishin*," *Idō no Nippon Magazine* 35, 11, 387:36–40, 1986; and Hosho K., "Effects of the *Empishin*," *Idō No Nippon Magazine* 55, 4, 428:61–62, 1980.

STERILIZATION

Often the *empishin* needles come in unsterilized packets. To sterilize these needles, we recommend removing them from their original packet, placing them in cotton in another sealed packet which is suitable for autoclaving, and autoclaving them, rendering them ready for application. (Use of the PYONEX needles makes this additional step unnecessary.)

POINT SELECTION

Point selection is made in the same way as it was when using the intradermal needles. Pressure pain is sought at the point. To mark the point, use either a blunt probe such as a *teishin* to leave a small indentation at the point, or mark either side of the exact point with a pen. Once the point is located, wipe the point thoroughly with alcohol to ensure that the skin is clean, then insert the *empishin*.

INSERTING AND TAPING THE EMPISHIN

Since the *empishin* needles are quite small, use tweezers to insert them. If you are using needles that are not preattached to tape, hold the handle of the needle firmly with the tweezers and place the tip of the needle at the exact point to be treated.

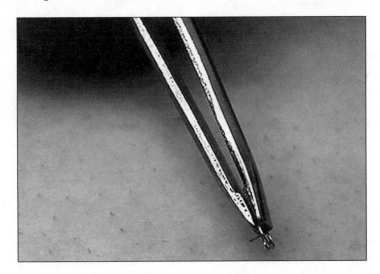

Hold the handle of the needle firmly with the tweezers.

As the patient exhales, apply pressure so that the needle penetrates the skin at the point.

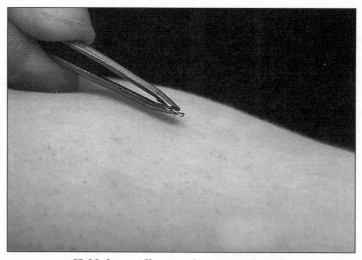

Hold the needle over the point selected.

Then let go of the needle with the tweezers and, using the pad of the forefinger, apply firm but gentle pressure to the needle to ensure a complete insertion.

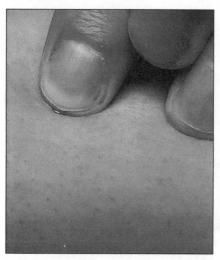 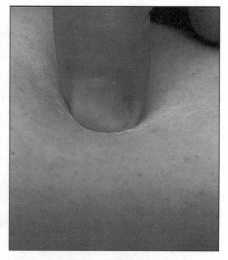

Apply firm pressure to the needle. Press the needle handle firmly with the forefinger.

The needle should be inserted as far as possible. We recommend that the pressure of the forefinger not be applied by merely pushing against the needle, but rather that a light rubbing pressure be applied, while holding the finger firmly on the needle handle.

This rubbing pressure ensures that the needle penetrates more easily and completely through the tissues and it is more distracting to the patient; this way, the patient receives minimum sensation from inserting the needle.

If the needle is preattached to tape, hold the corner of the tape with the tweezers and place the point of the needle at the acupoint in the manner described above.

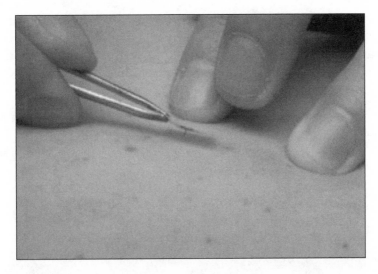

Hold the corner of the tape to position the needle over the point.

Then press the tape and needle onto the point firmly.

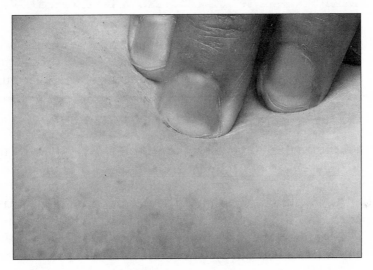

Press firmly over the needle and tape.

EMPISHIN FOR CHILDREN

To insert *empishin* on children, it is a good idea to stick the *empishin* handle to the tape first, and then apply the needle and tape at the same time. This way the child does not have to see the needle and is less likely to be disturbed by the procedure.

TAPING THE EMPISHIN

If you are using an *empishin* that is not preattached to tape, we recommend using a single large piece of tape. As with intradermal needles, the MICROPORE tape seems to work well for *empishin*. It is important to make sure that the tape has made a good contact with the handle of the needle and the skin immediately around it in order to keep the needle as secure as possible at the point.

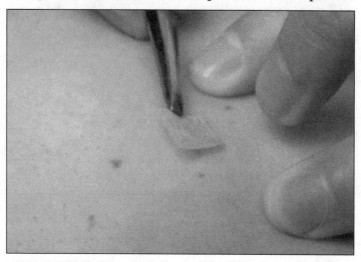

Stretch the skin slightly before pressing tape over the needle.

After placing the tape, use your index finger to secure it to the skin and needle. Again, we recommend the use of the MICROPORE tape, or the precut pieces of tape, to secure the needle placement.

RETAINING AND REMOVING THE EMPISHIN

As with intradermal needles, the length of time that the needle is retained depends on a number of factors. Most authors recommend that *empishin* be removed or replaced after three to four days. The patient should either remove the needle at home or return to the office to have it removed. Removal is quite simple; peeling back and removing the tape will either remove the needle or leave it exposed so that it can easily be removed. The patient should be advised of this so that it is not retained for too long. Occasionally, *empishin* have been left for longer without mishap, but it is better as a safety precaution to remove them after three or four days. During the summer, it is better to remove *empishin* a little sooner because of the increased heat and humidity which might increase the risk of infection. As with intradermal needles, patients should be advised not to wash or rub the taped area too vigorously, and, if the *empishin* should cause any discomfort, to remove it.

The *empishin* needle should not be used over bony areas because this will cause irritation. It also should not be used on skin areas that take a lot of pressure or friction, such as the soles of the feet or the tops of the knees. It is easiest and safest to use these needles on areas that have underlying muscle tissues.

Further precautions and restrictions for the use of the *empishin* are similar to those for intradermal needles. Be careful using them on diabetic patients or any patients with circulatory disorders. Be very careful using *empishin* on patients with immunological problems such as AIDS. Be careful when using them on patients who are particularly sensitive, e.g., very weakened and run-down patients, and children (especially infants). See the section on precautions with the use of intradermal needles in Chapter 6 for more details.

SOME SUGGESTED USES FOR EMPISHIN

The following list of suggested treatments comes primarily from papers by Shiozawa. As usual, treatment points or areas are indicated by sensitive responses to palpation. Treat with insertion and taping of *empishin* on the reactive points.

Blepharoptosis (drooping of the upper eyelid)

In the area superior and lateral to the eyebrow (TB-23, GB-14). A single *empishin* is often effective.

Bell's palsy

Focus on the number points or areas. The most commonly used points are: BL-2, GB-14, TB-23, ST-1, ST-2, ST-7, ST-6, ST-5. Select two or three points. If used after general treatment, which should involve treatment of the neck and shoulder regions to release tension and tightness there, good effects will be achieved.

Stiff shoulder

Focus directly on the most painful points, both those indicated by the patient on movement, and those found by pressure.

Stiff painful shoulder (50-year shoulder)

After general treatment, palpate about 1cm lateral to the shoulder joint, in the concave anterior joint where the head of the humerus meets the acromion. Treatment of this point seems able to make the symptoms lighter.

Shoulder and upper back pain

Treat on the most painful points.

Lumbar pain

For mild cases BL-23 and BL-35 bilaterally are usually sufficient (BL-52 is sometimes used in place of BL-23). In stubborn and chronic cases, effectiveness is seen only after appropriate general treatment, often with bloodletting.

Intercostal neuralgia

Palpate in the intercostal spaces and treat those points with clear pain or pressure pain. Because the *empishin* needle is short, it can be used even on very skinny patients without problems such as pneumothorax (caused by puncture of the lung.

Neuralgia of the upper arm

Focus on the points reported by the patient as being painful and those found to be clearly painful with pressure.

Sprain

Empishin treatment can be effective for acute or chronic problems resulting from sprain. For an abduction sprain of the ankle, palpate and treat GB-40.

Sciatica

Select and treat two to five points that the patient complains of as being painful or that show clear pressure pain. The most commonly used points are: Onodera's buttock point (located approximately 5cm below the high point of the PSIS), GB-30, BL-37, Sawada's *daigeki* point (3 finger-widths superior and lateral to BL-37, on the line joining GB-30 and BL-39), BL-58, BL-59, and, if lumbar pain accompanies the sciatica, BL-23 and BL-25. Appropriate treatment can reduce pain and speed up the healing process.

Whiplash

After light general treatment, palpate between BL-10 and BL-11, and treat the points that manifest strong pressure pain. Also check SI-15, TB-15, GB-21. If there is fatigue of the upper limb, check TB-9, LI-10.

Fullness or a "stuck" feeling in the epigastrium

Insert up to four *empishin* to points such as CV-12, ST-20, ST-21, depending on pressure reactivity.

Bloated abdomen

Insert about three *empishin* on the abdomen on points that were palpably reactive and uncomfortable.

Trichomonas infection (vaginal, bladder or urethral)

Treating the reactive points around CV-3 and KI-12 with *empishin* can help reduce the itching.

Cystitis

CV-3 and KI-12 as above.

Infantile asthma

Around ST-9 and KI-26 bilaterally.

Rhinitis, congested nose

Insert *empishin* at the point in the juncture of the nasal bone and cartilage of the nasal septum. For children, try leaving the *empishin* only 5 minutes or so every day or every other day.

Knee joint inflammation, hip joint problems

Focus on the points that the patient reports are most painful. Use from 2 to 6 *empishin*.

Chapter 8
Ryū—Press-Spheres

Ryū, a "press-sphere" or "metallic grain," is used in Japan where it has gained in popularity for simple and effective treatment of myofascial-type pain problems. In Japan the press-spheres are used mostly on body points.

Although the press-spheres are used in China, use of different kinds of seeds taped onto treatment points is a more common observance. Small seeds and herbal substances, such as *Semen Vaccariae, Semen Sinapis Albae,* and *Semen Brassicae Oleiferae,* are taped onto points, especially auricular points, in order to produce the desired therapeutic effects. In such treatments, it is primarily the pressure on the point that produces the effects, with suggestions of possible secondary pharmacological effects from the seed. (See, e.g., Wang Tianjun.) The seeds are typically used on auricular points for the treatment of disorders of a more internal nature.

While we can point to no clinical evidence that press-spheres taped on auricular points produce the same results as seeds taped to the same points, we feel it reasonable to assume that the mechanisms of action are very similar and that the press-spheres have the same efficacy.

Different types of press-spheres are available. In his discussions on the use of the press-spheres, Mr. Hyōdō recommends that the sphere not be bigger than 2mm in diameter.[1] The standard is a simple stainless steel press-sphere. In addition to this kind, there are plated press-spheres, such as those coated in silver and gold or other metals in a bimetallic manner.

---

[1]Much of the following information comes from M. Hyōdō, *Itami no Atarashii Chiryō (New Treatment Methods for Pain),* pp. 48-51, and *Shiranakatta Itami no Hanashi (Unknown Stories of Pain),* pp. 118-119. Some information derives from K. Akabane, *Hinaishin Hō (The Method of Hinaishin),* and some is derived from Chinese publications on the applications of pressure to auricular points, using seeds instead of press-spheres.

Currently in the U.S. the ACU-PATCH stainless steel press-sphere is available, as are the MAGRAIN gold and silver-plated press-spheres.

The following picture shows a strip of press spheres in a packet and a single press-sphere in comparison to a U.S. 10-cent piece (1.7cm). The press-sphere is secured to a circular piece of tape and ready for application.

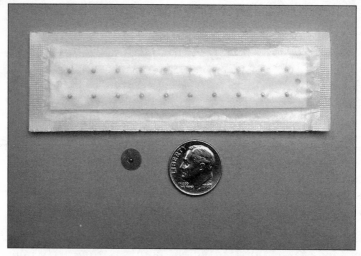

A press-sphere on a piece of tape next to a U.S. 10-cent piece (1.7cm).

For general uses the stainless steel press-sphere is more appropriate, although the MAGRAIN spheres can be used singly, not in a bimetallic application. If you have not studied the uses of bimetallic contact therapy, we do not recommend placing a gold-plated press-sphere on one point and a silver plated press-sphere on another point.

With a stainless steel press-sphere, the reactions are due primarily to the pressure applied at the point, with possible secondary effects due to the interactions of the metal with the skin. These secondary effects are probably minor for most individuals. With the gold- or silver-plated press-spheres, however, the effects are probably due as much to the metal plating as to the pressure at the point, especially if a gold press-sphere is placed on one point and a silver press-sphere on another.

TAPE

Hyōdō considered it important to use the appropriate kind of tape with press-spheres, firstly in order to eliminate hyper-allergenic tape reactions and secondly in order to provide sufficient pressure to the metal spheres so that they give adequate stimulation to the points without causing pain. When adequate pressure is given in this manner to an appropriately selected point, remarkable and surprising results can be obtained.

LENGTH OF APPLICATION

Usually press-spheres are placed on the desired points and retained for a maximum of three to four days. Longer application causes the effect to diminish, as the body apparently adapts to the stimulus provided by the pressure from the sphere. To counter this, Hyodo developed a routine of changing the press-sphere every three or four days, placing the new one at pressure pain points in roughly the same location as the previous points. He reported that in this fashion the same effects obtained with the first treatment could be maintained.

On occasion, a press-sphere may be irritating to a patient. Perhaps this is due to an allergic sensitivity to the tape or the metal grain itself, or because of excessive pressure at the point which can cause an irritated indentation in the skin. It is important to instruct the patient that if they experience irritation, the press-sphere should be removed.

GENERAL INDICATIONS

Hyōdō conducted controlled studies to investigate the utility of the press-sphere.[2] He found a 2-1 ratio (60% to 30%) of effectiveness in favor of the press-spheres versus a placebo patch of tape. Based on this study and the clinical uses of the press-spheres, press-spheres are considered effective for the following types of problems: mild myofascial-type lumbago; muscle pain; the pain of tendonitis; stiff, painful shoulders; and referred pain from the internal organs. Hyōdō found press-spheres ineffective for severe neuralgias, such as sciatica or trigeminal neuralgia. He recommended the use of the press-spheres on very sensitive patients or children, where normal treatments cannot be used because the patients are excessively sensitive. Akabane also recommended the use of the press-spheres for very sensitive patients in place of the intradermal needles. Akabane noted that because some painful conditions are too painful for much local stimulation, the placement of press-spheres locally in such cases can be an effective alternative procedure. (See Chapter 6 on intradermals for references.)

Some practitioners in Japan use the press-spheres much more to affect or support the *honchihō* root or general treatment. In the Toyohari style of treatment, at the end of treatment, when the patient is sent home, some practitioners will place press-spheres on points relevant to that patient's condition. For example, for a patient with a vacuous lung channel, after supplementing the lung

---

[2]See M. Hyōdō, *Shiranakatta Itami no Hanashi (Unknown Stories of Pain)*, pp. 118–119, for a summary of this.

channel, a press-sphere is often placed on GV-12. If the patient has more indications of spleen vacuity, the press-sphere is often placed on CV-12. If the patient shows weakness of the lower burner, a press-sphere may be placed on CV-6 or CV-4. The purpose of this kind of usage is to affect key points in order to reinforce the treatment. Another usage sometimes seen is that of placing a press-sphere on a point where an intradermal needle might have been placed, but because one has already been placed on the same channel stream, another intradermal would be inappropriate. For example, if an intradermal were placed on CV-12, and stimulus on CV-4 were also required, a press-sphere could be used instead of the intradermal. This allows milder stimulation of the same channel, and avoids stimulus overdose.

METHOD OF APPLICATION

The method of application is very simple. Apply pressure to the sore or affected area. After finding a distinctively sore point, place a press-sphere at the point, making sure to apply firm pressure to ensure adequate contact of the tape to the skin and adequate pressure of the press-sphere to the point. Usually the press-sphere has a milder stimulation effect than the *hinaishin* or intradermal and thus its effects are not seen quite as quickly as when using an intradermal needle. Often you will see the desired effects within five minutes of application of the sphere. As with almost everything else we have described in this text, the "less is better" principle applies. The fact that the amount of stimulation given is less doesn't mean that more points can or should be stimulated. It is best to try to use as few points as possible.

There are distinct advantages to the use of the press-sphere.

•They are safe and easy to use; there is almost no possibility of any complication if the proper points are selected.

•They represent a very useful form of home therapy. If a patient would benefit from the continuous treatment of a number of points, and neither moxa nor needles are appropriate, press-spheres may be used instead. Send the patient home with a package of press-spheres and instructions to replace the ones placed during the clinic treatment after three days or so. This use of press-spheres allows for a mild but continuous stimulation of the desired treatment points.

•For patients where intradermals are not indicated or are contraindicated, such as patients with AIDS who are very run down, press-spheres can be placed at the desired treatment points. The danger of infection is virtually non-existent.

•They are ideal for treating children, where the basic treatment approach in *shōnishin* is "much less is better." Frequently for children, needles are not inserted at all, especially in children under the age of five. A simple, effective, and safe support to treating children in the clinic is to use press-spheres at indicated points. The child's parent can easily be instructed to replace or remove the press-spheres.

•For those patients with extreme oversensitivity, where almost any stimulus seems too strong or too much, press-spheres can be useful as supportive therapy. In such patients, try to choose only one or two key points. Observe the "much less is better" approach to the treatment. Usually the press-spheres are best used to apply smaller but continuous stimulation to a point or points, or to use as a secondary symptom control therapy and home therapy.

•Press-spheres can be very useful when applied to points in different micro-systems such as the auricles[3] or Korean hand points.[4] As supportive therapy, stimulus of the auricle points has proven very helpful. Place the press-spheres at the points where you would normally needle or use intradermals. Some patients have very sensitive auricles and intradermals in the auricles cause too much sensation or discomfort. With such patients, the press-spheres are usually a good alternative, but be careful to check with the patient to see how well the press-spheres are tolerated.

The same is true of the use of seeds taped to auricular points— small stimulation is given continuously to the treatment points. A number of Chinese studies using seeds taped to auricular points describe remarkable results in the treatment of cholelithiasis, enuresis, neurasthenia, abnormal fetal position, and weight loss. A discussion of these studies and their results can be found in Appendix 2.

The predominant response mechanism to the taping of seeds to the points in the auricles appears to result from the pressure at the points. This is similar to the mechanism of action of the press-spheres on body acupoints. Because of this, we think that the use of press-spheres in the auricles can be as effective for the same conditions as the use of various small seeds.

POSSIBLE SIDE EFFECTS

While the studies discussed above show a somewhat limited clinical range of pressure effects on the acupoints, they are certainly illustrative of the potential efficacy of the use of press-spheres in the auricles. If you wish to use the press-spheres extensively in the auricles, we advise a little caution in the degree and

[3]See Y. Manaka, K. Itaya, and S. Birch, *Chasing the Dragon's Tail* pp. 219–223.
[4]*Ibid.*, pp. 223-227.

frequency of pressure applied to the points by the patient. The press-spheres leave indentations that are more clearly defined than those left from the placement of seeds. Thus they might be a little more irritating. Since we promote the "less is better" general approach, we think that it is better to cause less irritation or discomfort at the points.

With this in mind, the use of press-spheres or seeds to the auricles can be a very useful adjunct to treatment. Also, in the last Chinese study described in Appendix 2, a cautionary word is given about the potential side effects that can occur with pressure to points in the ears, including fainting, chest distress, dizziness, and nausea. These need to be taken into account, and a decision made about the appropriateness of this treatment method on each patient. For example, for the extremely vacuous or sensitive patient, this may prove to be too much stimulation and cause some side effects. Removal of the press-spheres from the auricular points will quickly stop these side-effects.

Chapter 9
Kyūkaku—Cupping

Cupping therapy has a long history as part of East Asian medicine and as an adjunct to the practice of acupuncture. Cupping, often referred to as "horn therapy," was mentioned in the *Wu Shi Er Bing Fang* text from the Mawang Dui graves, dating from 168 B.C.,[1] but seems not to have been used systematically until around 300 A.D. as attested in the work of Cui Jin and Zhang Guangqi.[2]

Since these early beginnings, cupping therapy has been used variously both in acupuncture and herbal practices as an adjunctive therapy. Its application involves the use of various cupping instruments which apply suction to the body surface. The action of creating a partial vacuum inside the cupping instrument draws skin and flesh up inside the cup, stimulating the blood circulation and the underlying musculature. The primary use of cupping therapy seems to have been for blood stasis conditions which led to the alternate name, blood stasis therapy.[3] Developing along with acupuncture and herbal medicine over the centuries, cupping therapy has been used for a wider range of disorders than has blood stasis therapy alone,[4] but cupping therapy is thought to be especially good for problems of blood stasis.

In Japan today, cupping therapy is used not only by professional acupuncturists, primarily as an adjunctive technique, but also by lay practitioners who specialize in the treatment and prevention of disease. These lay practitioners run clinics where cupping therapy,

---

[1]See P. Unschuld, *Medicine in China, A History of Ideas,* p. 93; and Wang Fengyi and Ren Huan Zhao, *Kyūgyoku Ryōhō (Cupping Therapy).*

[2]Cui Jin. and Zhang Guang Qi., "A Survey of Thirty Years of Clinical Applications of Cupping," *Journal of Traditional Chinese Medicine* 9(2):151–154, 1989.

[3]*Ibid.*

[4]*Ibid.*

used in very general treatment patterns, is the sole method of treatment. This specialization has allowed for the accumulation of detailed information on the uses of cupping therapy.

In this chapter we will describe different types of cupping therapy, a simple general methodology, general rules and precautions, uses of cupping on various body points, and the treatment of disorders using cupping therapy alone.[5] Our focus will be almost exclusively on the retained and momentary cupping methods. Indications, restrictions, and precautions combine the regular information coming from China, and the specialized information from Japan.

CUPPING METHODS

A variety of cupping methods are employed in China and Japan. While we will be describing a basic approach to the use of cupping and cupping in conjunction with bloodletting, it is worthwhile to briefly describe the other forms of cupping.

There are three forms of orthodox cupping where cupping techniques only are employed. These three forms differ according to the length of time the cups are left on the skin. With the "retained cupping" method, cups are left for a moderate to lengthy period of time; with the "momentary cupping" method, the cups are retained for a very short period of time; and with the "moving cup" method, the cups are moved about over the surface of the skin.

The retained cupping method involves applying the cups to the selected points or areas, and retaining them for one to ten minutes before removing them. This is probably the most commonly used cupping method and is widely employed for many different disorders.

The momentary cupping method involves applying the cup to the selected point or area and then almost immediately releasing the pressure; the process is repeated until the desired result is achieved. This method is good for drawing local congestion to the surface and is used mostly for disorders involving some kind of malfunction such as of underlying organs.

The moving cup method requires that petroleum jelly or some similar oily substance is first spread over the affected area. Then the cup is applied and moved over the oily skin at a moderate pace. This method is particularly useful for stimulating larger areas and should be used over relatively thickly muscled areas of the body such as the back.

---

[5]Much of this literature is drawn from A. Meguro, *Kyūkaku Ryōhō (Cupping Therapy),* a relatively popular book on cupping, and secondarily from Wang Feng Yi and Ren Huan Zhao, *Kyūgyoku Ryōhō (Cupping Therapy),* as well as from Y. Manaka, *Kyū to Hari (Moxibustion and Acupuncture).*

In addition to orthodox cupping, there is the "prick cupping" or cupping and bloodletting method, the "inserted needle" cupping method, the "boiled herb" cupping method, and the "stored herb" cupping method.

The "prick cupping" or bloodletting and cupping method involves pricking or piercing the skin with a special lancet at selected points or sites followed by cupping over the sites that were pierced. The vacuum helps draw blood out of the points thereby giving both beneficial bloodletting and cupping effects. This technique is good when cupping would seem useful and when signs of blood stasis, such as vascular spiders, are also present. The combination of bloodletting and cupping is described in detail in Chapter 10.

The "inserted needle" cupping method uses cupping over an inserted needle. The technique is usually applied over needles that are relatively deeply inserted which is the normal needling technique in most Chinese acupuncture approaches. In this method the cups are retained for about ten minutes or for as long as the needles are in place. This method is said to be useful for conditions such as rheumatism and disorders with accompanying pain conditions. Essentially, it combines the effects of cupping with the effects of the needle. Since the Japanese-style acupuncture we describe does not rely on deep needle insertion, we do not describe this technique further.

The "boiled herb" cupping method uses cups that are quickly taken out of a pot of selected boiling herbs, shaken, and then rapidly placed over the selected points or areas previously pricked with a lancet. The cups are retained for about ten minutes. This method combines cupping with bloodletting and small amounts of external herbal therapy. It is mostly indicated for conditions such as rheumatism, and is noted here, but not further described.

The "stored herb" cupping method uses cups that have been stored in liquids such as ginger liquid, pepper liquid, or wind-damp sake. The cup is removed from the liquid, shaken off, and then rapidly applied to the points or areas selected for therapy. This method is used mostly for conditions such as rheumatic pain, cough, flu, and gastric disorders, and is noted here, but not further described.

A final method mentioned in the literature employs very small cups constructed of plastic medicine bottles that have had the bottoms cut off and made smooth. The air is then withdrawn with a syringe stuck through the lid which is usually a rubber stopper. This method has the advantage of allowing cupping techniques to be applied to very small areas. New cupping sets, originally intended for the cupping of insect and snake bites, can also be used like this. An example of these devices is the "extractor," which is now commercially available.

TYPES OF CUPS

Modern-era cups are made of four different materials: bamboo, ceramic, glass, and plastic.

The bamboo cups come in three different sizes, and are made from trimmed pieces of bamboo. The bamboo cup is light and easy to use, is sturdy, and is readily obtained throughout East Asia, though less so in the West. Though good for most forms of cupping, it is best avoided when using "prick" cupping, where bloodletting is simultaneously employed (see Chapter 10).

Ceramic cups come in several sizes and can provide good suction, but have the disadvantage of not being as strong as the bamboo cups and thus more likely to break. However, the ceramic cups can be used with bloodletting because they are easier to sterilize.

Glass cups have the same advantages as the ceramic cups, but also have the further advantage of being transparent and allowing the practitioner to see changes in skin color, blood color, and the amount of blood. This allows for considerably more control during the treatment and fosters better decision-making concerning the amount of stimulation to be used. The following picture shows some of the different sizes of glass cups.

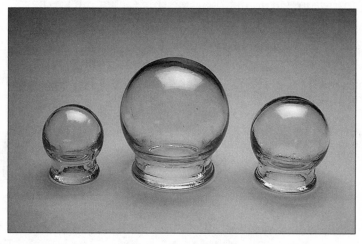

Glass cupping devices.

Plastic cups allow the same advantages as the glass cups but they are difficult to heat-sterilize because they can melt.

Traditionally the partial vacuum and suction necessary for cupping is obtained by placing either a lighted object inside the cup or igniting a thin film of flammable liquid, for example, alcohol, inside the cup. Then the lighted cup is applied rapidly to the skin. This is the "hot-cupping" or "fire cupping" method. As the small fire inside the cup burns up the available oxygen, a partial vacuum is produced which gently draws the skin and flesh up inside the cup.

More recent technological advances have allowed for appreciable refinements of technique. Cups are now available with built-in valves which are vacuum pumped, allowing for creation of a vacuum either manually or by means of a machine. Electric pumps are also available.

The small manual pump is like a bicycle pump, except that it draws rather then pushes the air. The degree of control is attained by the number of pumpings and the length of the strokes of pumping applied. The electric pumps can be preset to deliver specific amounts of pressure thus allowing very exact control over the amount of stimulation delivered.

In Japan, the use of a manual or electric pump with valved cups is by far the most prevalent form of cupping. The primary advantage of this method is that the amount of suction and thus the amount of force applied to the skin can be precisely controlled. This allows for considerable control over the amount of stimulation applied. As with virtually all other acupuncture and related techniques in Japan, the refinement of methods allowing greater control over the amount of stimulation delivered is characteristic of practice.

In our discussions in this text, it is important to note that when we describe cupping methods, either alone or in conjunction with bloodletting, we are referring exclusively to the valved pump cupping method. When using cupping extensively in the context of a comprehensive treatment, where the technique is usually adjunctive for symptom control, the amount of pressure delivered for each patient is very important. This degree of control cannot be achieved with the hot-cupping or fire-cupping technique.

The following pictures show a set of plastic valved pump cups and a set of glass valved pump cups.

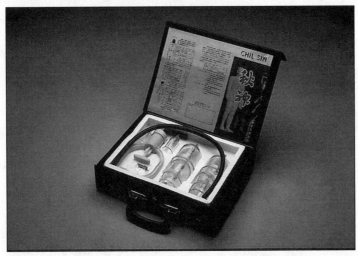

A plastic set of valved pump cups.

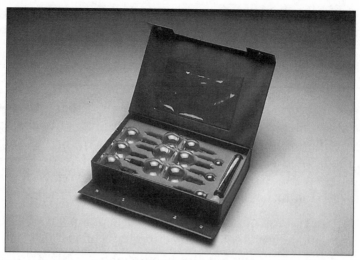

A glass set of valved pump cups.

To responsibly and routinely use the cupping and bloodletting treatment methods described in this text, we recommend purchasing one of the various pumped cupping sets available.

If you do not possess pump cups, we recommend that you not use them in conjunction with a comprehensive treatment. What permits so many steps to be applied in a single treatment without overstimulating the patient is the application of small and controlled stimuli at each step. If you cannot control the amount of stimulus, it is better not to employ the full panoply of steps.

INDICATIONS FOR ORTHODOX CUPPING THERAPY

Cupping therapy is indicated for a wide range of disorders. As mentioned above, some practitioners in Japan have adapted the methods so that they are suitable to all patients, and use them extensively. In general, cupping techniques are considered useful when muscle tightness is present because it is known to loosen tight muscles. It is also highly effective when blood stasis is clearly present because cupping is known to be a good therapy for increasing blood circulation. It can be used on patients who have conditions of repletion or conditions of vacuity.

Cupping can be effective for a wide range of conditions, including disorders of the neurological, digestive, circulatory, urogenital, respiratory, endocrine, gynecological, head, eye, ear, nose and throat, genital, and locomotor systems, as well as inflammation in general. It is considered effective for chronic disorders, but is also useful in some acute disorders such as the flu. The condition of the patient dictates the number of points utilized as well as the amount of pressure and length of time applied. Provided you follow the precautions and general rules outlined below, cupping therapy is a safe and easily applied form of treatment.

CONTRAINDICATIONS FOR ORTHODOX CUPPING THERAPY

Cupping is contraindicated on the abdomen or lower back of pregnant women. It is acceptable to use cupping for menstruating women, but in lower doses.

Do not use cupping methods on patients with inflamed organs or on patients whose organs could be or have perforated. For example, do not use cupping on the abdomen or back of patients with appendicitis, peritonitis, or gastric or duodenal ulcers–especially if bleeding is present. Do not use cupping on patients with colitis, especially if bleeding is present. If you are not sure or suspect that cupping might be inappropriate, refer the patient to the appropriate specialist to confirm the diagnosis. The physical pressure of the cupping could cause perforation of the affected organs.

Do not use cupping methods on patients with organic cardiac problems, such as valvular disease. Because cupping changes blood flow in the body, it can place a temporary stress on the heart. In patients with valvular problems, the increased stress could lead to temporary problems of cardiac insufficiency.

Do not use cupping methods on patients with diseases of the blood vessels such as thrombosis, aneurysm, or advanced arteriosclerosis.

Do not cup on the throat region.

Do not use cupping on patients with severe anemia or patients who are in an extremely weakened condition. Cupping can easily fatigue the patient, thereby causing inappropriate and unwanted reactions to treatment. Also, because cupping therapy alters blood flow in the body, the treatment could cause temporary cerebral hypotension with symptoms of dizziness and nausea. It is better to not use cupping on someone more disposed to developing this temporary problem.

PRECAUTIONS FOR ORTHODOX CUPPING THERAPY

Before applying cupping therapy, always explain clearly and thoroughly to the patient what it entails and what kind of marks might remain afterwards. After cupping therapy has been applied, marks and discoloration of the skin can be seen. These visible marks will disappear in 4 to 10 days depending on the degree of discoloration and the individual patient. Generally, with a healthier patient, the marks will be brighter red and they will disappear sooner. The more replete the patient and the more blood stasis present, the darker the discoloration and the longer it will persist. Some patients are very upset by the unattractive appearance of the discolored skin after cupping, and some are very disturbed by the pressure and sensation of the cupping. Inadequate explanation can unnecessarily upset patients and inhibit the advantageous therapeutic effects of the treatment.

As with most acupuncture methods, do not apply cupping methods within one hour of eating, exercising, or taking hot showers or baths.

It is not advisable to employ cupping therapy directly over traumatized or contused areas because it might cause discomfort for the patient. If you want to use cupping for traumas or contusions, it is better to use it outside the edges of the traumatized and contused areas.

Most patients do not like cupping on the face because it frequently leaves visible signs that look like bruises. Thus, the most commonly used points or areas are on the torso. However, if cupping is applied on the face, the momentary cupping method can be used.

If a number of cups are employed at the same time, do not place them too closely to each other because the skin will be pinched up too tightly between them, thereby causing unnecessary discomfort for the patient.

Always release the pressure from the cup before trying to remove it. With the valved cups this is easy; you merely release the valve which will release the vacuum in the cup. With the non-valved cups, you should hold the cup gently, pulling it slightly to one side, and with the fingers of the other hand, apply gentle pressure slowly to the raised skin on the opposite side of the cup. This should release the vacuum in the cup.

Always begin conservatively, with lighter doses of stimulation. Pay close attention to assess patient response and reaction.

Immediate and temporary side effects that might be seen with cupping overstimulation are symptoms of dizziness, dimness of vision, discomfort in the chest, nausea, and facial palor. In more serious cases, there may be coldness of the four limbs, cold sweat, minute pulse, and low blood pressure. Any of these signs or symptoms indicate that the patient has received too strong a dose. These side effects are most often seen in very sensitive patients, when assessment of the patient's sensitivity has been mistaken; in patients who are hungry or fatigued; or when cupping stimulation is too strong.

When any of these side effects do occur, they are almost always due to a temporary anemia of the brain. Have the patient lie comfortably on the table and apply *chinetsukyū* repeatedly to GV-14 if the patient is able to lie prone (on the belly), or to CV-6 if the patient is only able to lie supine (on the back). If these measures do not seem effective, apply *chinetsukyū* to the cupped areas also.

Longer-term side effects that usually do not become apparent until after the treatment include feeling excessively fatigued or drained, and on very rare occasions, the patient might complain of new symptoms. These different side effects are usually due to placement of too many cups, too lengthy application, and/or applying too much pressure to each cup.

Be careful. It is easy to overdose the patient!

Doses

We must again emphasize the importance of accurate assessment of the condition of the patient and appropriate adjustment of the doses of stimulation. This is especially important when treatment follows the multi-step approach described earlier in Chapter 2, the basic treatment modality that is representative of Japanese acupuncture. If you are treating a patient solely with cupping, it is still important to regulate the doses of stimulation, though generally you can apply somewhat higher doses of stimulation. Either way, it is crucial to observe the precautions and contraindications described above.

Adjustment of the dose of stimulation is made by considering three different variables in the cupping technique. First, consider the number of points or areas cupped; second, consider the amount of pressure applied with each cup; and third, consider the length of time each cup is retained. For the patient with extreme vacuity, it is better to apply only a few cups with very light pressure for short periods of time. For the patient with marked repletion, you can apply more cups with more pressure and for longer periods of time. Further adjustments can be made according to the patient or the target areas.

Altering the number of cups and length of time retained is a relatively straightforward variable from the technical perspective. Controlling the amount of pressure is simple, too, but it is the variable to which one must direct the most attention.

When working with the medium or small cups, the number and length of the strokes are fewer and they need to be adjusted accordingly. For the normal patient, who is neither markedly vacuous nor replete, you can cup about 5 to 7 points or areas, using the average number of strokes (around 3) and producing the following general amount of suction:

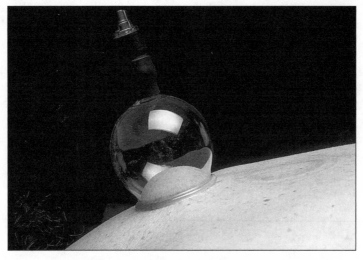

Medium stimulation (after three pump strokes).

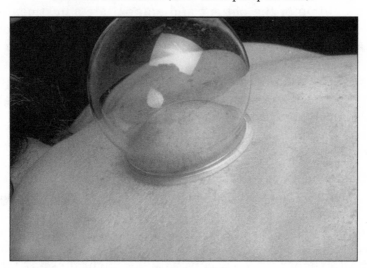

A close-up view of medium stimulation after three pump strokes.

The cups should be left in place for 3 to 10 minutes, with 3 to 5 being the most common length.

For the patient with vacuity, only two or three points or areas should be cupped, using lighter pressure, i.e, two normal or smaller strokes. The cups should be left in place for less time than for a normal patient, in a range from 20 seconds to two minutes.

Applying two lighter strokes only will raise the skin and flesh less (closer to 30cm of mercury) which will result in a much lower dose of stimulation:

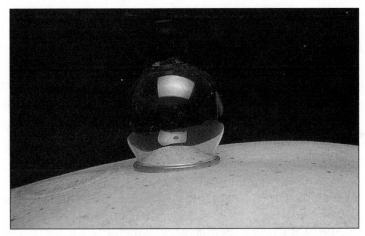

Lighter stimulation (after two pump strokes).

For the replete patient, you should cup between seven to ten points or areas. Apply stronger pressure, using three to four strokes, and leave the cups for slightly longer periods of time, usually between five to ten minutes.

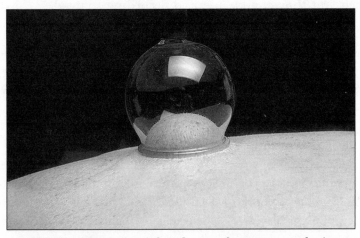

Heavier stimulation (after three or four pump strokes).

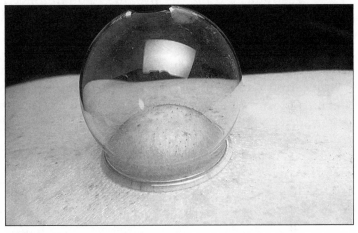

Close-up of heavier stimulation (after three or four pump strokes).

If you have an electric pump cupping set, the amount of pressure is preset on the machine. If you are using the manual cupping set, the amount of pressure is regulated by the number and length of strokes applied. The pressure should generally range between 30 to 50cm of mercury. Usually on the larger cups, three to four full strokes will give an appropriate amount of pressure (probably closer to 50cm of mercury, although this will vary according to the altitude).

Usually, if you work somewhere between the 30–50cm range, the results will be sufficient to regulate the degree of pressure. There are some body areas where more than four strokes are required to get sufficient pressure, such as on loose skin. On elderly and/or vacuous patients, two strokes can be too much. You must always consider each patient and body area individually in order to deliver appropriate doses of stimulation.

The following recommendations come from Akinobu Meguro, and are most relevant to his whole-body or root treatment approach, but they can be adapted according to need.

Supplementation Methods for Vacuous Patients			
METHOD	LOWEST DOSE	LOW DOSE	AVERAGE DOSE
Fire Cupping (40cm Hg)	5 seconds	20 seconds	40 seconds
Manual Cupping (50cm Hg)	5 seconds	20 seconds	40 seconds
Electric Cupping (60cm Hg)	3 seconds	10 seconds	20 seconds

Draining Methods for Replete Patients			
METHOD	MEDIUM DOSE	HIGH DOSE	HIGHEST DOSE
Fire Cupping (40cm Hg)	1 minute	2 minutes	3 minutes
Manual Cupping (50cm Hg)	1 minute	2 minutes	3 minutes
Electric Cupping (60cm Hg)	30 seconds	1 minute	90 seconds

The pressures indicated for the fire, manual, and electric cupping methods are the approximate maximum pressures. We can further adjust these doses by altering the pressure applied. If, for example, the manual cupping pressure is reduced by using fewer strokes with the pump, it is possible to leave the cups on longer to achieve the desired end. Thus for example, if the pressure were around 35cm Hg (low to moderate pressure), each cup could be left on for longer periods. It works out approximately as follows:

Approximate Ranges of Stimulation			
SUPPLEMENTATION		DRAINING	
Lowest	10 seconds	High	4 minutes
Medium	2 minutes	Average	60–80 seconds
Low	40 seconds	Highest	6 minutes

To gain a clear picture of the different effects achieved by varying the numbers and lengths of the pumping strokes and amount of
time, and to truly understand these differences, we recommend
practicing these cupping techniques on different body areas on
yourself or your friends and family. In addition, we recommend that
during initial treatments employing the cupping methods, you
apply slightly less stimulation than you might normally use in
order to assure that the possibility of overdoses is minimal.

APPLICATION GUIDELINES

The general indications we have just described should be considered when using cupping therapy as a symptom control treatment,
that is, as part of a whole treatment plan. Specialists in Japan who
use cupping therapy exclusively for all their patients will often use
many more cups in one session because they are not applying any
other therapy. This is especially so when they apply their whole
body "root" treatment which is used to promote and maintain
health, rather than to target specific symptoms. We describe both
approaches below, but recommend that when following the root
treatment procedures referred to throughout this text, it is preferable to err on the side of safety and use the lower doses we have
described.

Normally, if the cup causes pain, it is an indication that for the
particular patient the pressure is too much. The appropriate procedure is to release the pressure and reapply the cup using less
pressure. Sometimes the area of cupping is painful, feeling somewhat bruised after treatment. If done correctly, the cup will feel
tight but comfortable while on the body.

In judging the correct time of cup retention, the amount of discoloration that comes up with the cup is often a good indication.
When clear discoloration has come up, this is usually a good time to
remove the cup, especially in the range of patients with normal to
vacuous conditions.

The colors that come up can vary considerably from patient to
patient and area to area. Sometimes redness comes up with the
cup. Usually this color vanishes within a few minutes after removal
of the cup. Sometimes the area turns darker in color, usually a dark
red to purple color. These colors usually persist for a few days after
treatment. Darker colors often reflect a patient with a more replete
condition, or a condition of considerable blood stasis.

Sometimes where the cup was placed will turn yellowish or
greenish after a day or so; this effect presents no problem, and usually indicates that excessive pressure was used with the cup. After
removal, some amount of discoloration usually remains at the site

of cupping. As mentioned above, it is important to warn the patient beforehand that some discoloration might persist. On rare occasions, the discoloration may persist for several weeks. Most likely this effect is the result of having applied excessive pressure on a patient with considerable blood stasis.

It is advisable to apply cupping techniques to patients who are lying down rather than sitting or standing. Most points or areas that are indicated are on the torso, so it is best to have patients lying supine for the abdominal and chest points or areas, and prone for the back points or areas. For points or areas that are more on the side of the body, we recommend having patients lie on their sides such that the side to be treated is uppermost. It is preferable to have patients remain motionless while the cups are on since motion may displace the cups. In addition, it is a good idea to stretch or spread the skin slightly before applying the cups since loose skin may break the seal of the cup and release the vacuum.

When working on thin patients, you may find that the cups will not adhere well on the shoulder, back, and lumbar regions. In such cases it is often advantageous to have patients lie on their sides; this usually helps the cups adhere better.

On areas of the body where the skin is thicker, such as the soles of the feet, you may need to moisten the area first with a wet towel, to allow the cups to adhere better. When cupping over areas with weak and soft skin, with clearly visible blood vessels beneath, apply the cup for less time, removing and reapplying it repeatedly. By doing this on-off application repeatedly, you can keep the cup on the area for the appropriate amount of time.

ESSENTIAL TREATMENT POINTS FOR COMMON DISORDERS

Usually the point to be cupped will exhibit some pressure pain, tightness, and/or tension of the muscles. To select appropriately between a number of indicated points, palpate and select the points based on their responses.

The following general treatment patterns are taken from *Kyūgyoku Ryōhō (Cupping Therapy.)*

Disorders of the entire body

GV-14, GV-12.

Disorders of the lower half of the body

GV-4.

Respiratory disorders

BL-12, BL-13, BL-20, LU-1, CV-17.

Circulatory disorders

BL-15, BL-16, BL-17, BL-20, GV-11, GV-10, CV-14.

Gastric disorders

BL-17, BL-18, BL-20, BL-21, CV-12, CV-13.

Intestinal disorders

BL-20, BL-22, BL-25, ST-25, CV-4.

Liver disorders, gallbladder disorders

BL-18, BL-19, BL-20, CV-12, GV-9, LR-14, *ashi* points.

Genital and urinary organ disorders

BL-18, BL-20, BL-23, BL-28, 8 *liao,* CV-4, CV-3.

Endocrine disorders

BL-13, BL-15, BL-18, BL-20, BL-25, CV-12, CV-14.

Neurological disorders

BL-15, BL-14, GV-11, GV-10, BL-18, BL-20, BL-23.

Disorders of the cerebral blood vessels

BL-15, BL-14, BL-18, BL-20, GV-11, GV-10.

Locomotor disorders–upper limbs

LI-15, SI-9, SI-15, SI-14, *ashi* points.

Locomotor disorders–lower limbs

BL-23, 8 *liao* points, BL-54, GB-30, BL-37, ST-32, GB-31, *ashi* points.

Lumbar pain

GV-4, BL-23, BL-20, GV-3, BL-37, *ashi* points.

High fever

GV-14, GV-12, BL-15, BL-18, BL-13, BL-12.

Gynecological disorders

BL-18, BL-20, BL-23, BL-25, CV-4, CV-3, 8 *liao* points, *ashi* points.

Disorders of the five sense organs

BL-12, BL-13, BL-18, BL-20, BL-15, BL-23.

Dermatological disorders

BL-12, BL-13, BL-18, BL-20, *ashi* points.

SPECIFIC SYMPTOMATIC TREATMENTS FROM KYŪKAKU RYŌHŌ

The author recommends the use of treatment of one area on one day and another area on the next day, with alternation back and forth on alternate treatment days.

Gastric disorders
(chronic gastritis, gastric atony, gastric hyperacidity)

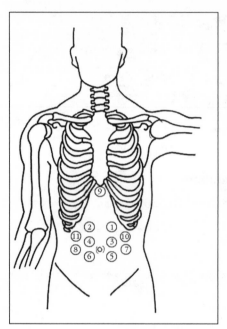

Abdominal region (day 1)

Apply #1 to #9 in consecutive numerical order. Initially leave #9 for about 20 seconds, then gradually increase the length of retention to 2 minutes.

Remove #9 first. Then remove the rest in the same order as they were applied.

#10 and #11 are for the patient with repletion.

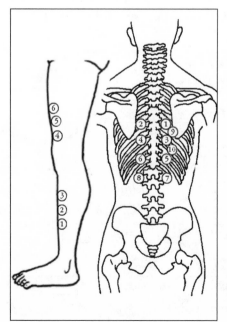

Back and leg regions (day 2)

It is usually better to use fewer cups or leave them for a shorter period of time according to the degree of vacuity of the patient.

Apply #1 to #8 on the back in consecutive order. Remove the cups in the same order as applying them.

Apply #1 to #6 on both legs to the points shown.

When removing the cups on the lower limbs, remove them in the reverse order. Add #9 and #10 for patients with accompanying liver disorders.

Intestinal disorders

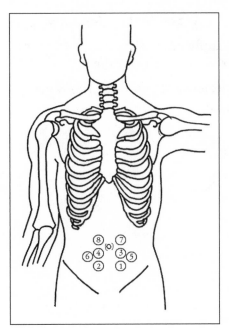

Abdominal region (day 1)

Apply cups #1 to #8 in consecutive numerical order.

Remove the cups in the same order as applying them.

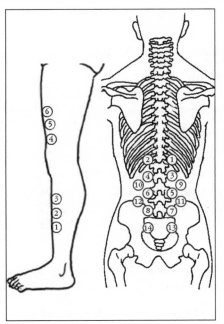

Back and leg regions (day 2)

Apply cups #1 to #12 consecutively in numerical sequence.

For thin patients with vacuity, do not cup #1 and #2 on the back. Instead place them at #13 and #14.

Remove the cups in the same order as applying them.

Apply #1 to #6 on both legs to the points shown.

Remove the cups in the reverse order as when applying them.

Hemorrhoids

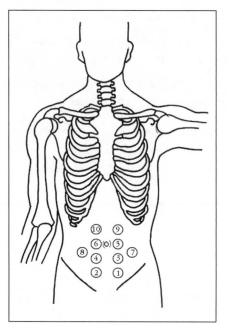

Abdominal region (day 1)

Apply cups #1 to #10 in consecutive numerical orders.

Remove the cups in the reverse order.

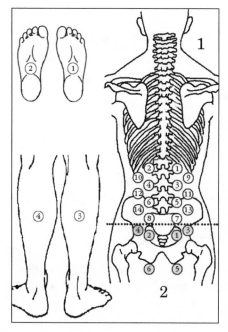

Back and leg regions (day 2)

First apply cups #1 to #4 in consecutive numerical order to the soles and around BL-57.

While these cups are on, apply the cups in consecutive numerical order to section 1 (above the line) on the torso.

Remove the cups from section 1 in the same order as applied, then apply them in consecutive numerical order to section 2 (shaded points below the line) on the torso.

Remove the cups from section 2 in the same order as applied.

Remove the cups from BL-57 and the feet in the reverse order as applied. If the cups fall off the soles of the feet, keep reapplying them until the end of treatment.

Chronic constipation

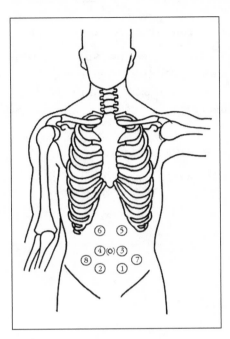

Abdominal region (day 1)

Apply cups #1 to #8 in consecutive numerical order.

Use the supplementation technique if the patient has vacuity; otherwise use the draining technique.

Remove the cups in reverse order as applied.

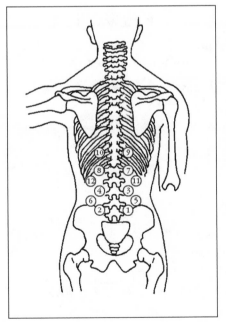

Back region (day 2)

Apply cups #1 to #10 in consecutive numerical order.

Remove the cups in reverse order.

Apply cups to #11 and #12 if there is accompanying lumbar pain or whole body fatigue.

Diarrhea

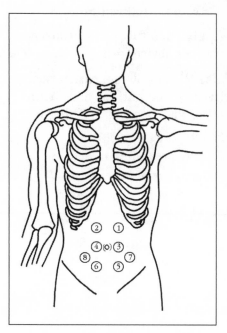

Abdominal region (day 1)

With diarrhea, the supplementation technique is used, even if the patient's condition is replete overall.

Apply cups #1 to #8 in consecutive numerical order.

Remove the cups in the following order: 6, 5, 8, 7, 4, 3, 2, 1.

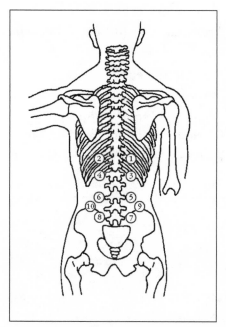

Back region (day 2)

Apply cups #1 to #10 in consecutive numerical order.

Remove the cups in reverse order.

Intercostal neuralgia

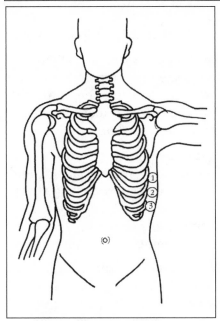

Chest region (day 1)

Treat #1, #2, and #3 on the diseased side.

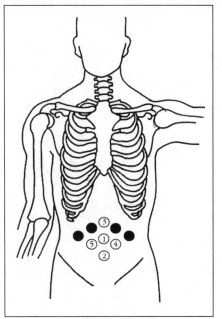

Abdominal region (day 1)

Cup points #1 to #5 in consecutive numerical order.

If the patient is very replete, add the shaded abdominal points shown.

Remove all cups in the order applied.

Back region (day 2)

Treat the diseased side, starting at the area of the pain and removing that cup last.

Apply cups #1 to #10 in consecutive numerical order.

Remove cups #6 to #10, then #4 and #5, then #1 to #3.

In acute attacks, do this treatment immediately before doing the chest and abdominal regions.

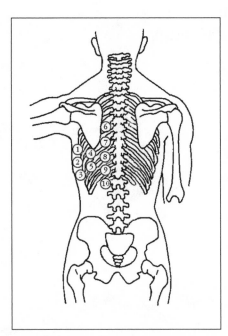

Sciatica

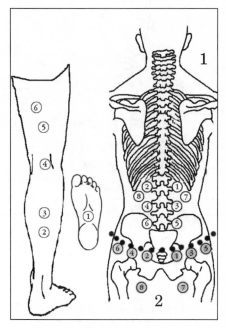

Low back and leg regions (day 1)

Apply cups to region 1 (torso above the line), region 2 (shaded torso points below the line), and region 3 (leg and foot) in consecutive numerical order.

Place the cups on the areas of pain first; then treat the leg and buttock regions, removing these cups last. Lastly, cup the low back regions (region 2, the shaded points below the line).

When removing the cups from the buttock region remove in reverse order. Remove cups from the leg in reverse order. Treat the region on the lateral portion of the thigh only if the pain is severe.

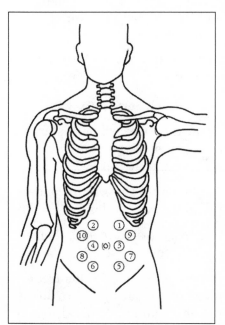

Abdomen region (day 2)

Apply the cups in consecutive numerical order.

Remove the cups in the order of application.

Stiff shoulders

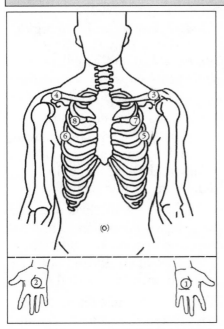

Chest and arm regions (day 1)

Cup #1 and #2 in the center of the palm of each hand, then cup #3 to #8 on the arms and chest in consecutive numerical order.

Remove in reverse order.

Back and shoulder regions (day 2)

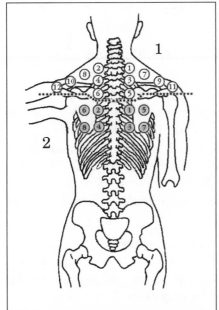

Apply cups #1 to #12 in the upper section (above the line) in consecutive numerical order. Do the same for cups #1 to #8 in the lower section (shaded points).

In replete patients, cup all the areas, leaving the cups on for slightly longer periods of time.

For patients with vacuity, do not cup #11 and #12 in the upper section 1, and #5, #6, #7, and #8 of the lower section 2.

Remove the cups in the order of application.

Head, nose, and eye problems

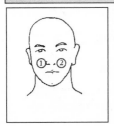
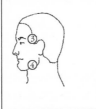

Cup the same regions as in the treatment of stiff shoulders, and add the facial regions shown.

For poor vision, add cupping of the abdomen, especially of the navel.

High blood pressure, stroke, and arteriosclerosis

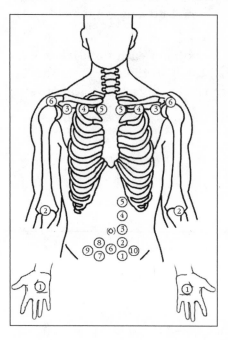

Chest, abdomen, and arm regions (day 1)

Cup #1 to #10 on the abdomen. While those cups are on, cup the chest and arm regions.

Remove the chest cups in the order #5, #4, #3, #6. Next remove #9 and #10 then #8 to #1 on the abdomen. Remove #2 and #1 from the arms and palms.

In the case of high blood pressure and arteriosclerosis, treat the chest and arm regions bilaterally. In the case of stroke and hemiplegia, treat only the affected side.

Initially leave the cups on for about forty seconds each. Gradually increase the length of time to three minutes per cup.

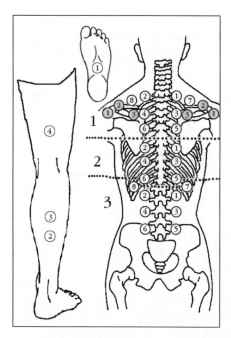

Back, shoulder, and leg regions (day 2)

Place cups #1 to #8 and shaded cups #1 to #3 (bilateral) in section 1. When removing the cups from section 1, remove in this order: #8, #7, then #1 to #6 of the medially placed cups, then #3 to #1 of the laterally placed (shaded) cups.

Place cups #1 to #6 in section 2, and remove the cups in the order of application. Place cups #1 to #4 on the legs and foot before #1 to #8 of section 3 (lower torso). Remove the cups from section 3 in order: #8, #7, then #1 to #6; then from the leg and foot, #4 to #1.

In conditions of high blood pressure and arteriosclerosis, treat the shoulder and leg regions bilaterally. With strokes and hemiplegias, treat the affected side only.

Bronchial asthma

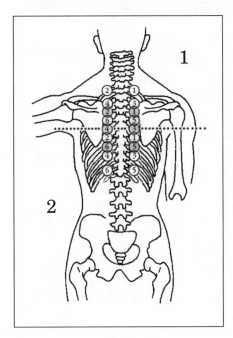

Back region

On Day 1 apply cups to #1 to #6 in section 1 (upper torso). Then apply cups to #1 to #6 in section 2 (lower torso).

On the next day, alternate by using the shaded points #1 to #6.

Use this treatment at the time of an attack. Apply cupping repeatedly.

If the patient is replete, use the draining method.

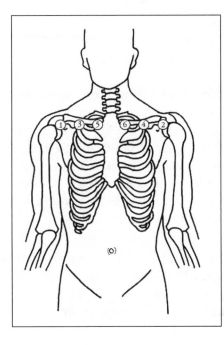

Chest region

Apply cups #1 to #6 in consecutive numerical order.

Remove the cups in the order in which they were applied.

This treatment can be used when there is no asthma attack in process. If the patient cannot tolerate the treatment, shorten the time that the cups are retained, but try to keep them for at least thirty seconds.

Gynecological disorders
(abnormal menstruation, painful or irregular menstruation, menopausal syndrome)

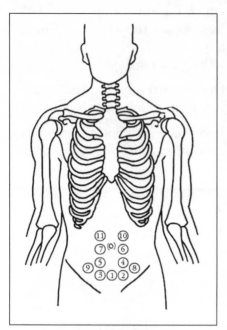

Abdominal region (day 1)

Apply cups #1 to #11 in consecutive numerical order.

Do not use #10 and #11 on patients with vacuity. Use supplementation or draining techniques according to the condition of the patient.

If there is abdominal pain, place cups at the painful areas first and remove these last.

Otherwise, remove #10 and #11 first, then #7, #6, #9, #8, #5 to #1.

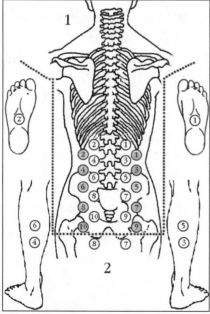

Back and leg regions (day 2)

Apply cups #1 to #8 in section 2 on the buttocks, legs, and feet in numerical order. Next, apply the cups #1 to #10 in section 1 on the upper torso. Apply the cups to the shaded points #1 to #10 on the upper torso of section 1. However, **do not** use the shaded points on patients with vacuity conditions.

Remove the cups from section 1 first, in the order of application. Remove the cups from #1 to #8 in section 2 on the buttocks, legs, and feet in the reverse order of application.

When beginning treatment, use from 6 to 8 cups at first on section 1, and slowly increase the number over consecutive treatments. Do not have more than 10 cups on at once. To apply more than 10 cups in a single session, remove those already applied before applying subsequent cups. Leave the cups in the buttocks region of section 2 for a little longer.

Kidney disorders (frequent urination, urgent urination)

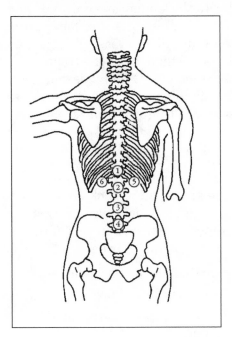

Back region (day 1)

Apply cups #1 to #6 in consecutive numerical order.

#1 is placed at the level of T12. Remove the cups in the order of application.

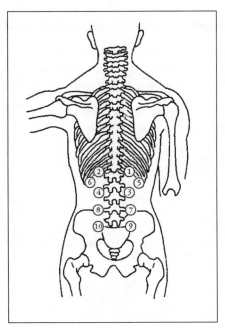

Back region (day 2)

Apply cups #1 to #10 in consecutive numerical order.

Remove #5 and #6 last, after removing the other cups.

CUPPING: A GENERAL HEALTH MAINTENANCE APPROACH[6]

The doses of stimulation are similar to those mentioned above. For the more vacuous or sensitive patient, use less pressure for shorter periods of time; for the replete patient, use more pressure for longer periods of time. If the patient feels comfortable after the treatment, it is usually a sign that the doses were correct. Cupping is done regularly for general patterns on the abdominal and back regions. There are two general treatment patterns that can be alternated on different visits.

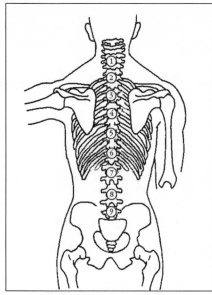

First Treatment Pattern

For the first treatment pattern, the areas on the back all lie along the spine. Treatment involves applying the cups in sets of three in the following order:

Starting on the back, cup #1, #2, and #3.

After removing these, cup #4, #5, and #6.

After removing these, cup #7, #8, and #9.

Observe that the procedure applies the cups continuously down the spine.

When finished on the back, have the patient turn over.

Cup #1, #2, and #3 on the abdomen.

After removing these, cup #4, #5, and #6.

After removing these, cup #7.

---

[6]Taken from Y. Manaka, *Kyū to Hari (Moxa and Needle Therapy)*, pp. 250–252, describing the lay practitioner's approach to cupping therapy.

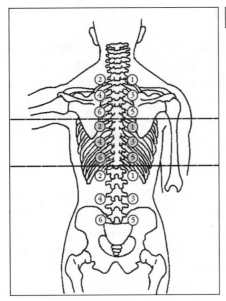

Second Treatment Pattern

The areas on the back are all paravertebral, running from top to bottom on the back.

Step One: Back Region

Place #1 to #6 in the upper region.

Remove these cups and cup #1 to #6 in the middle region.

Remove these cups and cup #1 to #6 in the lower region.

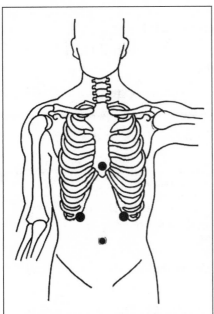

Step Two: Front Region

After removing the cups on the dorsal side of the body (Step One), have the patient turn over.

Cup the following points as shown—CV-17, LR-14, and around the navel.

When done correctly, the cups should feel comfortable and should be left for the appropriate length of time specific to each patient's condition. When the patient is familiar with cupping procedures and finds them to be comfortable, you can apply all the cups on the back at once, and then all the cups on the front at once.

As with most of our recommendations in this book, it is important to try to regulate the doses of stimulation as much as possible. If you are using this procedure as the entire treatment, you can apply a little more pressure for longer periods of time (again within the limitations of what is appropriate for the patient.) The procedure can be repeated once weekly on all areas for each treatment block. If the cupping treatment follows other stimulation therapy, or is part of the treatment procedure outlined earlier in Chapter 2, remember that lower doses must be applied. You should use much less pressure for shorter periods of time, or you should apply the cups in blocks for different appointments. A theoretical example follows, outlining treatment occurring over 6 sessions that can be repeated starting with Session 1 as deemed necessary.

By using a method such as this, you cup all the treatment areas and points over a period of time, thereby allowing greater control over the doses of stimulation given. Manaka recommended that when applying this therapy regularly, over a long period of time, occasional breaks in the procedure should be scheduled so that the body would have the opportunity to adapt to the stimuli.

First treatment pattern	
Session 1	Cup #1, #2, and #3 on the back and #1, #2, and #3 on the abdomen (p 208).
Session 2	Cup #4, #5, and #6 on the back and #4, #5, and #6 on the abdomen (p 208).
Session 3	Cup #7, #8, and #9 on the back and #7 on the abdomen (p 208).
Second treatment pattern	
Session 4	Cup #1, #2, #3, #4, #5, and #6 on the upper portions of the back, and then perhaps CV-17 on the chest (p. 209).
Session 5	Cup the mid-back areas, #1, #2, #3, #4, #5, and #6; then LR-14 on the abdomen (p. 209).
Session 6	Cup the lower #1, #2, #3, #4, #5, and #6 areas on the back along the periumbilical area (p. 209).

Chapter 10
Shiraku—Bloodletting

The practice of bloodletting in acupuncture has a long history. Some have argued that it may have been the earliest form of acupuncture representing a less systematized therapy.[1] Bloodletting is a commonly referenced treatment method in the famous Chinese acupuncture classic, *Huang Di Nei Jing Su Wen,* where its basic importance is stated in many contexts. Chapter 20 described its use for letting out apparent blood stasis before regulating vacuity (by supplementation techniques) or regulating repletion (by draining techniques).[2]

With the rise of the popularity of the *Nan Jing,* a later, more systematic text, where the practice of bloodletting was not mentioned at all, and where the concepts of qi circulating in the channels was clearly solidified,[3] the use and practice of bloodletting became less popular. However, it has survived in modern acupuncture practice. Many current books cite the use of bloodletting, though it has usually taken the status of one of a number of auxiliary techniques available to the practicing acupuncturist. With this limited usage naturally come restrictions on the general uses of bloodletting, so that it can be fit into the framework of the whole method of practice. For example, in current Chinese literature, bloodletting is generally cited as useful for a narrow range of disorders. *Chinese Acupuncture and Moxibustion* cites the following indications for bloodletting:

> *Blockage of the meridians; blood stasis; excess syndrome and heat syndrome, such as high fever, loss of consciousness, sore throat, local congestion or swelling.*

---

[1] For an interesting and well-documented discussion of the early history of the use of bloodletting in acupuncture, see D. C. Epler, *Bloodletting in Early Chinese Medicine and its Relation to the Origin of Acupuncture.* See also M. Maruyama, *Shinkyū Igaku to Koten no Kenkyū (Research Book of Acupuncture and Moxibustion Medicine and the Classics),* p. 61.

[2] M. Maruyama, *Ibid.,* pp. 60-61.

[3] D. C. Epler. See footnote 1 above.

This text also states that bloodletting is good when used at specific points for acute vomiting, conjunctivitis, carbuncles, and erysipelas.[4] *Acupuncture, A Comprehensive Text* gives the following indications:

> ...*Acute and chronic tonsillitis, neurodermatitis, allergic dermatitis, acute sprain, heatstroke, abscesses, febrile diseases, headache, rhinitis, acute conjunctivitis or keratitis, numbness of the fingers or toes, erysipelas, eczema, lymphangiitis, phlebitis, hemorrhoids and coma.*[5]

With the advent of the Meiji Restoration in Japan, and the restriction of the use of bloodletting to physicians, the practice of bloodletting in Japan became the purview of the Western medical acupuncture community. Two physicians, interested in practicing acupuncture, read the *Huang Di Nei Jing Su Wen* and were struck by the extent of the use of bloodletting in that text. These two, Masao Maruyama and Kunimasa Kudō, started practicing and researching bloodletting in their clinical practice. For many years they treated all their patients using bloodletting as the primary form of therapy. Kudō supplemented this with the use of *kyūtōshin*, the moxa on the handle of the needle technique, but bloodletting was clearly the focus of both doctors' treatment methods.

Kudō and Maruyama wrote several books together and singly on the use of bloodletting. Much of the content of these books focussed on studies of the nature of blood stasis and scientific experiments to explore the physiological effects of bloodletting. Juxtaposed with this scientific data was a considerable amount of clinical data, enough to write a book.

In their clinical emphasis on bloodletting, Maruyama and Kudō constantly refined and controlled their techniques so that bloodletting produced markedly favorable results on virtually *all* their patients. Consequently, the restrictions placed on the use of bloodletting in other styles of acupuncture, such as modern T.C.M., do not apply to the information given here. Provided proper attention is paid to judging the correct doses of bloodletting for each patient, and provided it is not clearly contraindicated, bloodletting is a safe and effective treatment method. Problems identified as being at the blood level are relatively deep problems and thus typically stubborn. When the correct visible signs are present, or when you have clearly identified the presence of blood stasis in a patient, the use of bloodletting can speed up the healing process in the patient dramatically, providing both symptomatic and systemic effects.[6] We

---

[4] See Cheng Xin-Nong, *Chinese Acupuncture and Moxibustion*, pp. 333-334.

[5] D. Bensky and J. O'Connor, *Acupuncture, a Comprehensive Text,* p. 429.

[6] See Y. Manaka *et al.*, *Chasing the Dragon's Tail,* pp. 128-131, for more detailed discussions of the nature, signs, and treatment of blood stasis *(xue yu).*

have observed many cases where stubborn, slow-responding complaints improved immediately following the application of bloodletting and the removal of a few drops of blood.

The information presented below represents the core of Kudō and Maruyama's clinical experiences, translated mostly from their book, *Shimpan Shiraku Ryōhō (Bloodletting Therapy)*. The information deals with the contraindications of bloodletting; a brief statement regarding their thoughts on the nature and formation of vascular spiders or spider nevi, called *sairaku;* bloodletting techniques for these vascular spiders *(sairaku shiraku)*, including the additional use of cupping; indications for the uses of *sairaku shiraku* on different body areas, especially those where vascular spiders are commonly found; and indications and applications for cutaneous bloodletting *(hifu shiraku)*, which includes *ranshi hō*, bloodletting on local cutaneous regions, and *mattan shiraku,* bloodletting on the extremities, including the uses of bloodletting on the *jing* points at the nail corners on the fingers and toes. In addition, we have added information on how to ascertain and determine the exact dosage of bloodletting for each patient, and how to correct problems associated with removal of too much blood.[7]

CONTRAINDICATIONS FOR THE USE OF BLOODLETTING

Obviously any patient who suffers from hemophilia should not be bloodlet. Also patients who are taking blood thinning medications such as COUMADIN™ should not be bloodlet.

Some authors have recommended against the use of bloodletting on patients suffering from anemia or low blood pressure. However, Kudō and Maruyama state that one cannot say for sure that bloodletting is so contraindicated. According to Dyes (1887), bloodletting has distinctive effects on pernicious anemia and chlorosis (a form of anemia). Van Noordes also suggested that a small amount of bloodletting would stimulate the blood-forming organs with good results. In their experience and research, Kudō and Maruyama found that many patients with severe anemia recovered using repetitive bloodletting in small quantities. It is thus hard to concur with authors who advise against bloodletting on anemic patients. With regard to low blood pressure, their research and experience showed that bloodletting was able to regulate blood pressure, a finding that would actually recommend rather than contraindicate its use. Of course, what is important is to regulate the amounts of bloodletting for both these conditions.

---

[7]This information is derived from the lectures of Kudō's student, Kōei Kuahara, based on the work of Kudō and the researches of members of the Tōyōhari Association, of which he is a member.

A few other restrictions should be mentioned:

•In certain cerebral conditions such as cerebral embolism, it is contraindicated to do much bloodletting, although bloodletting at the nail corners in small quantities can be helpful for the overall condition.

•In patients with cardiac disorders, it can be contraindicated to use bloodletting techniques, especially with patients who have had a myocardial infarction. The contraindications are for any bloodletting on the upper back or back of the shoulder; this can be extremely dangerous. Bloodletting in small quantities from the nail corners can, on the other hand, be quite helpful for cardiac conditions, with no risk of worsening the condition.

•Bloodletting is contraindicated in various forms of tuberculosis, particularly because the patient is often exhausted and run down. Any bloodletting on the torso should be avoided, but bloodletting distally in small quantities can be helpful for the relief of symptoms.

•Bloodletting is contraindicated in patients in the last stages of a malignant tumor or any conditions of extreme weakness.

More details of the restrictions and doses of bloodletting according to each patient's condition are given below. We would add a few precautionary words about the use of bloodletting techniques on pregnant patients and patients with complicated disorders and highly contagious diseases, such as hepatitis, AIDS, etc.

Usually any acupuncture technique or treatment on a pregnant women should be more gentle and at a lower dosage than usual. Certain acupoints or areas of the body are contraindicated for needling. There are similar restrictions or precautions that need to be followed when using bloodletting techniques. Pregnant women tend to be very sensitive to treatment, so it is important to avoid certain areas and techniques and to carefully regulate the dose of bloodletting. Bloodletting with cupping and bloodletting of the *jing* points are both considered to be too strong for pregnant women, and better avoided. If bloodletting is to be used, it should be only by the squeezing method, either after piercing a vascular spider or applying small cuts to a skin area. It is better to avoid the low back area. Usually bloodletting is only used when varicose veins need to be addressed as a common complication of pregnancy. In such instances, small vascular spiders are selected on the legs for bloodletting and moxa cones are used afterwards (see below for details).

Provided that you avoid the use of bloodletting with cupping, that you avoid bloodletting the *jing* points, and that you follow the guidelines for treatment on the legs only, bloodletting on pregnant women should be safe. But apply this technique with great caution. If the patient has any other health issues, such as difficulty walking or a history of miscarriages, it is better not to use the bloodletting techniques when treating a pregnant woman.

When treating a patient with diabetes who is suffering from peripheral neuropathy, be careful about the techniques employed. While it is not necessarily contraindicated to use bloodletting on such a patient, there are certain guidelines to follow. If, for example, the neuropathy is in the toes, it would be ill-advised to use bloodletting on the toes or feet; likewise on the hands or fingers, if the problem were on the fingers. It is perhaps better either to use no bloodletting on a patient suffering from peripheral neuropathy, or to use low-dosage bloodletting on the torso only.

If the patient is diabetic, but without peripheral neuropathy, you must still be extremely careful. Focussing the use of any bloodletting techniques on the torso would be better. Though use of the fingers or toes would not be contraindicated, great care must be taken and decisions based on a case-by-case analysis. For example, if the patient has no problem healing from accidents, small cuts, or contusions, then it is relatively safe to proceed with low-dose bloodletting on extremity points. But, it should also be remembered that many diabetics apply small amounts of bloodletting on themselves on a regular basis, for the purposes of measuring their blood sugar levels. Typically, this is done on the fingertips. If patients are applying such techniques to themselves already, this is a good sign that there should be no problem with using bloodletting techniques at least on the fingers.

As we will see below, bloodletting can be used on patients who have hepatitis, but the practitioner must be extremely careful when handling bloodied materials from such patients because some forms of hepatitis are *very* easily transmitted. When treating patients with AIDS or patients who have tested positive for the HIV virus, the same precautions need to be taken when handling bloodied materials.

Some practitioners in the West feel that it may be better not to use bloodletting techniques on patients who have tested HIV-positive even if they have no symptoms. We think that in the symptomless state and provided the general condition of the patient is good (see discussions below regarding judgement of correct dosage), bloodletting can be used at the nail corners very carefully and in small dosage when it is clearly indicated. But in patients who have an advanced AIDS condition with multiple symptoms and signs of vacuity, bloodletting likely should not be used.

There is no real hard and fast rule here; we do not have sufficient experience to judge clearly one way or the other. For a patient who is HIV positive, bloodletting, like the insertion of any needle, represents a break in the patient's defensive layers which are already weakened by the viral infection and its complications. Thus extreme caution should be taken; the numbers of points stimulated should be kept down and dosages of bloodletting should be very carefully regulated.

PRECAUTIONS WHEN USING BLOODLETTING TECHNIQUES

One problem any acupuncturist faces when treating patients is the lack of knowledge of whether a patient is actually carrying an infectious disease such as hepatitis or HIV. As such, practitioners must always employ the "universal precautions" approach, where every patient is approached as a potential carrier of a highly infectious disease. This approach is already observed by most acupuncturists in the West but it is even more important when practicing bloodletting techniques because of the deliberate work with a body fluid. ***You should always wear disposable surgical gloves for protection when bloodletting.***[8]

When handling bloodied materials, such as cotton balls, gauze, cups, and needles, always retain the gloves, and always place these bloodied materials on clean surfaces, such as a tray, so that they may be cleaned or sterilized later. If any blood is spilled or any bloodied objects touch other surfaces, such as the treatment table, always clean and sterilize that surface before any other contact with it. If gloves become contaminated, that is, if there is some blood on the gloves, be careful not to touch any other objects or surfaces other than those one is working on. If any objects are touched, the same cleaning techniques must be applied.

To dispose of bloodied materials, such as cotton balls, gauze, and protective gloves, use the same containers and follow the same procedures as for disposal of used needles. Do not throw them in the trash. Instead, place them in a special container kept for disposing of used acupuncture supplies. Needles should be disposed of separately. A good technique to help seal the bloodied materials and ensure that none are dropped is to hold all contaminated materials

---

[8]Recent reports of studies examining the effectiveness of different gloves as barriers to disease-carrying organisms have shown that polyethylene and polyvinylchloride latex gloves can let the AIDS virus through in 20 to 40% of cases. (See, for example, a report in the October 10, 1990 issue of the *New York Times*.) This suggests that if you want to use these gloves for protective purposes, they should be worn in double layers. Regular latex gloves fared somewhat better, but the Occupational Safety and Health Administration (OSHA) recently came up with recommendations to double up on the use of any latex glove. Rubber gloves, which are thicker and non-porous, can be worn in single thickness.

in one hand, and, with the other, peel the glove off inside out, so that everything that was held in the hand is now inside the inverted glove. Then hold the glove containing the materials in the other hand and peel off the second glove so that the first, with its contents, is placed inside the second glove. Dispose of the gloves and their contents in the contaminated materials disposal container.

There are a variety of cleaning agents that can be used for cleaning or sterilizing surfaces where blood has been spilled or where bloodied objects have made contact. Perhaps the easiest to use is a bleach solution. Until recently a 0.5% bleach solution was recommended. More recently a 1% bleach solution is recommended. It is a good idea to check the concentration of the commercial bleach before proceeding. Bleach that is commercially available for laundry purposes usually has a 5 to 6% concentration. In order to make a 1% solution for sterilization, mix one cup of the commercial bleach with four cups of water. This 1% solution is approved both in Japan and in the U.S. as being sufficient to kill all bacteria and viruses, including the hepatitis virus.

Objects that have had contact with blood, such as the suction cups used with the bloodletting in order to increase blood flow, should be soaked in the 1% bleach solution for approximately one hour. However, before any object, such as a cup, is placed in the bleach solution, it should be thoroughly wiped with alcohol swabs in order to remove all debris, dried blood, etc., from the surfaces. If the object is not wiped clean first, the bleach will not clean off the surface; it will only kill all living organisms that might be in the blood.

After soaking the object for one hour in the solution, rinse the object thoroughly in hot running water, then dry it. Wear sterile gloves when wiping the cups or other objects with alcohol and placing them in the bleach solution. When removing an object from the bleach solution and rinsing it in hot water, consider wearing gloves again, since the bleach is deleterious to your skin.

If cleaning up spilled blood, such as on a table surface, place some of the bleach solution on the contaminated area after wiping up as much of the bloody debris as possible. Leave the solution on the surface for up to one hour, then wipe and rinse it off. If you want to achieve the same effect in less time, use a stronger bleach solution, e.g., the undiluted commercial bleach, for 20 to 30 minutes.

METHODS OF BLOODLETTING

There are two primary methods of bloodletting described in this book:. The first, *sairaku shiraku,* involves piercing and draining out quantities of blood from very small superficial visible blood vessels called spider nevi or vascular spiders. The second, *hifu shiraku,* has two types: *ranshi hō,* or bloodletting from relatively replete cutaneous regions (used more for conditions of repletion, with palpable skin texture changes) and *mattan shiraku, or* bloodletting from the extremities such as the ears, nose, crown of the skull, and fingers and toes (*jing* points).

There are specific findings and symptom patterns associated with each of these techniques, with further specificity according to the area or digit worked on. Additionally there are general guidelines regarding the amount of blood to be drawn with each technique, as well as techniques that should or should not be used.

In their books, Kudō and Maruyama also described venesection, or the opening and draining of blood from veins. We do not recommend venesection, and do not describe it here.)

SAIRAKU SHIRAKU—BLOODLETTING VASCULAR SPIDERS

Maruyama and Kudō said the following about distinguishing between normal (non-pathological or physiological) vascular spider formations and abnormal (pathological) vascular spider formations.

> *From our observations over many years, we can say that vascular spiders do not only form in the presence of some pathological condition, they can be seen in healthy individuals too. It is true that they appear during pregnancy, liver cirrhosis, stomach ulcer, duodenal ulcer, pituitary tumor, syphilis, hypertension, bronchial asthma, cardiac diseases, all forms of tumor or cancer, etc., but they are also found, with careful inspection, in virtually all chronic diseases and even appear in acute disorders, and on occasion can be found in people with no specific disorder. In fact, they have been found in about 30% of all school children inspected. They frequently appear on the backs of infants who have particularly pale skin, especially in the lumbar region, even when healthy.*
>
> *We can also add that the appearance of vascular spiders seems to depend in part on seasonal influences. In general, during the winter, especially January and February, and during the summer, especially July and August, or during periods of extreme heat, they do not frequently appear. But they do appear with highest frequency during the weeks before and after the equinoxes in March-April and September-October.*

Vascular spiders appear as "wiggler like" angiomas. They can be very small, thinner than downy hair, or they can be thicker, with a width as much as 1mm. In general, those that are thought of as more non-pathological are thinner, while those that are pathological are thicker. They can appear in a variety of lengths and spirally shaped with branches like a spider's web (hence the name "vascular spiders") or they can appear as straight lines. They can appear in bunches in a local area or singly. Those that appear in healthy bodies are always bright light red, while those that are thought pathological can have a variety of colors, from light red to dark purple. In many cases, congestion can also be recognized in the surrounding skin.

It is possible to distinguish between the physiological and pathological vascular spiders according to the criteria provided above. But to distinguish them more accurately, examine the color of the blood once it has been drawn from the spider. When physiological, the amount of blood that flows is small, limited to only a couple of drops, and its color is bright red with luster. When pathological, the blood flows much more easily so that larger quantities flow out and you can see distinctive changes in the quality of the blood, e.g., it is darker or more viscous.

AREAS OF VASCULAR SPIDER FORMATION

On the face. They usually form in the zygomatic arch area, the cheek area, at the tip of the nose, and the wings of the nose.

In the occipital region. They usually form behind the auricle, on the auricle, and on the region at the back of the neck.

On the back of the body. They usually form at the back of the shoulders (especially between C6 and T4 and between the scapulae); around the acromion process; in the lumbar-sacral region (L4 to sacrum); and in the hip region.

On the front of the body. They normally form in the pectoralis major region and in the subcostal-lower costal region.

On the lower extremities. They usually form in the femur region, popliteal fossa region, sides of the lower legs, and foot joint region.

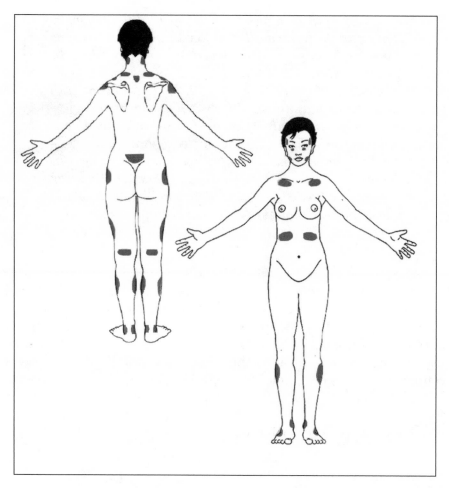

Areas of vascular spider formation.

FINDING VASCULAR SPIDERS

Natural bright light is the best light for looking for vascular spiders. Fluorescent light is usually the worst. Usually you can see the vascular spiders with simple visual inspection. In these cases, you should focus on and bloodlet only the slightly thicker and darker vascular spiders. But many times these spiders are not easy to find. Usually you can locate them by carefully stretching the skin. Thus it is always a good idea to stretch the skin for a more thorough inspection.

METHODS AND DOSAGE FOR BLOODLETTING VASCULAR SPIDERS

There are two methods for bloodletting vascular spiders. The first is to pierce the vascular spider and squeeze out the appropriate amount of blood. The second is to pierce the spider and then apply cupping techniques to enable the blood to flow more easily and profusely.

To determine the appropriate dosage of bloodletting for each patient, you must have a good idea of the patient's overall condition. You must determine whether the patient is relatively normal or average (i.e., not too replete and not too vacuous), relatively vacuous, or relatively replete. Often this judgment is based on the patient's overall appearance as well as diagnostic palpation. Is the patient thin, weak-looking, normal-looking or large-framed and well muscled? Are the radial pulses relatively weak, relatively normal or relatively strong and bounding? Does the area to be worked on look normal when touched and examined? Does it look weak, with soft loose skin and muscles? Does it look replete, with firm skin and muscles? Is the skin soft to the touch, relatively normal and healthy to the touch, or firm and full to the touch? Are the muscles thin and weak, normal or full, or hard to the touch?

Based on the overall assessment of the patient and the assessment of the local area to be worked on, you can select one of three general categories for each patient: vacuous, normal, or replete. For each kind of patient, different bloodletting techniques have different doses of stimulation. However, if you are not completely sure whether or not a patient is relatively normal or somewhat replete, it is preferable to err on the side of the "less is better" principle. There will always be a milder reaction to a treatment if you use milder bloodletting. When in doubt, play it safe and use the lower dosage.

For bloodletting vascular spiders, the approximate range of dosage for these three categories is as follows:

•For a relatively normal patient, select up to 5 to 7 vascular spiders for treatment. Pierce and then cup them.

•For the relatively vacuous patient, select only 2 to 3 vascular spiders for treatment. After piercing them, use only the squeezing techniques to remove blood.

•For the relatively normal and especially for the relatively vacuous patient, after bloodletting the vascular spiders, it is a good idea to use the *chinetsukyū* technique afterwards (see below for details).

•For the relatively replete patient, select up to 7 to 10 vascular spiders for treatment. Pierce them and cup them. Unless too much blood has been removed, there is no need to use the *chinetsukyū* technique after bloodletting the more replete patient.

BLOODLETTING TOOLS

There are a variety of bloodletting lancets available. We recommend the diabetic "medi-lancet" that is available in pharmacies, as it is disposable and easily handled, and can be used with a device that applies the technique for painless insertions (suitable only for *jing* points; see below). The lancet appears as in the following photo:

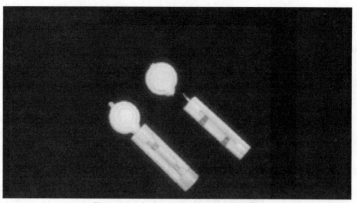

Lancets for painless insertion.

RECOMMENDED TECHNIQUES FOR BLOODLETTING VASCULAR SPIDERS

We recommend the following procedures and techniques for blood-letting vascular spiders:

1. Make sure that the light in the room is adequate.

2. Prepare paper towels or tissues, cotton swabs, alcohol, and a tray or other surface in advance; this is important because on occasion, a vascular spider may yield a couple of cubic centimeters of blood which will need to be swabbed up immediately as you remove the cup. Otherwise you might spill the blood on the patient, their clothing, or the table surface.

3. Holding the lancet in one hand between the forefinger and thumb, stretch the skin around and over the vascular spider with the other, in order to better expose the vascular spider.

4. Choose the vascular spider you wish to bloodlet.

5. Place the point of the lancet at the skin directly over the widest part of the chosen vascular spider, making sure that the beveled edge of the blade of the lancet is roughly perpendicular to the direction of the vascular spider.

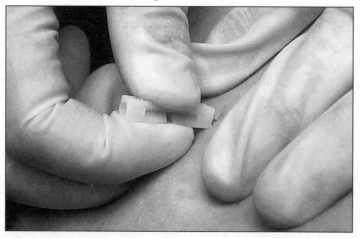

Place the lancet point directly over the widest part of the vascular spider.

6. Using a rapid in-and-out technique, pierce the skin and vascular spider.

If done properly, a drop of blood will well up around the cut.

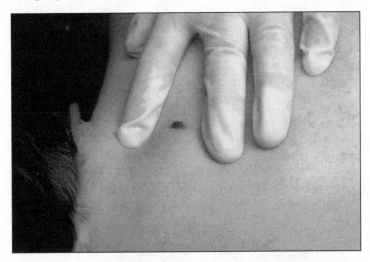

Once the lancet pierces the skin and spider, a drop of blood will well up.

If the cut is too shallow, very little bleeding will occur. If it is too deep, it can bleed quite well, but afterwards subcutaneous hemmorhaging will be apparent, since the blood leaves the vessel both in upward and downward directions. It is therefore very important to precisely control the depth of insertion of the point of the lancet. Ideally, the lancet will pierce the spider nevi but will not penetrate through it. How you hold the lancet should be your main focus. You should hold the lancet in such a fashion that the needle point only protrudes a little beyond the end of the fingers grasping it.

It is also important that the cut be made quickly. The blade of the lancet is relatively thick and if it is inserted too slowly, or retained for too long, it can be quite painful. This is completely unnecessary and avoidable. If no blood flows, the problem is either that the cut was not good enough, or that the vascular spider was deeper than calculated. Usually treatment should focus on the very superficial spider nevi. This is the reason we use the skin stretching techniques to expose them. If you feel that the blood did not flow because the lancet was applied too superficially or for other reasons to do with poor technique, try lancing the vascular spider again.

7. Once the cut is made, apply either the suction cup or the manual squeezing method.

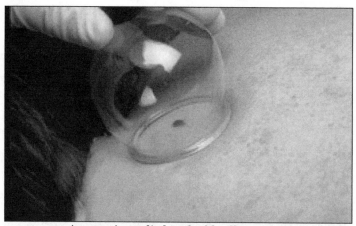

A pump is applied to the bloodlet spider.

With cupping, two to four strokes of the pump will be sufficient.

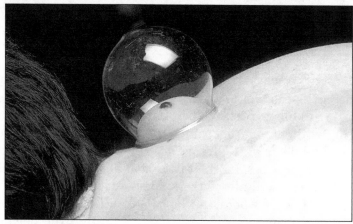

Effect of two to four strokes of the pump.

For a more replete patient, four is probably better. For a more vacuous patient, two to three strokes of the pump is better. What is important is that the cupping no cause pain.

8. Remove the cup after blood has finished flowing and has gathered around the base of the cup.

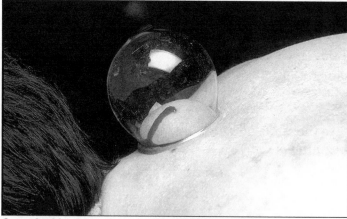

Once the blood has flowed around the base of the cup, remove it.

If the the blood that flows seems dark, and the vascular spider seems to want to keep bleeding, and if the patient is not in the category of vacuity, wipe up the blood with dry towels, tissues, or swabs, then with alcohol-moistened swabs, then reapply the cup.

If you feel that one application of the cup is sufficient, either because the blood turned lighter with the application, or because sufficient quantities flowed, then soak up the blood with dry towels, tissues, or swabs.

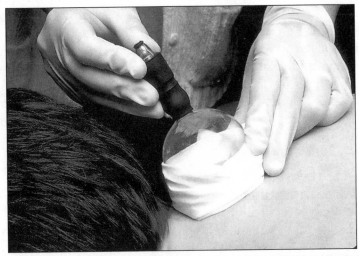

Use towels, tissues, or swabs to contain the blood flow.

When removing the cup, apply a paper towel as shown in the picture. Release pressure from the cup, tilt the cup back, and lift it off. At the same time, soak up the released blood with the paper towels.

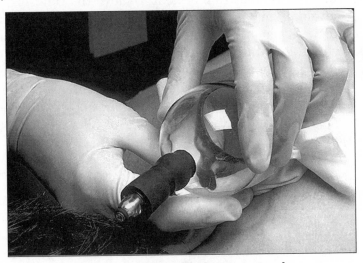

Soak up the blood with dry paper towels.

Wipe the skin surface well with alcohol-moistened swabs and then dry it off with a clean towel, tissue, or swab.

If you have used the squeezing method, squeeze in order to draw a few drops of blood, and clean the area as above.

On occasion, the vascular spider will "spout" like a geyser. Often when this happens, the blood is darker-colored and it is a sign that the right spot was lanced. If the blood does spout, so that it strikes the inside of the cup, be more careful about dosages of stimulation because the blood is flowing out at a greater rate.

9. Depending on the patient, repeat the technique on other vascular spiders. If you are a beginner, it is probably better to apply this technique to only one vascular spider at a time. Sometimes cups have poor valves and lose their suction. In such cases the cups may loosen and fall off, spilling their bloody contents. It is better to avoid this! Using the technique on only one spider at a time ensures that this does not happen. Also, cleaning up blood from more than one cup requires that you move quite quickly to avoid spillages. Beginners might be too hesitant to deal with this optimally.

If using the cupping technique in combination with the bloodletting, and with automated cupping devices, the cup pressure should not exceed 45cm of mercury; usually 30 to 45cm of mercury is better. The more vacuous the patient, the lower the pressure, and vice versa for a more replete patient. If the cup pressure causes pain for the patient, it is too much.

The *chinetsukyū* or cone moxa method can be used at the site of bloodletting after the procedure is finished. Place the cone over the point of insertion of the lancet blade, light the cone, and when the patient feels a light sensation of heat, remove the cone. This technique is not necessary if the patient is relatively replete. In relatively normal or vacuous patients, it is a useful technique, and often necessary. If the point of the lancet blade insertion will not stop bleeding, it is usually a sign of some vacuity condition and/or blood stasis. In such cases, burning a moxa cone repeatedly at the site of insertion usually stops the oozing of blood. If this still does not stop the oozing, place a small adhesive bandage or plaster over the point of insertion.

INDICATIONS FOR BLOODLETTING VASCULAR SPIDERS (SAIRAKU SHIRAKU) ACCORDING TO THE REGION

Back of the shoulders

The area between C6 and T4 and between the scapulae has the highest incidence of vascular spider formations on the trunk of the body. This is an important area because it relates to the movement of the upper limbs and tends to develop circulatory problems easily.

Clinically, this region has the highest value, being effective for all problems on the upper half of the body. Together with the next region, the lumbosacral region, which is the equivalent lower half body area, these are the two major areas on the trunk of the body for locating vascular spiders.

Look for vascular spiders on the back of the shoulders when treating patients who present with the following symptoms:

•Patients whose main complaints are accompanied by stiff shoulders and heaviness of the head, or high blood pressure, menopause, chronic gastritis, or beriberi.

•Patients whose main complaints are headache or dizziness (including Meniere's disease).

•Patients whose main complaints are accompanied by palpitations, such as cardiac asthma or Basedow's disease. However, bloodletting is contraindicated in cases of myocardial infarction.

•Patients whose main complaints are accompanied by difficulty breathing, expectoration, and problems such as bronchial asthma and chronic bronchitis.

•Patients whose main complaints are problems of the eyes, ears, nose, face, neck, and throat.

Lumbosacral region

This region extends from L4 to the sacrum and is effective for problems of the lower half of the body, especially a wide variety of chronic problems. In some cases, with repeated bloodletting, we can obtain unexpected improvements. In this region, when we cannot find vascular spiders, we look for *small* superficial venules. They seem to function the same as the vascular spiders. Consider treatment here for patients whose complaints or conditions are of the types listed below:

•Patients with an accompanying complaint of pain in the lumbar region, for example, lumbar pain, sciatica, and other neuralgias of the lower limbs.

•Patients with inflammation of joints in the lower extremities (arthritis), such as articular rheumatism of the knee, rheumatoid arthritis, simple arthritis of the knee, arthritis of the ankles and toes; also inflammation of the coccyx.

•Patients with gynecological problems, dysmenorrhea, amenorrhea, endometritis, salpingitis, oophoritis, menopausal disorders, abnormal bleeding, and chronic leukorrhea.

•Patients with problems of the urogenital system, cystitis, urethritis, and pyelitis.

•Patients with prostatic hypertrophy or orchitis.

•Patients with colitis, proctitis, and hemorrhoid problems.

•Patients with essential hypertension.

•Patients with skin problems on the lower body.

•Female patients experiencing a feeling of cold in the lower half of the body.

The region of the acromion

This is an area extending from the acromion process to the superior ridge of the scapula. This region has the second highest number of vascular spiders in the upper back region. Cupping this region would be effective for patients presenting with the following conditions:

•Stiff shoulders, stiff painful shoulder ("50-year shoulder"), or neuralgia of the upper extremities.

•Paralysis of the upper extremities.

•Mastitis.

•Skin diseases (with especially good results for urticaria).

The face

Vascular spiders most often appear in the area from the zygomatic arch to the cheek. If the cup will not stick well in this region, use the squeezing techniques instead. Bloodletting in this region is effective for patients whose main complaints are as follows:

•Headaches, hypertension, eye problems (these last being especially effective if accompanied by headache).

•Trigeminal neuralgia, Bell's palsy, facial spasm.

•Eye disorders.

•Nasal disorders.

•Dental problems.

•Apoplexy.

The region around the head of the fibula

This region manifests the appearance of vascular spiders, especially in women. It is effective for patients whose main complaints are as follows:

•Gynecological problems, especially chronic leukorrhea.

• Bleeding disorders such as stomach or duodenal ulcers, hemorrhoids.

• Lumbar pain, sciatica.

Other areas of the body

Vascular spiders can appear on other areas of the body, each having its own clinical significance; bloodletting can be applied on them as the need arises. In these cases, taking into account concepts such as the neural dermatomes, the channels, and acupoints can make the application of bloodletting in these regions broader and more effective.

We mentioned above treating pregnant women with varicose veins. In such cases, look for several small dark vascular spiders on the legs, in the region of the varicosities, and bloodlet those, using only the squeezing technique and removing only a few drops of blood from each. Finish with the precautionary moxa techniques described below. Taking a little blood at each visit, in conjunction with root or general treatment, should help the varicose veins.

RANSHI HŌ, BLOODLETTING FROM CUTANEOUS REGIONS

This method is different from bloodletting vascular spiders. With *ranshi hō*, instead of piercing small visible blood vessels to remove blood, we apply small cuts to areas of skin. Once the skin area has been selected and the small cuts applied, either the squeezing or the cupping techniques can be used to aid in blood flow.

This method has been in use both in the East and West since ancient times. Leeches were a common method of drawing blood, but today are not entirely practical, although they have seen a minor resurgence in hospitals for the use of returning blood flow to reattached fingers and other body parts. Today we can use the small bloodletting lancets sold in pharmacies (see p. 222).

When bloodletting vascular spiders, the same needles are used, but the cuts are shallower (0.5-1.0mm deep) because if vascular spiders are chosen correctly, the cut should be very superficial. When bloodletting on cutaneous regions, it is important to make sure that a sufficiently deep cut is applied to get the blood flowing. Usually 1.5mm to 2mm deep is most effective.

JUDGING THE CORRECT DOSAGE OF BLOODLETTING BY RANSHI HŌ

Usually *ranshi hō* is used for more replete conditions, where no vascular spiders can be found, and when bloodletting seems to be indicated. The doses of stimulation described above for vascular spider bloodletting, and the restrictions applied at each level, do not apply here. Since this technique is used only in cases of local repletion, applying only the doses for more replete patients is appropriate. When working with this technique on a clearly replete area on a clearly replete patient, select up to seven areas to treat. Pierce and apply cupping to these areas. If the patient shows signs of some vacuity with local area repletion, use the same techniques but on fewer points. Lower the doses further and use the squeezing technique instead of the cupping techniques.

SELECTING THE AREA TO BE TREATED

Selection of the area to be treated should be based on the local stiffness of tissue as well as signs of congestion of blood, pressure pain, and pinching pain. You can also use the indications of local or neighboring acupoints to help decide selection.

PROCEDURE FOR RANSHI HŌ BLOODLETTING

1. Make sure that there is adequate lighting.

2. Prepare paper towels, tissues or swabs, etc. in advance.

3. Use the same methods of holding and applying the bloodletting lancet as described above for the vascular spiders except that the needle point should protrude slightly further.

4. Apply cuts quickly and relatively superficially in the area chosen to bloodlet. Usually five cuts are applied, often one in the center and four around the central cut.

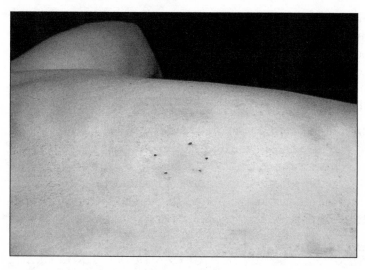

Usually five cuts are quickly applied.

5. Apply cupping or squeezing techniques.

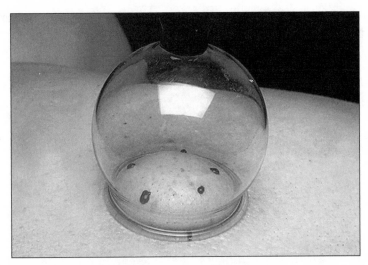

Apply cupping techniques.

It is important that the cuts be placed close enough to the central cut so that all five will fit into the space covered by the cup. Generally the *ranshi hō* method is used in conditions of relative local repletion where no vascular spiders are present. (The cupping method is more often used with vascular spiders.) However, if the patient is relatively vacuous, with some local repletion in an area and no clear vascular spiders present, this technique can be employed with the squeezing method so that less blood is removed. Because the area chosen in this method manifests a relative repletion condition, it is better to not use supplementing *chinetsukyū* or cone moxa at the site of insertion, unless you removed too much blood with *ranshi hō* and the patient is showing some kind of reaction such as fatigue or faintness.

Once the cuts are cupped, the released blood gathers at the base of the cup.

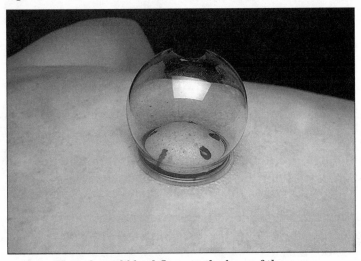

The released blood flows to the base of the cup.

Once the blood has stopped flowing, the cup can be removed using the procedure described above (p 225).

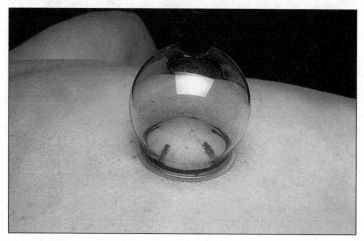

When sufficient blood has flowed, remove the cup.

The suction from the cupping leaves a mark on the skin that can take several days to dissipate.

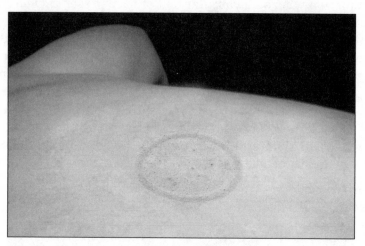

Suction from the cups leaves temporary markings on the skin.

LOCATIONS AND INDICATIONS FOR USING RANSHI HŌ

Note that this technique can be used on many more areas and for many more conditions than the representative ones listed below.

Stomach problems, gynecological problems (especially menopausal disorders), stiffness of the neck and shoulders, toothache, problems of the eyes and ears

Bloodlet the region on the top of the shoulders, the area above the supraclavicular fossa, and the anterior ridge of the trapezius muscle.

Headaches, hypertension, cerebral hemorrhage, problems of the ears and nose, stiffness of the neck

Bloodlet the occipital region at the posterior portions of the neck–at the border of the hair and in the area posterior to the tendon of the trapezius muscles.

This region is frequently reddened in appearance on patients who have an elevated blood pressure and who suffer from headaches, or who have had a cerebral hemorrhage.

When pinching this area, as well as the reddened appearance, the tissues will feel thick. They will be hard to pinch up and often the patient will feel pain from the pinching. Bloodletting in this area using *ranshi hō* is vital for patients with these conditions. This treatment also has great utility when used preventively.

Hypertension, cerebral hyperemia, cerebral hemorrhage, Meniere's disease, problems of the eyes, ears, and nose, Bell's palsy, trigeminal neuralgia

Bloodlet the region at the inferior border of the mastoid process.

Mastitis, insufficiency of milk, stiff and painful shoulder (50-year shoulder), rheumatism of the upper extremities, facial furuncle

Bloodlet the region at the inferior fossa of the scapular spine.

MATTAN SHIRAKU—BLOODLETTING FROM THE EXTREMITIES

Mattan shiraku is an important and frequently used bloodletting method, partly because it often deals directly with the channels, vis-a-vis the *jing* points, and partly because the blood circulation is easily impaired at the extremities. For example, frostbite most often affects the toes, fingers, and auricles.

METHODS AND DOSES OF MATTAN SHIRAKU

To assess the appropriate dose of bloodletting at the *jing* points for each patient, first determine if the patient's condition is relatively normal, vacuous, or replete, according to the descriptions above. For a relatively normal patient, you can bloodlet 4 to 5 points and remove up to 10 drops of blood from each. For a relatively vacuous patient, you should only bloodlet 1 to 2 points and remove 1 drop of blood from each. For a relatively replete patient, you can bloodlet from 7 to 10 points and remove up to 15 drops of blood from each. Vary the amounts within this range according to the overall assessment of the patient. A patient who shows some signs of vacuity can be bloodlet at 3 to 4 points, removing 5 or so drops of blood from each point.

It is important to try to regulate the amount of blood as indicated. This requires exerting very fine control over the actual insertion of the bloodletting lancet and the depth of the cut it makes. Overly deep cuts tend to bleed much more and the correct dosage can be easily surpassed. Thus, the technique of bloodletting needs to be quite exact, as should the squeezing method that is used to squeeze out each drop of blood.

The technique for bloodletting the extremities is a little different from the *sairaku shiraku* technique used on vascular spiders or in the more general *hifu shiraku*. Because you should try to control exactly the amount of blood removed from each point (i.e., number of drops), more precision is necessary. Furthermore, since the extremities tend to be very sensitive, especially at the nail corners or *jing* points, a delicate and deft technique must be used to prevent unnecessary pain and discomfort for the patient. For example, it is ill-advised to use this technique on a two-year-old child unless you can do it painlessly.

A simple method that can be used is to place the bloodletting lancet in the autolancet device available from pharmacies for individuals who need to check their blood sugar levels. This device delivers a very quick and relatively painless insertion which allows you to squeeze out a few drops of blood.

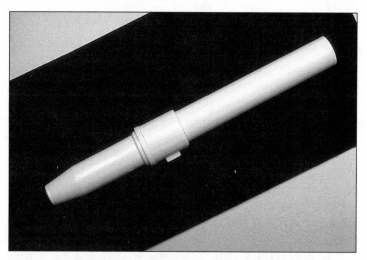

An autolancet device readily available from pharmacies.

The drawback with this device is that it will need to be thoroughly cleaned and sterilized before use on another patient, a process requiring employing the bleach-cleaning solutions and methods previously described. Another option is to keep an autolancet for each patient for whom this form of bloodletting is used, though this might cause cost and storage problems. We recommend mastering the manual technique of lancet application using the diabetic "medi-lancet" (p. 222). This method is simple and safe, and with skilled use can be painlessly applied with great regularity.

After selecting the point to be treated, e.g., a *jing* point, rub the point with firm pressure before wiping it with alcohol, holding the finger firmly with your thumb, index, and middle finger.

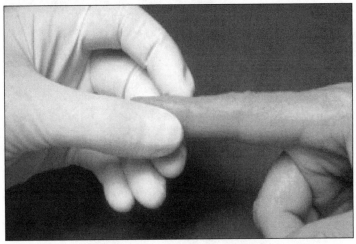

Hold the finger securely as shown.

Place the tip of the lancet at the point, holding the lancet at about 45° to the skin. Be certain that the point of the lancet does not protrude beyond the tip of the finger and thumb holding it.

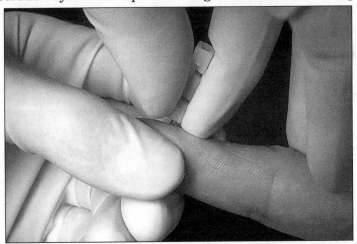

Position the point of the lancet as shown.

Then, in a single swift motion, rotate the lancet up to and past the 90° angle, to a roughly 45° angle on the other side of the point, removing the lancet from the point as it rotates onto the other side of the point. As the lancet is taken through this rotation, it should very briefly pierce and leave the point.

This motion requires some practice, and, if done well, is completely painless. The advantages of this technique are that there is almost no downward motion of the lancet into the point, which allows for a shallow penetration of the point. The motion is very quick; the lancet penetrates the point for only a fraction of a second. If applied correctly, the penetration is both painless and shallow, allowing for a greater degree of control over the amount of blood removed from the point. A drop of blood usually wells up at the point.

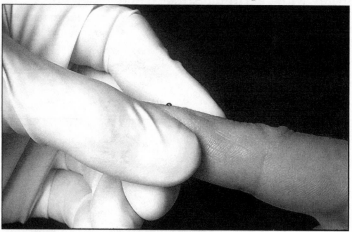

A drop of blood will appear once the point is pricked.

The squeezing techniques employed are important, especially for the bloodletting of *jing* points. Sometimes, even though the point has been pricked by the tip of the lancet, no blood may flow out of the point until you begin to squeeze. The number of drops that come out of the point depends on the number of times you squeeze the point. When bloodletting the *jing* points, it is important to squeeze with your middle finger, index finger, and thumb of the left hand. Your middle finger should be held across the last joint of the digit being treated, which is held by the index finger and thumb as follows:

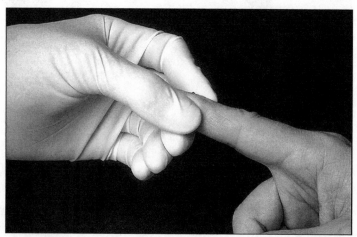

Position your thumb and fingers around the pricked point as shown.

The thumb and index finger of the right hand are held on the digit, proximal to the cut.

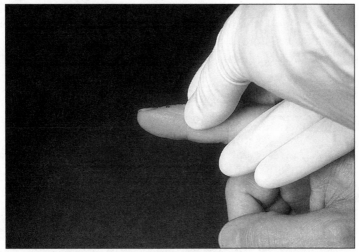

The thumb and index finger are held on the digit.

Squeezing is best achieved by a simultaneous pushing of the three digits of the left hand and two of the right hand. Care should be taken not to squeeze the nail itself because it can cause unnecessary pain and discomfort for the patient. With each squeeze, a drop of blood should well up which should then be wiped off with a cotton swab.

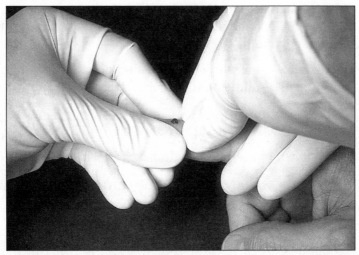

With each squeeze, a drop of blood wells up and can be swabbed off.

For the one or two drops of blood removed from the point of a patient with a vacuity condition, use a dry cotton swab. If removing as much as ten to fifteen drops from the point, the blood will flow more easily if it is wiped off with an alcohol-moistened swab. If you are unable to get the blood flowing, try pulling the five digits away from each other. This should have the effect of opening the cut. If, at the same time, you apply a little downward pressure, the blood should flow quite easily. With practice, this technique is simple, safe, and effective and it allows for relatively precise control over the amount of blood removed from each point. If, however, the initial cut is too deep, the blood may flow excessively. To ensure that this does not occur, hold a dry cotton swab with pressure over the point until it stops bleeding.

LOCATIONS AND INDICATIONS FOR MATTAN SHIRAKU

Insomnia, cerebral hyperemia, hypertension, neurosis, rachiodynia (spinal irritation)

Bloodlet the region on the crown of the skull.

This is the area around the meeting point of the line of the *du mai* or governing vessel and a vertical line joining the tops of the auricles, around the acupoint GV-20. In cases of insomnia or cerebral hyperemia, the skin will be loose here.

Apoplexy, speech disorders, shock

Bloodlet the sublingual area.

Cerebral hemorrhage, hypertension, cerebral hyperemia, tinnitus, frostbite of the auricle

Bloodlet the auricles. Look for an area that is distinctively red or dark purple. Sometimes vascular spiders are found at the edge or back of the auricles. These can be treated in the same fashion, though they tend to bleed very easily.

These vascular spiders have the same indications as above, and are indicated additionally for headaches.

Problems of the nose, hypertension, cerebral hemorrhage, rosacea (drunken nose).

Bloodlet the tip of the nose, including the wings of the nose.

Apoplexy, *jing* point symptoms, cardiopulmonary disorders, hormonal problems

Bloodlet the corners of the fingernails.

The areas at the corners of the fingernails are the most frequently used areas on the extremities. Bloodlet by applying a single cut and then squeezing the patient's finger with your fingers. There are cases such as apoplexy where bloodletting can be applied to all the fingers as a form of first-aid. There are also cases where bloodletting is applied to specific fingers. In such cases, select the points to be treated according to the finding of red swollen nail corners, pressure pain at the nail corners, symptoms associated with each nail corner *jing* point, and symptoms associated with the channels that start or stop on that finger or at that nail corner. You can also use the Akabane testing procedure to select the point to be blood-let.[9]

If we think of the physiological mechanisms that might be associated with bloodletting the nail corners of the fingers, we can speculate the following. The fingers are controlled centrally by the motor regions of the cerebral cortex, which occupy relatively large regions of the motor cortex. It is easy to see how a sizable effect on the reflexes of the nerves can be obtained by effecting a small change in the flow of blood at the ends of the fingers.

Regarding the effects on the cardiovascular system of bloodletting at these points, we can further speculate as follows. In certain cardiopulmonary disorders, such as congenital heart disease, mitral valve disease, and bronchiectasis, we find "drum stick" fingers, or discoloration of the nails, as seen in conditions of cyanosis. Additionally, pain can radiate to the little finger in angina pectoris. From these facts, we can guess that improving the circulation of the fingers by applying bloodletting there can have direct effects on the activities of the heart. Further, when thinking of the acromegaly seen in abnormal hormonal secretion of the pituitary gland, we can think about the effects on the hormonal system of bloodletting the distal parts.

Bloodletting from the fingertips is very important for the treatment of acute and urgent disorders, especially a fit of apoplexy. In such cases, bloodletting is applied on all the fingertips of both hands. If much blood gushes out and normal color and vitality are seen to return to the face, this is a good prognostic indication.

INDICATIONS FOR THE NAIL CORNERS OF THE FINGERS

Thumb (mainly the radial corner, LU-11): Good for tonsillitis, pharyngeal catarrh, mumps, bronchial asthma, and teething fevers of infants. (Can be applied at both corners.)

Index finger (mainly the radial corner, LI-1): Good for lymphadenitis of the neck region, bronchial asthma, and toothache of the lower jaw.

Index finger (radial corner, PC-9): Good for palpitations, neurosis, paralysis of the median nerve, and diseases with high fever.

Index finger (ulnar corner) (some say related to the diaphragm): Good for difficulty swallowing, hiccups, and stiff shoulder.

---

[9]K. Akabane, *Chinetsukando Niyoru Shinkyū Chiryōhō (Acupuncture and Moxibustion Therapy by the Heat Sensitivity Method)*.

Fourth finger (mainly the ulnar corner, TB-1): Good for headache, congestion of the brain, dizziness, congestion of the eye, and pharyngeal pain.

Little finger (radial corner, HT-9). Good for unconsciousness, shock, various heart disorders, dyspnea, and neurosis.

Little finger (ulnar corner, SI-1). Good for unconsciousness, shock, various heart disorders, dyspnea, rheumatism, pharyngeal pain, convulsive disorders.

INDICATIONS FOR THE NAIL CORNERS OF THE TOES

These are interesting areas for the application of bloodletting techniques. Though they are not as frequently used as the fingernail corners, they do have wide application and distinctive effects for the indicated symptoms. Their indications are as follows:

Big toe (medial corner, SP-1): Indigestion, acute gastroenteritis, and infantile seizures.

Big toe (lateral corner, LR-1): Good for eye problems (especially those accompanied by severe pain), convulsive disorders, frequent urination, and genital organ disorders.

Second toe (mainly the lateral corner, ST-45) Good for toothache of the upper jaw, beriberi, beriberi-like symptoms, and gastroenteritic disorders.

Third toe (mainly the lateral corner): (Usually related to the stomach channel because a branch of the stomach channel runs here.) Good for pain in the heel bone, eye problems, lumbago, and sciatica.

Fourth toe (usually the lateral corner, GB-44): (Sometimes the medial corner is very effective.) Good for headache, eye pain, ear pain, flank pain, and dizziness.

Fifth toe (lateral corner, BL-67): Good for hemorrhoids, nasal obstruction, lumbago, headache, and intercostal neuralgia.

Don't forget that selection of points should be based on the finding of appropriate signs at the *jing* point, such as redness, swelling, and pressure pain, as well as associated symptoms.

In cases of contusions and sprains, applying bloodletting to several points in the local area can be extremely helpful to reduce the swelling, inflammation, and pain. The blood usually flows quite easily in such cases. If you find vascular spiders, these should be some of the points used. If one or more channels are clearly involved, based on the location of the problem and the trajectories of the channels, bloodletting the associated *jing* points is usually helpful, especially when the problem is more distal, as in the case of a sprained ankle.

RECOGNIZING ILL EFFECTS FROM BLOODLETTING OVERDOSE

If too much blood is taken from a patient, the patient can become dizzy and may faint. This usually happens as soon as the procedure is finished. It is relatively easy to remedy, though the best cure is prevention. Always try to judge what is the appropriate dosage of bloodletting for each patient before starting the procedure. Sometimes excessive bloodletting can cause patients to feel very heavy the next day, so heavy that they feel as though they cannot move. It can also occasionally aggravate the patient's symptoms.

Besides trying to limit the amount of bloodletting according to the assessment of overall condition, you can monitor the patient's radial pulses and the changes of blood flow and color. If the pulse starts to become fast, floating, and weak or empty, it is definitely time to stop the bloodletting procedure and use some of the moxa techniques suggested below to remedy the problem.

For patients who are very weak, and for whom you would want to use much lower levels of bloodletting, if the blood is very dark and viscous to begin with, do not wait for the blood to become lighter and less viscous. Apply the general rules described above about the limits of bloodletting according to the patient and the technique used. Use the bloodletting procedures repeatedly over a number of treatments to get the appropriate effects. This is much better than to do too much at once and make the patient sick.

If the patient is in the normal to replete range, you can usually keep the blood flowing until it becomes lighter and less viscous. So long as you monitor the radial pulses in order to ensure that too much blood has not been removed, judging the correct time to stop the procedure by the changes of blood flow is usually a safe monitor.

To help prevent any reactions to treatment, use *chinetsukyū* at the site of bloodletting of skin areas or vascular spiders. If the patient seems in the weak to very weak range, it is a good idea to use one *chinetsu* moxa cone on each site where the cut was made. It is generally thought that the bloodletting can cause a temporary weakness at the site. Using the light heat sensations of the *chinetsukyū* technique can supplement the point sufficiently to prevent any possible reactions. In this sense, the *chinetsukyū* technique is used preventively. If the point where the bloodletting technique was applied will not stop bleeding, as sometimes happens in patients with qi vacuity or blood stasis, apply the *chinetsukyū* technique directly at the site of bloodletting to stop the blood flow. If you are proficient in the use of moxa, remedying the rare reaction to treatment is usually easy and effective. However, if it is not enough, hold a dry sterile cotton ball with pressure to the point until it stops bleeding.

If the patient begins to show reactions to the treatment, or if you observe pulse changes in response to the procedure (i.e., fast, floating, and weak), you should undertake one or more of the following methods.

•Use *chinetsukyū* cone moxa repeatedly at GV-14 *(dazhui)* with a small amount of heat felt each time until the pulse qualities reverse and/or the patient feels better.

•Use *chinetsukyū* cone moxa or salt moxa repeatedly on CV-8 (the navel).

•Use thread-size direct moxa repeatedly at GV-20 or ST-36 .

With the moxa procedures described above, the pulses will become slower, deeper, and stronger. You should continue with moxa treatment until this happens.

It is usually a good idea to inform your patients that a mild sensation of fatigue after bloodletting is a normal experience. Suggest that they take things easy for a time after the treatment. If they seem particularly fatigued following treatment, use one or more of the above moxa correction techniques, and have them rest at your clinic for thirty to sixty minutes before leaving.

After bloodletting, either by the squeezing or cupping method, if some mark or bruise remains, it will usually disappear within three days. It is a good idea to inform your patients of this possibility, and again discuss any concern they might have about such a mark. If the patient's blood stasis condition is severe, the mark may take up to a week (or longer) to disappear.

Following the above recommendations will contribute to a safe and effective practice. When correctly and appropriately applied, bloodletting procedures can be markedly effective in addressing stubborn chronic problems, and can also provide quick resolution to many acute problems.

Chapter 11
Manaka's Wooden Hammer & Needle

Manaka's wooden hammer and needle technique[1] can be used almost anytime and anywhere to improve the patient's health. There are no contraindications or restrictions on its use and the technique has proven helpful when used on a daily basis. It is particularly effective for relieving the stresses and tensions that would otherwise accrue daily in the body and predispose patients to health problems. It has also proven useful in the treatment of different health complaints including headache, toothache, gastrointestinal discomfort, constipation, stiff shoulders with restricted mobility, lumbar pain, knee pain, and nasal problems.

Earlier in the text, we mentioned a little of the history of needle therapy in Japan, including the Mubunryū style used in the imperial court in the late 1500s. This form of traditional therapy, where gold needles were held at reactive points on the abdomen and lightly struck with a wooden hammer at a rhythmic rate, is a uniquely Japanese form of therapy. Isai Misono, who originated the Mubunryū approach, used thick gold needles with a hammer made of ebony.

This hammer and needle set was reproduced by Baba Hakkō of Kyushu prefecture. The gold needle was 1.5mm thick and 27mm

---

[1]The information in this chapter is compiled from the works of Yoshio Manaka and Kazuko Itaya. It comes from two papers they wrote: one was published a number of years ago in a popular Japanese health journal and made available through the Shinkyū Topology Association in Kyoto; the other was written, but not published, with the assistance of Hiromasa Okusada. We are indebted to Mr. Okusada for his assistance in the translation of these papers. There is a brief discussion of the use of the wooden hammer and needle treatment method in *Chasing the Dragon's Tail* (c.f. pp. 193, 243–3, 253–258). This form of therapy was used often by Manaka, but not at all by more traditionally oriented therapists such as Fukushima or Shūdo. We think that this treatment method is very useful as a supportive therapy because it is so safe and easy to use. The practitioner may choose to utilize these treatments at the time of the clinic visit, or to teach patients to use the hammer and needle as a simple form of supportive home therapy.

long, weighing 2g. The hammer, made of ebony, was 95mm long with a 20mm diameter head, weighing 12.8g. The interior of the head of the hammer was weighted with a little gypsum; the part of the hammer used for striking the needle was padded with leather with gold leaf on the opposite surface.

More recently, Fujimoto Rempu of Nara Prefecture reproduced the hammer and needle for modern use, making the following modifications. He fabricated both silver and gold needles that were 80mm long and 3.5mm thick with a blunted point and a weight of about 8g. The hammer was constructed to a weight of 35g, a length of 150mm and a 30mm diameter head. The design of the thicker, heavier, blunted needle and the heavier hammer allowed for a firmer percussive action with no insertion of the needles.

Manaka's hammer is an extension of Fujimoto's design such that the layperson can use it. The needle is made of a relatively light wood and is 10mm thick and 120mm long, weighing 7.2g. It has both ends blunted but one is slightly more pointed. The hammer is 160mm long, with a head 35mm in diameter and a weight of 32g. It has a leather patch on the striking surface of the head. These modifications facilitate either firm tapping or very light tapping which may be required on sensitive patients or sensitive surfaces such as hard or bony surfaces where the thicker end of the wooden needle is held at the skin. When Manaka's hammer and needle is used correctly, the blow is quite resonant.

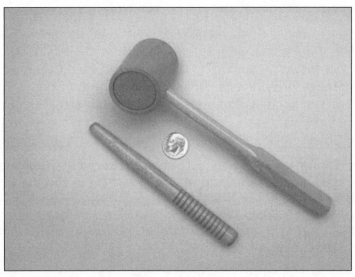

The Manaka wooden hammer and needle, relative in size to a U.S. dime (1.7cm).

Manaka thought that a wooden hammer with a blunt wooden needle would be a useful tool because many people are needle-phobic, and because many patients in the modern city are unable to make regular appointments. The wooden hammer and needle is not frightening, and it can be used by patients at home on a daily or regular basis. Besides these advantages, Manaka and his colleagues found that many people liked how the treatment felt. Even if used too much, the procedure never seemed to cause any fatigue or ill feeling. It is impossible to overstimulate with this procedure, unless, of course, you strike the needle too hard with the hammer and bruise the point.

HOME THERAPY

It is a common custom in Japan for practitioners to mark points on a patient and for the patient or a family member to moxa the point at home. Points can be marked for stimulation with the hammer and needle as well. This procedure can be an extremely useful tool for a stiff neck or shoulders, or fatigue in those areas. It can be performed anywhere at any time.

Manaka and Itaya reasoned that the effects of the wooden hammer and needle were similar to those of shallowly inserted needles. In some cases the effects are similar to those of more deeply inserted needles, especially when the patient gets distinctive sensations from the vibrations of the needle which are felt quite deeply. The simplicity and effectiveness of stimulating relevant acupoints using the wooden hammer and needle can be further enhanced by utilizing Manaka's metronome frequency relationships for each channel.[2]

Essentially, tapping the points at a rate corresponding to the channel on which the point lies tends to further enhance the tapping-stimulation effect. When using the metronome to reinforce the effects of treatment, the following are the frequencies in beats per minute:

METRONOME FREQUENCIES FOR WOODEN HAMMER AND NEEDLE			
YANG CHANNEL	RATE	YIN CHANNEL	RATE
Du Mai	104	*Ren Mai*	104
Gallbladder	120	Liver	108
Small Intestine	120	Heart	126
Triple Burner	152	Pericardium	176
Stomach	132	Spleen	132
Large Intestine	108	Lung	126
Bladder	112	Kidney	120

Usually quartz metronomes are easier to use and more precise in their timing. As can be seen, the rates of some channels are quite close to each other. Thus if using these rate correspondences, it is important to have good rhythm. To help develop good rhythm, we recommend that you practice on yourself until you can strike the

---

[2]These relationships and the manner of their discovery are described in Y. Manaka, K. Itaya, and S. Birch, *Chasing the Dragon's Tail*.

wooden needle at the correct frequency. In the text, where specific acupoints are mentioned, we include the metronome frequency in parentheses for quick and easy reference.

TAPPING TECHNIQUE

The wooden needle should be held loosely between either the thumb and forefinger or forefinger and middle finger. It should be held lightly to the point to be treated, using the other fingers, placed lightly on the skin, to secure the point of the needle.

With the hammer in the other hand, tap the more rounded and wider end of the needle lightly. The hammer has a soft leather pad on one surface; this is the surface that should be used for the tapping. Tapping should be done rhythmically and evenly, either in a randomly selected even-paced rhythm or at the corresponding rhythm for the channel. Correct tapping will allow the needle to vibrate slightly between the finger and thumb and transmit vibrations to the point treated. Each point should be tapped 10 to 30 times.

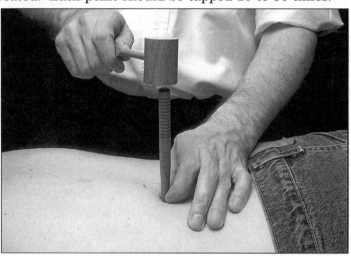

Proper grasping of the needle is important to stay on the point.

For elderly patients or others who might bruise easily, tap more lightly. Normal treatment should focus on acupoints or other points that are specified by palpation. For laypersons not familiar with the acupoints, treating the points found by pressure around the acupoints or in the same treatment area will often be sufficient.

Usually in a treatment, it is better to start with the acupoints on the feet and then slowly work up the body. If the desired effects are obtained from just a few of the selected points, without having treated all of them, it is good to stop treatment there. For example, menstrual difficulties such as dysmenorrhea often respond well to treatment of LR-3, LR-4, SP-10, SP-6, BL-32. If, after treating LR-3, LR-4, and SP-6, the pain symptoms are alleviated, there is no need to progress to SP-10, BL-32.

Holding the wooden needle incorrectly, by grasping closer to the tapped end, as shown below, may often create instability: the point of the needle is more likely to slip off the acupoint. Further, if the needle is grasped too tightly, the vibration at the acupoint is largely lost.

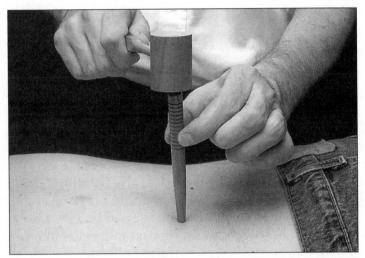

Incorrect technique: do not hold the needle this close to the tapping end.

When acupoints or points on the back of the body are to be treated, it is best to have another person administer the tapping. However, some patients might not have someone to help them at home. In such cases, treatment can be administered simply by holding the wooden needle firmly in one hand, placing it on the point to be treated, and rhythmically pressing it into the point then releasing it.

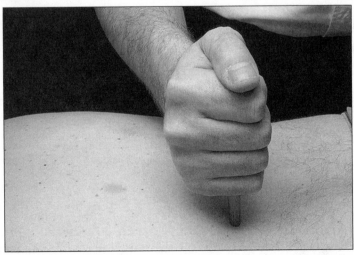

The one-handed technique, used when unassisted or on hard-to-reach points.

This vibration is a little different from the one when the needle is actually tapped, but good therapeutic effects can be had. When using this particular technique, the angle of application is often important. Use the angle that feels the most comfortable. Sometimes areas or points are hard to reach; in such cases, use the leather padded surface of the hammer to tap the point area. Do not tap too hard! The blow should be light and comfortable. It is best to instruct patients in each of these techniques and have them use what is easier and more comfortable.

TREATMENT OF SPECIFIC DISORDERS

Tapping with the hammer and needle rids the fatigue, tension, and stress that build and accrue daily. If you are able to relieve these things at the end of each day so that they do not build up, you will find it extremely helpful for the relief of symptoms, for the treatment of disease, and for general health maintenance. During the day, energy reserves are used up, stress is encountered, and the muscles tense up and remain tight into the next day. Day by day, these are very slight changes. But when these tensions occur asymmetrically, e.g., from repeated use of one hand in a particular movement at work, or occur repeatedly, they often accrue and can lead to pathological conditions.[3] Relief of these daily stresses by whatever method possible can be helpful as supportive therapy for the treatment plan for each patient. The wooden hammer and needle is specifically tailored for this purpose.

A simple general method that requires the help of a partner is as follows:

- •With the patient sitting, tap a point on either side at the base of the occiput, then 1 or 2 points on both shoulders.
- •With the patient lying supine, tap along two lines about 3cm apart on each side of the spine. Start at the upper back and work down the sides of the spine. Tap each point about 10 times, alternating sides as you move down each line on the back.
- •Have the patient turn onto their back and tap lightly from the inferior border of the sternum out along the costal arches.
- •Tap along the top of the pubic symphysis, then down the *ren mai* from the sternum to the pubis.
- •Tap down along the big muscles of the legs.
- •Tap each *jing* point on the fingers and toes about 10 times.

Altogether, this should take no more than 20 minutes. Since you are working on many body areas and not necessarily the channels, this tapping can be done without the aid of the metronome.

---

[3]See the discussion of Dr. Keizō Hashimoto's ideas about the origins of disease in our daily work and living habits in Y. Manaka, K. Itaya, and S. Birch, *Chasing the Dragon's Tail,* pp. 195-197.

The treatment of specific problems usually requires tapping at specific acupoints. This procedure can be reinforced by first applying the above general treatment and then tapping the specific acupoints. If you are following the treatment flow charts laid out in Chapter 2, you will have already performed a root or general treatment on the patient in the office before you use the wooden hammer and needle for symptom control therapy. In such cases, use the local treatments specified below.

If you recommend home therapy using the wooden hammer and needle, and a general stress-relieving treatment is indicated as well as treatment of the points specified for the symptoms, then demonstrate both forms of treatment for the patient, along with suggestions for frequency of application at home.

A few problems are listed below with suggestions for acupoints to treat.

Shoulder problems—pain, stiffness, limited motion

Usually it is important to release palpable shoulder stiffness and tension regardless of whether or not the patient is complaining of shoulder problems. The general treatment outlined above can be helpful; focussing treatment on the most reactive and tense points on the shoulders can also be very useful. To maximize the effects of this simple approach, try to determine which channel is involved and tap at the appropriate frequency.

Many acupoints are said to be good for shoulder problems. Manaka recommended palpating points on the large intestine, small intestine, and triple burner channels and then treating the most reactive points on each. He also recommended selecting from among the following general points: BL-10 (112), GB-21 (120), SI-14 (120), BL-43 (176/112), GV-12 (126), GV-5 (152), *jōsen* (104). He found these points to be very helpful. Check these points carefully and treat each if it is reactive.

If the shoulder is very stiff, inflamed, or has limited motion, it is better not tostimulate too much locally. Local points should be tapped more gently and it is better to look for distal points to treat. For instance, treat LI-10, LI-11, ST-38, and GB-34. If the patient shows signs of counterflow qi, such as a reddened appearance and excessive emotional responses, add BL-60 (112) and GV-14. GV-14 is the meeting point of the yang channels; thus it may be tapped at a number of different frequencies. Because counterflow qi conditions often involve the bladder, gallbladder, and stomach channels, it is advisable to tap GV-14 alternately at (132), (120), and (112) beats per minute, 10 to 20 strokes at each frequency.

Lumbar pain

There are many internal and musculoskeletal causes of lumbar pain. Whatever the cause, it is important to relieve tension in the musculature in the lumbar region. To achieve this end, you should use regular acupuncture and moxibustion therapy, exercise therapy, stretching therapy, and the wooden hammer and needle.

When using the wooden hammer and needle for lumbar pain, the first area to treat is along the musculature to the sides of the lumbar vertebrae, tapping at the tight, sore, reactive points. Very often BL-18 (108), BL-22 (152), BL-23 (120), BL-25 (108), and BL-52 (120) show reaction.

If the pain is acute, it is often liver-related. In this case tap at BL-18 (108) and GV-8 (104). To get maximal effects, it is better to combine the tapping procedure with *sōtai* exercise therapy.[4]

If the lumbar pain is chronic, it is often more kidney-related. In this case tap at BL-23 (120) and/or BL-52 (120). Useful distal points are GB-34 (120), BL-40 (112), BL-58 (112). Palpate and treat the reactive points. Unless combined with *sōtai* exercise, the best treatment of lumbar pain is to tap each point as many as 50 times.

Knee pain

Often, because of the complexity of the muscular and tendinous structures in the knee, it is difficult to clearly identify which are the most affected channels or muscles. Because of this a very general and simple approach is better.

Two simple treatment approaches are recommended. In the first, palpate around the acupoints ST-34 (132), SP-10 (132), SP-9 (132), and GB-34 (120) and select and treat the sorest points at their respective frequencies.

In the second, palpate around the swollen, sore, or reddened areas on the knee and stimulate reactive points. In this approach, we often use points in a circle around the patella. In such cases, do not use the metronome since many points are not channel points.

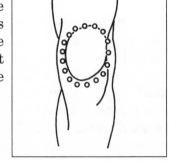

---

[4]This procedure is described in K. Matsumoto and S. Birch, *Hara Diagnosis: Reflections on the Sea,* pp. 381–384, and again as procedure C in Y. Manaka, K. Itaya, and S. Birch, *Chasing the Dragon's Tail,* pp. 200–201.

Joint pain

There are many forms and degrees of articular rheumatism. Relatively uncomplicated cases exhibit painful swollen joints and tight muscles around the joints. More complex cases, such as rheumatoid arthritis, exhibit painful, swollen, and deformed joints. Regular treatments with the wooden hammer and needle as home therapy can assist with symptomatic relief of much of the pain and swelling associated with this condition. Manaka and Itaya recommended a two-step approach when using the wooden hammer and needle.

First, stimulate a set of general points; then, work gently on each affected joint. The general treatment points are GB-21 (120), BL-18 (108), BL-20 (132), BL-23 (120), BL-52 (120), SP-10 (132), SP-6 (132), and KI-3 (120). Treat the reactive points. Then, for each affected joint, tap in circles around the joint. The tapping should be light and gentle. For small joints, tap at about a one-inch radius from the joint. For larger joints, tap at about a two-inch radius from the joint. If the tapping is too painful, widen the radius of the circle.

Headaches

For headaches caused by flushing up, that is, when the patient suffers from counterflow qi which usually gives a flushed appearance and often has a sensation of energy rising upwards, have the patient stand and tap at tender points around the Achilles tendons, especially at BL-60 (112). Then, with the patient sitting, tap at LI-4 (108).

Frontal headaches are often related to disorders of the eyes or nose. Thus it is a good idea to select from and stimulate BL-10 (112), GB-20 (120), GV-23 (104), GV-20 (104), LI-4 (108), LR-2 (108). For those points on the head, tap lightly and gently.

Migraines usually involve the liver and/or gallbladder channels. If there is tenderness along the gallbladder channels on the head, stimulate the back of the neck, for example, GB-20 (120) or BL-10 (112) and along the gallbladder channels on the leg. Tap from GB-31 (120) down the gallbladder channel, paying special attention to GB-34 (120), GB-38 (120), GB-40 (120) and GB-41 (120). You can also palpate and select from TB-3 (152), and TB-4 (152) because the gallbladder and triple burner channels are associated through their *shao yang* relationship. If there is tenderness on the liver channel, especially in the right subcostal region, then focus on the liver channel. You can select and treat from LR-3 (108), LR-4 (108), BL-18 (108), PC-6 (176). These methods will often reduce the migraine pain.

If a headache is present at the time of treatment, do not over-stimulate at the painful area. In general, for any headache, you can treat GV-20 (104), BL-10 (112) and GB-20 (120) very gently. You should also make sure to release any tension found in the neck and shoulder regions by tapping at reactive points.

Toothache

It is usually important to release neck and shoulder tension in order to diminish tooth pain. Treating pressure-sensitive points on the large intestine channel will often help with this. Check especially around LI-4 (108), LI-10 (108), and LI-11 (108), treating until the sensitivity at the points releases. LU-7 (126) is often helpful, also ST-37 (132). These points are usually effective for problems of the upper teeth. For problems of the lower teeth, focus instead on the stomach channel, especially ST-44 (132) and ST-39 (132).

Gastrointestinal disorders

ST-36 (132) can be treated for almost all gastrointestinal problems, and alone can often be effective in giving some relief. It can also be helpful to stimulate reactive points along the tibialis anterior muscle from ST-36 to ST-41. Also tap CV-12 (104/132). On the back, select from BL-17 (112), BL-18 (108), BL-20 (132), BL-21 (132). Palpate down along the edges of the spine at the *huato* level and treat where reactive.

In general, dietary problems and daily stresses also need to be addressed. The general treatment can be useful, especially for relieving neck and shoulder tension. For gastroptosis, treat ST-36 and add ST-41 (132). For chronic problems, especially with food allergies or sensitivities that can cause rashes, treat ST-36 and add BL-18 (108), BL-20 (132), BL-25 (108), SP-8 (132), SP-7 (132), and around both medial and lateral malleoli. For gastric or duodenal ulcers, treat along the gallbladder channels from GB-34 (120) down to the fourth toes, focussing especially on reactive points. For acute problems of stomachache or food poisoning, moxa on *uranaitei* is best.

Constipation

Increased fiber in the diet is often necessary as are general recommendations to improve the patient's dietary habits and exercise habits. As well as stimulating BL-25 (108) and ST-27 (108), it is useful to stimulate the abdomen in a clockwise fashion, moving from the lower right quadrant to the upper right quadrant to the upper left quadrant to the lower left quadrant and then back to the lower right quadrant. This can be done while sitting on the toilet. This should increase the motility of the intestines.

Hemorrhoids

Sitting with the legs pulled up, in order to cause retraction of the hemorrhoid, tap SP-7 (132), LU-6 (126), GV-2 (104) and GV-20 (104). GV-20 should be tapped lightly. For bleeding hemorrhoids, if the above procedure has not already helped and the anus seems to be spasming, use the fingers to stretch the anal muscles; this seems helpful in stopping the blood flow and retracting the hemorrhoids.

Liver disease

In East Asian medicine, the concept of liver disease is different from that in Western medicine. Western disease entities such as hepatitis are usually more advanced forms of the liver problems recognized in East Asian medicine. In both systems, problems of the liver usually present with tenderness and tightness over the liver in the right subcostal region, and on the back to the right of the spine, usually centering around right BL-18. Treatments that help soften up these regions are usually helpful for relieving the problem. Combining *sōtai* exercise and wooden hammer and needle tapping procedures referred to above[5] will be helpful for this purpose. For other general home therapy, stimulate the following points: right BL-17 (112), right BL-18 (108), right BL-20 (132), right LR-14 (108), CV-12 (104), SP-10 (132) and LR-3 (108).

Respiratory problems

For a patient in the early stages of catching a cold, with symptoms of headache, stiff neck and shoulders, weakened energy, and runny nose, try stimulating BL-12 (112), GB-20 (120), and GV-16 (104), and select from among the following points: BL-10 (112), BL-17 (112), LU-5 (126), and LI-4 (108).

This method can also be a helpful supportive therapy for bronchial asthma in both adults and children. For children up to age 10, treatment with the wooden hammer and needle can be helpful since they are generally more sensitive to therapy. Stimulate GV-12 (104) and GV-4 (104). Adding specialized *shōnishin* techniques for children to stimulate along all the channels is also helpful. In adults, selecting from and stimulating other points such as *ding chuan*, the *ding chuan* and sympathetic points in the auricle, and LU-7 (126) can be helpful.

For an acute asthma attack, select from and stimulate CV-22 (104), KI-25 (120), KI-26 (120), KI-27 (120), and the sympathetic and *ding chuan* points in the auricles. Using the regular wooden needle in the auricles is usually difficult. Use a toothpick instead, pressing rhythmically at the points.

---

[5]These are more fully described in Y. Manaka, K. Itaya, and S. Birch, *Chasing the Dragon's Tail,* and K. Matsumoto and S. Birch, *Hara Diagnosis: Reflections on the Sea*

Gynecological problems

For menstrual problems such as dysmenorrhea or irregular menstruation, make sure that LR-3 (108), LR-4 (108), SP-6 (108, 120, 132), Manaka's three-yin meeting point (2 finger widths above SP-10) (108, 120, 132) and BL-32 (112) are treated. In addition, treat sensitive points down the medial line of the thigh, in the inguinal region, and on the sacrum. BL-31 (112), BL-33 (112) and BL-34 (112) are also often stimulated if reactive. Usually it is important to begin treating these points 4 to 5 days before menses begins.

In cases where the problem has accompanying emotional symptoms such as irritability and emotional stress as seen in premenstrual syndrome, East Asian medicine tells us to focus on the liver channel. To do this, make sure to treat LR-3 (108), GB-39 (120) and GB-40 (120) as well as treating the points mentioned above. Treat according to the general treatment for overall relaxation.

Sexual dysfunction

For sexual dysfunction, such as impotence in men, select and treat from among the following list of points: LI-10 (108), BL-40 (112), BL-58 (112), KI-7 (120), LR-3 (108), LR-4 (108), GB-34 (120), SP-6 (108, 120, 132), SP-10 (132), CV-12 (104), ST-25 (132), CV-4 (104), GV-20 (104), GV-12 (104), BL-18 (108), BL-20 (132) BL-23 (120), BL-32 (112) and BL-33 (112), focussing especially on LR-3 (108) and the points on the sacrum and down the medial line of the thigh.

Lactation problems

Nursing mothers who are having difficulty breastfeeding their infants often respond well to a simple treatment. Use the wooden hammer and needle by palpating and stimulating from among the following points: CV-17 (104), GB-20 (120), and SI-11 (120).

Eye problems

For symptoms of bloodshot eyes or eye fatigue caused by overuse of the eyes, stimulate GB-34 (120), *tai yang* (120), ST-2 (132), and BL-2 (112) with gentle tapping. Stimulate a reactive point found just lateral to GB-20 (120); if the sensation from this point can be felt in the temples, this treatment will be effective. You can also stimulate BL-10 (112), TB-21 (152), SI-19 (120), and GB-2 (120), all of which are good points for eye problems.

Nasal problems

For conditions such as rhinitis, with symptoms of stuffy runny nose, nasal inflammation, and a feeling of heaviness around the nose and eyes, select from and stimulate GV-20 (104), GV-23 (104), GB-20 (120), BL-12 (112), ST-36 (132), LI-10 (108), and LI-4 (108).

Sinusitis

The condition of sinusitis is usually more difficult to treat than simple rhinitis. When pus is present in the paranasal sinus cavities of the face, many of the same symptoms of rhinitis can develop, but they are usually more severe, being both more chronic and stubborn in nature. Sinus headaches or a feeling of strong pressure in the forehead or in the paranasal region can develop, too. As supportive home therapy for this condition, the same treatment points as those for rhinitis are used. These points will need to be treated over a longer period of time.

Rehabilitation for hemiplegia following stroke

Rehabilitation of hemiplegia following a stroke can be difficult. Usually acupuncture, exercise, and massage can be helpful, especially if the treatment begins as soon as possible after the stroke. The wooden hammer and needle can also be helpful because it allows simple daily treatment, which is important in such cases. The dedication and determination of family members are vital in rehabilitation, for they can provide the regular therapy and caregiving that are required for recovery.

For the following points, palpate and treat bilaterally, regardless of the unilateral symptoms. Usually many points will be treated: LI-10 (108), LI-11 (108), TB-8 (108,120, 152), BL-40 (112), BL-58 (112), KI-7 (120), LR-3 (108), LR-4 (108), GB-31 (120, 112, 132), GB-34 (120), GB-38 (120), SP-6 (108, 120, 132), SP-10 (132), CV-12 (104), ST-25 (132), CV-4 (104), GV-20 (104), GV-12 (104), GB-7 (120), BL-18 (108), BL-20 (132), BL-23 (120), BL-32 (112), BL-33 (112).

When using the wooden hammer and needle, it is also a good idea to tap all the *jing* points on the fingers and toes, both on the affected side and the healthy side. When doing this, use the relevant frequency of tapping for each channel. If the patient has difficulty talking, stimulate the brain point in the auricles. If it is too difficult to use the wooden hammer and needle in the auricle, use a toothpick pressed rhythmically to the point.

Insomnia

Acupuncture and moxibustion used over a period of time are generally good for insomnia. The wooden hammer and needle method provides a useful adjunctive therapy. For the treatment of insomnia, it is helpful to be able to stimulate points just before going to bed. Many points can be stimulated.

Select from among the following points as a form of general therapy: LI-10 (108), BL-40 (112), BL-58 (112), KI-7 (120), LR-3

(104), LR-4 (108), GB-34 (120), SP-6 (108, 120, 132), SP-10 (132), CV-12 (104), ST-25 (132), CV-4 (104), GV-20 (104), GV-12 (104), BL-18 (108), BL-20 (132), BL-23 (120), BL-32 (112), and BL-33 (112). Finally, add KI-1 (120) and the insomnia point in the center of the heel.

It is best to do this treatment just before bedtime, or at least to treat these points sometime during the day, then treat KI-1 and the insomnia points just before retiring. If the patient suffers from very cold feet, tap at both corners of the nails of the feet (including the *jing* points), and tap the soles of the feet and rub the bottoms of the feet, too. This will often cause the feet to warm up. When cold feet have been disturbing sleep, this will help. If the upper parts of the body run warmer than the lower parts of the body (usually they will look redder), tap around the achilles tendon, especially BL-60 (112), as this will often help.

Traumas and contusions

The wooden hammer and needle can be helpful in the treatment of fractures, wounds, contusions, and sprains. It will not heal something like a fractured bone, but it can speed up the healing process. Typically a fracture, trauma, or contusion is accompanied by local swelling. This swelling will cause a decreased circulation at that area and thus slow down the natural healing process. If the swelling can be reduced, even for only a short period of time, the healing process will be greatly enhanced. The wooden hammer and needle can be useful in this regard.

Tap at sore points slightly distal and proximal to the swollen area. You can also tap around the swollen area. It is helpful to tap at the *jing* points on the fingers or toes, especially on the channels most affected by the injury and swelling. It is also helpful to tap at the meeting points in the affected area. On the lower legs, medial side, tap SP-6 (108, 120, 132); on the lower leg, lateral side, GB-39 or GB-35 (112, 120, 132); on the upper legs, medial side, Manaka's three-yin meeting point (2 finger widths above SP-10) (108, 120, 132); on the upper leg, lateral side, GB-31 (112, 120, 132); on the arm, dorsal surface, TB-8 (108, 120, 152); on the arm, palmar surface, Manaka's three-yin arm point (located on the channel point halfway between PC-3 and PC-7) (126, 176).

Treatment of a sprained ankle can be simple and effective. First palpate around the swollen ankle and tap gently at the more reactive points. Then tap at the *jing* points of the more affected channels; for example: tap GB-44 (120) and BL-67 (112); then tap at the meeting points such as GB-39 or GB-35 (112, 120, 132). It is sometimes helpful to treat on the opposite limb in the same area that is affected.

There are many possible uses for the wooden hammer and needle. The ones given above represent only a few simple suggestions for the relief of specific symptoms. Manaka, for example, used this method to relieve symptoms and occasionally for his general root treatment. He also employed it to stimulate the extraordinary vessel treatment points or the five-phase and source points. Many different treatment strategies can be devised and many point combinations can used with this method. It is easy, simple, effective, and safe.

Practitioners who regularly administer this technique like to have a number of sets of wooden hammers and needles in their clinic so that they may be loaned or sold to patients for home therapy. These tools are inexpensive enough to make this quite feasible. The metronomes are generally more expensive, though; other arrangements might be necessary.

Chapter 12
Case Studies

Case studies are perhaps the best indicators of the efficacy of clinical techniques and methods. We have described quite a range of different clinical techniques and methods. Most of these lie outside of the typical methods of practice of acupuncture currently employed in the West, exemplified by the modern Chinese approaches that use relatively strong stimulation.

In the materials above and in the general treatment methods described in Chapter 2, the use of "less is better" was strongly emphasized. For the reader unfamiliar with the information described in this text, and especially for the reader already practicing according to the modern Chinese approach, showing good clinical results is perhaps the best way to demonstrate the validity of the approaches described.

The following case studies are primarily taken from the work of authors whose books and papers we used to compile this text. In most cases, the specific techniques were the only techniques, or the primary techniques used, and are included to demonstrate the effectiveness of these techniques as the sole or primary form of treatment.

The rest of the case studies are taken either from our own work, or the work of the practitioners whose overall approaches were characterized in Chapter 2. For example, we have included case studies representing the approaches of the Keiraku Chiryō school and the Manaka style. These case studies are included to show the uses of the techniques as part of the overall treatment, thus demonstrating how and where they fit within the general scheme of things. Usually these techniques are administered as the "symptom control" part of treatment and are the last step in a series of simple treatment steps.

CHISHIN TREATMENTS

Case 1—an illustrative treatment[1]

MAIN COMPLAINT:

Kidney vacuity lumbar pain.

INDICATIONS:

Look for evidence of the following symptoms:
  —the lumbar region feels cold and painful.
  —the pulse is sinking and tight.
  —the third left deep (kidney) and first right deep (lung) pulses are weak.
  —Pain might extend from the neck to the buttocks.
  —Coldness of the lower limbs and lower abdomen and frequent urination may be reported.
  —The lumbar pain has a deep characteristic.

TREATMENT METHOD:

Use *chishin* methods at the following points, choosing location by palpation and leaving the needles on the lumbar region for 30 minutes: BL-23, BL-52, BL-25, CV-3, KI-10, LU-5, KI-3, KI-7, BL-60, BL-58, BL-40, BL-28.

Case 2[2]

PATIENT:

Female, age 27.

MAIN COMPLAINT:

Though the patient listed only migraine, headache, nausea, and stiff neck and shoulders as complaints, she actually had many other complaints, including dizziness, palpitations, shortness of breath, stomachache, lumbago, abnormal menses, and leukorrhea. Shūdo suspected that the patient had an imbalance of the autonomic nervous system which can present multiple symptoms like this.

OBSERVATION AND EXAMINATION:

The patient was perspiring from her forehead. She had a floating and fast pulse and she appeared to have a cold (it was the time of year when colds were very common.) She had a slight fever. Her migraines had started with menarche; she had bad migraines at

---

[1]From S. Okabe, *Shinkyū Keiraku Chiryō (Acupuncture and Moxibustion Meridian Therapy)*, p. 113.

[2]Taken from the case records of Denmei Shūdo, found in his contributions to *Idō no Nippon Magazine* 1987, 7:47-48, and 1987, 8:43.

every menses. Her condition included symptoms of the eyes; she was unable to open them and she wore a headband in an effort to relieve her headaches. She had a medical history that included nephritis, tonsillitis, and chronic gastritis, and earlier that year she had developed an acute asthmatic condition which had become chronic. She had tried multiple therapies and therapists, including prescription medications, injections, acupuncture, moxibustion, shiatsu, and massage.

Pulse diagnosis revealed a lung vacuity pattern with secondary liver repletion. The pulse quality was fast, and immediately after lying down on the treatment bed, it was floating and soft. Pressure pain was found on the abdomen at right ST-25 and ST-27, confirming the lung vacuity pattern. But the overall condition of the abdomen was not vacuous. Pressure pain was also found at GV-22, GB-5, BL-2, above BL-10, GB-12, GB-21, SP-6, BL-27, BL-59.

TREATMENT METHOD:

Chishin was applied to the dizziness point in the right and left auricles, GV-22, and right and left GB-5. *Chishin* was next applied to right LU-9 and SP-3, left LR-3, and left and right SP-6. After leaving the needles in for a while she was asked how she felt; she reported that she no longer had the headache or nausea. The needles were removed and an intradermal needle was placed at the right auricle point. Because pressure pain was then found at GV-9, moxa was applied 5 times. Then, with the patient sitting, moxa was applied 5 times to the right and left GB-21.

The patient returned 12 days later, at which time she reported that she had had no headaches until the day before, and that she had felt better generally. The primary diagnostic pattern was of liver vacuity so the same treatment was applied except that liver and kidney points were used in place of the lung and spleen points.

The patient returned eleven days later, complaining of a left-sided headache and nausea. The same treatment pattern was applied and she was sent home with an intradermal needle on left GB-5, and moxa was added on LI-10 and SP-6.

The patient did not return again for over five months. She explained that her condition had been good all this time, but on this particular day she had a headache, nausea, and dull pain from the lateral abdominal to lumbar region on the right. Pulse diagnosis revealed a pattern of liver and kidney weakness (liver vacuity), with repletion of the stomach and gallbladder channels. Pressure on the ileocecal region caused borborygmus and light pressure pain. Pressure pain was also found around the navel, especially to the left of the navel (confirming the liver vacuity pattern). Left ST-37 was drained, and the extra point lateral to right BL-25 was needled and then moxa applied 10 times for the abdominal pain. Otherwise the treatment was the same as before.

The patient came again about five months later. At this time she reported that her condition had been good, but that three days before, she had started feeling unwell, with no appetite, and had a headache on the right side that started the day of the treatment. A similar treatment protocol was employed again.

The patient returned for treatment since then only to deal with seasonal or weather changes, reporting that overall her symptoms were much improved. Shūdo stressed that he felt her condition involved blood stasis and an imbalance of the autonomic nervous system. He thought that her primary pattern was liver vacuity with LR-3 and GB-12 being significant points for her condition.

Case 3[3]

PATIENT:

Female, age 49.

MAIN COMPLAINT:

Depression. The patient complained of headaches, heavy-headedness, feelings of anxiety, and disinterest in everything. She had been diagnosed in a local hospital as being menopausal. She also had poor appetite.

OBSERVATION AND EXAMINATION:

Pulse diagnosis revealed a slow, slightly sinking pulse, with a primary pattern of kidney vacuity. Pressure pain was found on GV-10, GV-11, and SP-6.

TREATMENT METHOD:

Treatment was applied by the *chishin* method to right and left KI-7, CV-6, right and left BL-23, above right and left BL-10, around right and left GB-12, right and left GB-21, GV-22, and the dizziness point in both auricles. Moxa was also applied to GV-10, GV-11, and bilaterally to SP-6.

Over the next ten days the patient had four more treatments before she returned to her hometown. During this time, her insomnia initially was worse, but improved with the needling of GB-12. Her headache disappeared, and her pattern changed to a liver vacuity pattern. But her appetite and general disinterest in things did not change much. Shūdo commented that for patients who have a tendency towards depression, this style of treatment administered for only a short period of time is not likely to be completely successful.

---

[3]*Ibid.*

Kyūtōshin Treatments[4]

Case 4

PATIENT:

Female, age 60.

MAIN COMPLAINT:

Chronic diarrhea, unknown etiology. She had tried a long course of conventional therapy with no success, and was now rather underweight from the diarrhea.

OBSERVATION AND EXAMINATION:

There was considerable tenderness at KI-16, ST-25, ST-27, CV-12, CV-10, CV-4, GV-4, *jōsen,* BL-52, and BL-25.

TREATMENT METHOD:

Kyūtōshin was used on all these reactive points, with the addition of direct moxa *(okyū)* to ST-36 (10 times). This treatment was applied seven times after which the diarrhea was completely cured. This patient had suffered for a considerable amount of time and was greatly relieved by the treatment effects. (This case describes a reasonable approach for patients suffering from severe chronic diarrhea, as can be seen, for example, in HIV infected patients.)

Case 5

PATIENT:

Female, age 40.

MAIN COMPLAINT:

Severe leukorrhea, with blood in the discharge, lumbar and lower abdominal pain, and difficulty walking. The family physician had a suspicion of cancer, and she had received regular therapy at the hospital, but without improvement.

OBSERVATION AND EXAMINATION:

Lower abdominal pain was evident even with normal walking, and the lumbar area was extremely sensitive and painful to the touch. However, since the characteristic odor of cancer[5] was not present, Akabane decided to try treating the patient.

TREATMENT METHOD:

The *kyūtōshin* technique was applied only to the pressure pain points on the abdominal and lumbar areas, with direct-thread moxa *(okyū)* bilaterally to SP-6. After a course of ten treatments all the symptoms disappeared.

---

[4]Akabane described several interesting cases where the *kyūtōshin* method was used almost exclusively. The following cases (#4–#9) are taken from his *Kyūtōshin Hō (Moxa on the Handle of the Needle).*

[5]This is Akabane's description and observation. No further reference is provided.

Case 6

PATIENT:

Male, age 54.

MAIN COMPLAINT:

Left sided sciatica. The patient had undergone surgery on the lumbar region for this condition the previous year, but the condition had recurred.

OBSERVATION AND EXAMINATION:

There was a large scar on the lumbar region that was very tender to the touch, with tenderness on all the lumbar vertebrae and radiating discomfort to the whole left leg.

TREATMENT METHOD:

The following points showed particular sensitivity and were treated with the *kyūtōshin* method: BL-22, BL-23, BL-52, BL-25, pressure pain point on the left buttock, BL-37, BL-40, BL-56, BL-57, GB-39. Treatment was applied daily or every other day. After three weeks of treatment, the pain was much reduced and, after a few more treatments, it was gone. On a five-year follow up, the condition had not recurred.

Case 7

PATIENT:

Female, age 55.

MAIN COMPLAINT:

Duodenal ulcer. The patient had been hospitalized for a long time, but with only slight improvement; the doctors had advised that surgery probably would not cure the condition.

OBSERVATION AND EXAMINATION:

Both shoulders and both areas from the mid-thoracic vertebrae down were very stiff. The abdominal skin was loose and the muscles of poor tonus, with a bloated lower abdomen (characteristic of gastroptosis). The patient also had a tendency towards constipation.

TREATMENT METHOD:

Initially treatment was applied by the *kyūtōshin* method to 18 pressure pain points on the shoulders, back, and abdomen every day for a period of three weeks. Then the patient started developing nausea and anemic symptoms, which forced reducing the number of points treated to fewer than half of the original number; the abdominal and back points were split up in order not to do too much in a single treatment. After this treatment the latter symptoms disappeared, and within another six weeks, the condition was completely cured, with no recurrence years after the fact. It was noted that care should be taken not to overdose with the *kyūtōshin* method.

Case 8

PATIENT:

Male, age 60.

MAIN COMPLAINT:

Lumbago. The condition had developed four years before, and the patient had suffered constant pain, with no relief from Western therapy. He was unable to lift even the smallest things.

OBSERVATION AND EXAMINATION:

Any turn of the upper body was very painful. There were pressure pain at points on the lumbar region, especially BL-23, BL-22, BL-52.

TREATMENT METHOD:

Initial treatment was to apply *kyūtōshin* with five balls of moxa to each of these points and to some pressure pain points on the back of the legs. Treatment was applied daily. However, after three days, when it became evident that the patient was not feeling heat penetrating through to the abdomen, the number of moxa balls was increased to six. This caused the heat sensation to penetrate through to the abdomen. After four more days of treatment, the patient reported being able to rise in the morning with much less pain. After another week of treatment, this pain had disappeared completely. At the end of a month (total) of daily treatments, the patient was completely free of pain.

Case 9

PATIENT:
Female, age 42.

MAIN COMPLAINT:

Prolapsed uterus. The woman, a mother of eight, had suffered a prolapsed uterus about six years before. She had been to many hospitals and had tried many different therapies with no success. Finally she was told that surgery was the only remaining option. Since she did not want surgery, she came for acupuncture.

TREATMENT METHOD:

Treatment focussed on the use of the *kyūtōshin* method on pressure pain points on the lumbar region and CV-2. However, despite daily treatments, no heat was felt penetrating to the lower abdomen until after three weeks of treatment. As soon as the heat started being felt in the lower abdomen, the prolapse started improving. Two weeks later, the prolapse was completely recovered.

OKYŪ TREATMENTS[6]

Case 10

PATIENT:

Male, age 25.

MAIN COMPLAINT:

Gastric atony. This patient had originally been a strong healthy individual involved in agriculture studies. However, he had developed gastric atony, with accompanying symptoms of poor appetite, poor sleep, fatigue, palpitations, heavy-headedness, dizziness, dulled mental capabilities, and poor memory. He had progressed to a point where he was now unable to work and had the appearance of a cripple. A year after the onset of the problem, he came to Shirota for treatment.

OBSERVATION AND EXAMINATION:

Abdominal palpation revealed a soft and weak abdomen with the sounds of fluid accumulation in the stomach clearly present. There was pressure pain on CV-9, KI-16, and CV-6, especially on CV-9. Particularly acute pressure pain was found on BL-23, Sawada's GB-25 (BL-52), and especially on the left scapula near BL-43, where the area was swollen and hypersensitive.

TREATMENT METHOD:

Treatment was applied using moxa on the following points five times each: CV-12, left TB-4, CV-9, KI-16, ST-27, CV-6, GV-12, TB-15, left BL-43, 1.5 *cun* lateral to the intervertebral space between T8 and T9, BL-18, BL-20, BL-22, BL-23, Sawada's GB-25 (BL-52), BL-32, LI-11, ST-36, and Sawada's KI-3 (around KI-6.)

Aside from the points that were selected because of pressure pain, almost all the remaining points are points in Sawada's *taikyoku* or general moxa treatment protocol. This treatment is indicated for severely run down patients who are difficult to treat. After Shirota had applied moxa to all these points, the relatives of the patient, who had brought the patient in for therapy, were instructed in the use of moxa and directed to moxa the same points daily.

---

[6]These cases (#10–#12) are from Bunshi Shirota, *Kyūryō Zatsuwa (Miscellaneous Lectures on Moxibustion Therapy)* and *Shinkyū Chiryō Kisogaku (Fundamentals of Acupuncture and Moxibustion Therapies)*. Shirota's case studies are extensive, covering many years and a much broader range of therapeutic options than the limited range of moxa treatments described in the moxibustion section above. We have tried to select a few cases that are clearly illustrative of the uses of the treatment techniques described there.

The patient returned twenty days later. He had been receiving moxa therapy daily, but had developed some reactive symptoms, such as diarrhea, headache, and vomiting, and was unable to describe any progress.

The patient returned thirteen days later, during which time he had received daily moxa therapy at home. He reported that he was able to sleep better. Moxa on ST-27 was discontinued and started on ST-24 and right ST-21 instead because of the presence of pressure pain on those points. The rest of the points remained unchanged.

The patient returned again three weeks later, again having received daily home moxa treatments. During this time he had diarrhea only once and reported that he had been feeling better. A slight alteration of the points was made, and the patient received moxa therapy at home for another two months before returning again to Shirota. On this visit, he reported that he had gained weight, his appetite was improved, and that he generally felt much healthier, "the best I've felt for years." Because the heavy-headedness was unexpectedly stubborn, moxa was also applied to pressure pain points 1/2 *cun* lateral to GV-16 and slightly above BL-10.

After another six months of repeated therapy, he completely regained his health and strength, and was able to return to work.

Shirota commented that while the patient had been diagnosed as having gastric atony, many of his symptoms fitted well with a diagnosis of neurasthenia. In such cases, pressure pain frequently appears around left BL-43 and BL-45. He also noted that the *mengen* or what we have now call the "healing crisis" occurred as the treatment process began. While this is not a common occurrence in moxibustion therapy, it is definitely not a sign of inappropriate treatment and we should not be swayed to change the treatment, as it will naturally improve with continued treatment.

Case 11

PATIENT:
Female, age 47.

MAIN COMPLAINTS:

Rectum-bladder leakage. Four years before, the patient had undergone surgery for a myoma of the uterus, which appeared to cure the condition. However, about one year after the surgery, the patient started having severe abdominal pain, but on returning to the original surgeon, was told that nothing was wrong. Since the pain did not improve and was quite severe, the patient finally underwent an exploratory abdominal surgery. The surgeon found that there was residual infection from the surgery a year before, since some gauze had been left in the abdomen by accident. The infection was so severe that at that time the surgeon decided to leave the wound open so that it could be drained. But the infection spread instead and finally caused adhesions between the rectum and bladder, with an eventual ulcer formation between the rectum and bladder so that fecal matter started passing into the bladder. The patient's urination was very cloudy with fecal matter in it. Further medical interventions at that time were of no help. When the patient visited Shirota, her main complaints were of tension of the lower abdomen, discomfort of the bladder, and cloudiness of the urine.

OBSERVATION AND EXAMINATION:

The patient was of a relatively strong constitution and the abdominal scar was well healed. Pressure pain and resistance was found in the region over the bladder, and pressure pain in the lumbar region and above the sacrum.

TREATMENT METHOD:

Moxa was applied five times to each of the following points: CV-12, left TB-4, CV-3, GV-12, BL-18, GV-8, BL-20, BL-23, GV-4, LI-11, HT-3, ST-36, SP-6, Sawada's KI-3 (around KI-6.) Relatives of the patient were instructed to apply moxa daily to the same points.

The patient returned two weeks later. After the daily treatments, the cloudiness of the urine had disappeared, her frequency of urination was decreased, and the feeling of tension in the bladder was almost gone. The patient was instructed to continue moxa therapy at home.

The patient returned two months later, reporting that all her symptoms had disappeared with no recurrence. Shirota commented on this case that we can see how moxa is good for organic problems as well as functional ones, and that the "general" body treatment can be very helpful in such cases.

Case 12

PATIENT:

Male.

MAIN COMPLAINT:

The following case is rather anecdotal, but interesting and illustrative nevertheless. In 1931, a male patient complaining of severe acute abdominal pain visited his physician, who administered an analgesic injection. The pain was not relieved. The doctor examined him again and proclaimed that the patient had perforative peritonitis, and would probably be dead in several days, or perhaps in only one or two. The patient's guardian sent a telegram to Shirota requesting he come immediately to treat the patient.

OBSERVATION AND EXAMINATION:

The patient's abdomen was tight, full, distended, and had acute pressure pain, but in a different pattern than that which is usually seen in gastric ulcer. Shirota felt that it was neither perforative peritonitis nor appendicitis, and decided to try treatment in spite of not having a clear diagnosis.

TREATMENT METHOD:

Because ST-34 is the *xi*-cleft point of the stomach channel, and is therefore good for acute stomach problems, he used moxa on ST-34. After treating this point, the tension of the abdominal wall and distinctive pressure pain had reduced by 50%. Inspired by this change, he then applied moxa to CV-12, TB-4, CV-14, ST-21, ST-24, CV-9, CV-6, and ST-27, 20 times on each point, selecting all points by the presence of pressure pain. He also needled right LR-13 shallowly.

After treating these points, pressure on the abdomen showed almost no tension and no pressure pain. He then applied simple abdominal massage, during which the patient passed wind, and reported that his abdomen now felt comfortable. Shirota had the patient lie prone and palpated his back, finding distinctive pressure pain on BL-20 and BL-50. He shallowly needled BL-20, BL-22, and BL-50, and applied moxa to BL-23, Sawada's GB-25 (BL-52), BL-20, BL-50, BL-17, GV-12, BL-12, then LI-11, ST-36, GB-34, and Sawada's KI-3 (around KI-6.) Following this treatment, the patient reported that he was free of all discomfort and pain, and promptly fell asleep. He regained his health almost immediately after treatment. Shirota told of this case because he wanted to stress the great utility of ST-34 for the treatment of acute abdominal pain.

HINAISHIN TREATMENTS[7]

Case 13

PATIENT:
Female, age 26.

MAIN COMPLAINT:

Morning sickness. The woman was about six weeks pregnant, and was experiencing relatively severe morning sickness symptoms, including vomiting up all ingested foods.

---

[7]These cases (# 13–#17) are taken from the work of Dr. Matsuo Takaoka. Takaoka describes what is often the exclusive use of intradermal needles for the treatment of a variety of pain conditions in his book, *Ika no Tameno Itami no Hari Chiryō (Acupuncture Treatment of Pain for Physicians)*. Note the rather startling effectiveness in his case studies.

OBSERVATION AND EXAMINATION:

Because the patient's symptoms were much worse during the day, and alleviated at night, abdominal diagnosis was made with the patient standing up, her back to the wall. With the patient standing thus, pressure pain was found on a point midway between the inferior border of the sternum and the navel (around CV-12).

Palpation was continued on the patient's back, while the patient stood face to the wall. Pressure pain points were found to the right and left of the twelfth thoracic vertebrae (T12, around BL-21). Pressure pain was also found at bilateral points roughly six centimeters above the medial malleoli, on the posterior ridges of the tibia (around SP-6).

TREATMENT METHOD:

Intradermals were placed and taped on these five points. The patient immediately reported that the discomfort in her stomach had disappeared. Following this treatment, the patient was able to go out to a noodle store and successfully eat full servings of food, with no nausea or vomiting.

The patient returned twelve days later. She had been fine all this time. Having palpated the same points again, Takaoka decided to insert intradermal needles only at the abdominal and leg points; the only difference in treatment was that the needles were actually placed from 1 to 3mm distant from the original locations of these three points.

The patient returned one week later, reporting that she had experienced some symptoms of morning sickness and complaining that she believed that they had recurred because the back points had not been treated the last time. Her back was palpated again while she stood facing the wall. Pressure pain points were found lateral to the eleventh thoracic vertebrae (T11, around BL-20). Intradermals were then left in all five points, the same as had been done on the first visit.

The patient returned ten days later, with no complaints of morning sickness at all. Takaoka then removed all intradermal needles[8] and discontinued treatment. Later discussion with the patient confirmed that the morning sickness never returned.

---

[8] Occasionally some practitioners leave intradermal needles in place for more than the maximum recommended time of one week. We still consider a maximum of one week to be a valuable constraint.

Case 14

PATIENT:

Female, age 34.

MAIN COMPLAINT:

Eye strain. Recently the patient had been very busy at work, and was rather fatigued. About two days before, her right eye had started feeling heavy, tired, and uncomfortable.

OBSERVATION AND EXAMINATION:

Because the position of the patient has no influence in a case such as this, Takaoka palpated while the patient was in the supine position. The patient described an area superior and slightly lateral to her right eye as the focal point for this discomfort. Palpation of the area revealed reactions at almost the midpoint on the superior ridge of the right eyebrow (around *yuyao*), and on the superior ridge of the zygomatic arch in between the eye and ear, but slightly towards the ear.

TREATMENT METHOD:

Intradermal needles were placed at these two points. As soon as the intradermal needles were inserted, the heavy, tired, and uncomfortable feeling disappeared, and the right eye became clear. After ten minutes, the intradermal in the eyebrow was removed, and the one anterior to the right ear was taped and left in place.

The patient returned the next day and, since her symptoms had completely disappeared, the intradermal was removed. The symptoms did not recur.

Case 15

PATIENT:

Female, age 58.

MAIN COMPLAINT:

Bronchial asthma. The patient had been suffering from bronchial asthma for over forty years, and had been a patient of Dr. Takaoka for over ten years.

OBSERVATION AND EXAMINATION:

The patient had suffered asthma attacks about once a month which usually took about two weeks of injection and medication therapy to treat. On one occasion, she had a typical severe attack, but the usual injection and medication therapies didn't work to calm the symptoms down. In frustration, Dr. Takaoka decided to try intradermal needle therapy on her because, according to the acupuncture literature, asthma was supposed to respond to acupuncture therapy.

(Dr. Takaoka, principally a pain specialist, and utilizing intradermal needles only on pain patients, was not familiar with other acupuncture approaches for the treatment of asthma.)

TREATMENT METHOD:

After palpating on the back and shoulders of the patient, Takaoka placed intradermals at four bilateral points (roughly in the vicinities of BL-17, BL-13, TB-15, and GB-21). Sitting and talking with the patient, Takaoka noticed that about five minutes after the needles were inserted, her breathing began to improve. On examining her with a stethoscope, he found that the usual respiratory sounds characteristic of asthma had disappeared and that her asthma attack had completely subsided. He then taped the intradermal needles and sent the patient home.

On the next occasion the patient returned with the same symptoms. Takaoka tried the use of the intradermal needles as before, but this time the treatment had no effect. On subsequent attacks he tried the needles each time and found the same kinds of results: on some occasions, the attacks would stop, on others, no response was observed. Analyzing these experiences, Takaoka discovered that if her attacks were brought on as a consequence of allergic reactions, the needles were ineffective if used in this manner. But, as was often the case with this patient, if the attack was brought on by a stiffening in the patient's back and shoulders, this treatment was very effective.

Case 16

PATIENT:

Male, age 54.

MAIN COMPLAINT:

"50-year shoulder." One year before coming to Dr. Takaoka, the patient had developed the "50-year shoulder" syndrome on the right side.

OBSERVATION AND EXAMINATION:

The patient had symptoms of a stiff painful shoulder with limited range of motion. Over the last year, the shoulder had slowly improved, but he still had pain on raising the arm, which he had to do frequently since he commuted by train daily, and often needed to hold the straps above his head to support himself. The patient was asked to raise his arm to the position that caused the pain. The pain was fixed on the back of the upper arm. With the arm held in this position, pressure pain points were searched in the painful area. After a pressure pain point was found, the point was marked, and his arm was lowered.

TREATMENT METHOD:

With the arm lowered, an intradermal needle was inserted into the marked point; then the patient was asked to raise the arm again as before in order to see how the pain was. The pain had completely disappeared. The needle was taped with instructions that it be removed after two or three days.

Case 17

PATIENT:

Male, age 22.

MAIN COMPLAINT:

Lumbago. Nine months before, he had hurt his back lifting a heavy object. After massage at a bonesetting clinic, his back pain had improved, but the pain persisted (although to a lesser degree). Ten days before the first office visit, his back pain had flared up and was quite severe. It was diagnosed by an orthopedic specialist as a herniated disc. He had tried medication and traction for the condition, with no effect.

OBSERVATION AND EXAMINATION:

When walking, he had to drag his left leg, and he could not bend forward at all with the upper half of his body. When questioned, the patient indicated that he had spontaneous pain in the standing position in the left lateral lower back, lateral to L2 and L3. With the patient standing, face and chest to the wall, palpation at this area revealed two distinctive pressure pain points which were about two and half centimeters lateral to L2 and L3 (around BL-23 and BL-24). These were marked with a pen.

TREATMENT METHOD:

With the patient lying on his abdomen on the bed, intradermal needles were placed at these two pressure pain points. On rising, the patient said that the pain was lighter. Five minutes later, the patient reported that the pain was now vague, with a feeling of heaviness in the lower back. The patient was then asked to stand with his face and chest to the wall again. Palpation was applied again, revealing pressure pain points between L4 and L5, and between L5 and S1 (GV-3 and *jōsen*). The patient was asked to lie down on his abdomen again, and intradermal needles were inserted to these two points. On rising, the patient reported that the pain and heavy feeling had disappeared. These four needles were taped and left in place. Follow-up revealed that the patient's lumbago was cured by this one treatment!

EMPISHIN TREATMENTS[9]

Case 18

PATIENT:

Female.

MAIN COMPLAINT:

Sciatic pain.

OBSERVATION AND EXAMINATION:

An outbreak of herpes zoster lesions was found along the course of the sciatic nerve.

TREATMENT METHOD:

Placement of a couple of *empishin* along the sciatic nerve route, at reactive points, not only stopped the sciatic pain, but also helped clear up the herpes lesions.

Case 19

PATIENT:

Male.

MAIN COMPLAINT:

Herpes zoster.

OBSERVATION AND EXAMINATION:

This condition was found on the forehead, from the area of the left eyebrow to BL-4.

TREATMENT METHOD:

Three *empishin* were placed at reactive points at the borders of the outbreak. Changing the *empishin* daily over the next two days allowed the patient to experience complete relief of the herpes.

Case 20

PATIENT:

Male.

MAIN COMPLAINT:

Abdominal pain of unknown etiology.

OBSERVATION AND EXAMINATION:

The patient had received little help from his doctor.

---

[9]These brief anecdotal cases (#18–#21) from the work of Fumiyo Shiozawa describe successful resolutions to what can be rather difficult cases.

TREATMENT METHOD:

Empishin were placed at reactive points on the abdomen, at ST-27 and ST-28, with very good relief.

Case 21

PATIENT:

Female, age 32 months.

MAIN COMPLAINT:

Cerebral palsy.

OBSERVATION AND EXAMINATION:

At the initial visit, the patient had no strength in the neck, with instability of the head; no movement or strength in the arms or legs, such that they were dangling loosely; no facial expression; no communication skills; difficulty breathing, probably from the profuse uncontrollable drooling of saliva; inability to swallow correctly, with extreme difficulty being fed; and no sign of milk teeth.

TREATMENT METHOD:

Shiozawa treated the child every two to three days for about three months, using massage, special children's needle techniques and intradermal needles, but with little clear sign of improvement. He then decided to try the *empishin* needles. Continuing with the massage and special needling techniques, the treatment was changed by using *empishin* at LI-10 or TB-9 and ST-36, instead of the intradermals, to a total of four needles on the limbs, which were retained between each treatment. For the difficulty breathing and drooling, *empishin* were also used on special points one *cun* above ST-9, during the treatment on every other visit, but not retained. The child's family brought her two to three times weekly; members of the family routinely changed the *empishin* needles.

After a month, the child started moving both her upper and lower limbs, and her milk teeth started appearing. Within another three months, all the milk teeth had come out, and she had voluntary control of both arms and legs. In another two months, she was able to raise both her arms horizontally; she started showing a more normal facial expression, including the ability to smile. At this time her breathing difficulties were considerably improved and there was a distinctive decrease in the amount of drool. Her legs were strong enough to be able to stamp her feet, and she had gained sufficient strength to be able to hold her head up by herself. In another three months she had greatly improved motor control over her hands. Two months later, she could drink a cup of water on her own and could, without too much difficulty, turn her head from left to right to be able to follow movements around her.

Shiozawa admitted being quite surprised and pleased by these distinctive improvements in only one year of therapy; he was sure that the *empishin* needles had enabled this progress.

CUPPING THERAPY TREATMENTS[10]

Case 22

PATIENT:
Male, age 34.

MAIN COMPLAINT:

Chronic gastritis. For over one year, the patient had suffered repetitive attacks of left epigastric pain, with belching, noisy stomach, and weakness of the whole body.

OBSERVATION AND EXAMINATION:

Clinical tests showed a hypertrophy of the gastric mucosa, with a clinical diagnosis of chronic hypertrophic gastritis.

TREATMENT METHOD:

Treatment used cupping therapy every other day, with cupping on GV-14, CV-13 and BL-20 during the first treatment, then GV-12, CV-12, and BL-21 during the next, alternating between these two patterns for a total of ten treatments. After the tenth treatment, the patient was completely asymptomatic and considered cured.

Case 23

PATIENT:
Female, age 40.

MAIN COMPLAINT:

Meniere's disease.

OBSERVATION AND EXAMINATION:

The patient had been suffering for about two years from weekly bouts of dizziness with vomiting and tinnitus. She had already tried both Chinese herbal and Western pharmaceutical therapies without success.

TREATMENT METHOD:

Cupping therapy was applied a total of thirty treatments. The treatments alternated between GV-14, BL-15, BL-18, then BL-20, BL-23, and then CV-12; the cups were applied every other day. After a course of thirty applications, all the symptoms had completely abated and the patient was considered cured.

---

[10]Cases #22–#23 are taken from A. Meguro, *Kyūkaku Ryōhō (Cupping Therapy)*; cases #24–25 are from Wang Fengyi and Ren Huan Zhao, *Kyūgyoku Ryōhō (Cupping Therapy)*.

Case 24

PATIENT:

Male, age 32.

MAIN COMPLAINT:

Influenza.

OBSERVATION AND EXAMINATION:

Two days before, the patient had developed chills, and the next day he had headache, nasal congestion and runny nose, aching of the whole body, fever, dry mouth, throat pain, and a slight nonproductive cough. He had already tried herbal therapy, with some reduction in the symptoms that was followed by a flare-up of the symptoms. His body temperature was a little over 100° Fahrenheit.

TREATMENT METHOD:

Treatment was applied with cups to GV-14 and BL-12. A second treatment was applied later to GV-14 and BL-13. After these two treatments, the fever broke and the patient's symptoms disappeared.

Although the authors of *Kyūgyoku Ryōhō* specifies the use of the "prick" cupping method for the treatment of influenza, this case was treated with the cupping method with very good success. Perhaps this method was used because the fever was not too high.

Case 25

PATIENT:

Male, age 56.

MAIN COMPLAINT:

Urticaria.

OBSERVATION AND EXAMINATION:

The patient had itchy rashes over most of the body, especially bad on the four limbs. Anti-allergy medications had provided no relief.

TREATMENT METHOD:

Treatment was applied by cupping the navel area. In this treatment, the cup was applied for 3 to 5 minutes, removed, applied again for 3 to 5 minutes, then removed and applied again for 3 to 5 minutes. This made a total of three cuppings on that area. This pattern was applied daily. After two sessions, the itchiness began to abate, and the rashes became lighter. After four treatments, the condition was cured and all symptoms relieved.

SHIRAKU TREATMENTS[11]

Case 26

PATIENT:

Male, age 71.

MAIN COMPLAINT:

High blood pressure. At the age of 62 the patient suffered and recovered from a small stroke. At the age of 70 he had undergone surgery for a stomach ulcer. His blood pressure was slightly elevated but not problematic.

OBSERVATION AND EXAMINATION:

When the patient first came for treatment, he had experienced a spontaneous nosebleed four days before, and the night just prior to the nosebleed he had felt a distinctive cold sensation of the lower limbs. The patient's blood pressure was 210/110mm Hg, his face was flushed, and his shoulders were hard and painful when pinched. Further examination revealed vascular spiders both in the shoulder region and in the lumbosacral region.

TREATMENT METHOD:

Bloodletting and cupping techniques were applied to these vascular spiders, and 150cc of blood was removed. Following this treatment, no change in the blood pressure could be detected.

The patient came for treatment the next day and had a blood pressure reading of 190/100mm Hg. Bloodletting and cupping therapy were applied to the same regions, with 60cc of blood removed; the *jing* points of both hands were also bloodlet. Immediately after treatment, the blood pressure was 150/90mm Hg.

The patient came for treatment again the next day, at which time his blood pressure was 160/90mm Hg, and he said that he felt much better.

Case 27

PATIENT:

Female, age 69.

MAIN COMPLAINT:

Hypertension and mild stroke.

---

[11]The following cases (#26–32) are taken from the works of the bloodletting specialists, Kunimasa Kudō and Masao Maruyama, specifically from Kudō's book, *Zusetsu Shiraku Chiryō (Illustrated Bloodletting Therapy)* and Maruyama and Kudō's book, *Shiraku Ryōhō (Bloodletting Treatment Method)*. They often used bloodletting as their only treatment modality.

OBSERVATION AND EXAMINATION:

The day before, she had suddenly felt ill and was treated immediately by a doctor at the clinic who found that she had an elevated blood pressure and had suffered a slight stroke. She had a slight paralysis on the left side of the body, with disorders of the joints, especially the fingers of the left hand which could barely extend. The upper blood pressure reading was measured at that time to be 230mm Hg. When Kudō saw the patient, she was bed-bound, and examination revealed that she was rather overweight, red-faced, and had cold hands and feet, with stiffness of the left shoulder and body chills.

TREATMENT METHOD:

Bloodletting was applied to the corners of all the fingers and the corners of the toes on the left foot. From this treatment alone, the patient's ability to extend the fingers of the left hand improved. With the patient lying on her abdomen, bloodletting from the cutaneous regions was applied with cupping on the left shoulder and upper back regions; 30cc of blood was removed. Bloodletting was then applied on the face and auricle. After these methods, the stiffness of the left shoulder disappeared along with the body chills. The blood pressure was taken and found to be 190/90mm Hg.

The next treatment was three days later. Her blood pressure before treatment was 200/90mm Hg. The treatment was repeated.

The next treatment was five days later. The symptoms in the fingers and joints had almost all totally disappeared and the blood pressure was 190/80mm Hg. The same treatment was repeated.

The next treatment was administered a week later at which time her blood pressure was found to be 160/80mm Hg. Her progress had been very good, and she was now able to sit up in bed. Two weeks later, she was sufficiently recovered to be able to practice standing up and walking.

Case 28

PATIENT:

Male, age 37.

MAIN COMPLAINT:

Ankle pain.

OBSERVATION AND EXAMINATION:

About six weeks before visiting Kudō, the patient had suffered a skiing accident, severely spraining the right ankle. For the first couple of weeks the swelling and pain had been very bad, but for the last month or so, the difficulty walking was improved, though the swelling and pain levels were still bad. Examination revealed that the skin in the region was dark, and that edema could develop as high up as the lower thigh with walking. Pressure pain was also found in the regions underneath the internal malleolus and the external malleolus.

TREATMENT METHOD:

Bloodletting and cupping methods were applied to the pressure-pain areas and the area immediately around them. Dark red sticky blood in the amount of 15cc came out. The warming needle technique was then applied to SP-6. Following this the patient reported a sensation of lightening of his leg.

He returned for treatment four days later. At this time the swelling was considerably reduced, and skin color much improved. When bloodletting was applied the 10cc of blood that came out was a more normal color and consistency.

The patient reported later that his ankle healed very quickly after this second treatment and he required no further treatment.

Case 29

PATIENT:

Female, age 21.

MAIN COMPLAINT:

Asthma.

OBSERVATION AND EXAMINATION:

The patient's asthma condition started not long after her menarche. The condition had been progressively worsening, and had been unresponsive to a battery of different medical procedures. At the time of her first visit to Kudō and Maruyama, she was receiving daily adrenaline shots. Examination showed that while she seemed to have a relatively strong constitution, her skin had a darkened appearance and she had many vascular spiders on the shoulder and upper back regions, ranging down to the lumbosacral region. Stethoscopic examination revealed distinctive bronchial and whistling sounds; otherwise no other notable signs appeared.

TREATMENT METHOD:

Bloodletting and cupping were applied to the most distinctive vascular spiders on the upper back and shoulder regions and on the lumbosacral regions; about 70cc of blood was removed. Immediately the patient reported that her breathing difficulty was alleviated, and that this was more than any of the other treatments had been able to do for her.

She came for treatment two or three times a week, during which sessions, the same treatments were administered: less than 50cc of blood was removed on each occasion. After two weeks, the adrenaline shots were almost unnecessary, and her skin had taken on a more normal color and luster. Financial reasons forced the family to cut treatments back to once or twice a month, during which time she continued to improve. After a while she was able to go out and work as a company clerk. This was the first time she had been able to work.

Case 30

PATIENT:

Female, age 68.

MAIN COMPLAINT:

Trigeminal neuralgia.

OBSERVATION AND EXAMINATION:

The right-sided trigeminal neuralgia had first developed about three years prior to her first visit. Before that time, she had been relatively healthy, with no significant medical history. During this three-year period, the condition had shown many ups and downs, but generally seemed to get worse despite all kinds of medical therapies. Examination showed that she was relatively strong and healthy for her age, but that talking seemed to irritate the pain. Careful inspection of the facial region revealed vascular spiders on the cheek region and mandible.

TREATMENT METHOD:

Bloodletting was applied to these vascular spiders. This reduced the pain 50%. *Chishin* (leaving needle) was then applied to ST-5 and ST-6 for five minutes.

The patient came for treatment the next day. She reported that the pain was almost gone, but that there was some residual numbness persisting near the lips. After finding vascular spiders in the same regions again, bloodletting was applied on them and on the nail corner of the index finger (LI-1). This caused her symptoms to disappear completely. Followup revealed no recurrence of the neuralgia.

Case 31

PATIENT:

Male, age 53.

MAIN COMPLAINT:

Lumbar pain and sciatica.

OBSERVATION AND EXAMINATION:

The patient had no particularly significant medical history until about two months before, when he developed left-side lumbar and sciatic pain. For the last two months he had tried many different therapies, all of which were unsuccessful, and indeed, his condition had worsened. Examination revealed that his gait was off somewhat, that he had a reduced Achilles tendon reflex, and a distinctive Lasegue's sign. His posture was poor and slouched. It was speculated that his sciatic pain was caused by a herniation of an intervertebral disc due to a slight scoliosis.

TREATMENT METHOD:

Initially, the treatment focussed on the use of bloodletting from the small veins (venesection). The first procedure was to bloodlet from visible veins in the popliteal crease on the affected side, while the patient was standing. After about 100cc of very dark blood was removed, the patient was able to straighten his lumbar area and stand up straight; he reported that his left leg felt lighter. Then, with the patient lying on his abdomen, *chishin* (leaving needle) technique was applied to distinctive pressure pain points in the lumbar region, and direct moxa was applied seven times to BL-23.

The patient returned the next day for treatment, reporting that he had been able to sleep better and felt better overall, but he still dragged his left leg. The same treatment was performed, with the exception that only 80cc of blood was removed. The patient returned for treatment the next four days, during which sessions the treatments were almost the same as the first, but with a gradual reduction in the amount of blood removed. After the sixth treatment, the walking disturbance had considerably improved, and the spontaneous pain was much better. The patient returned for treatment every other day for seven more visits. Each time, the same treatment was done; after this, he was completely cured.

Case 32

PATIENT:

Female, age 46.

MAIN COMPLAINT:

Rheumatic joint pain.

OBSERVATION AND EXAMINATION:

Except for a bout of pneumonia 25 years earlier, the patient had been fairly healthy until two years before, at which time she had started developing rheumatic pains of the joints of the right arm, fingers of the right hand, and both knees. At first the pain had not been too bad, but recently it had worsened considerably. She was only able to come for treatment after having a strong analgesic injection.

The patient was of weaker constitution, and showed signs of melanin pigmentation which are characteristic of chronic rheumatism around the affected joints. Very clear vascular spiders were observed, both on the upper back and shoulder region and on the lumbosacral region.

TREATMENT METHOD:

Bloodletting and cupping were applied to both of these areas, with *chishin* at BL-40 and SI-11. After treatment, the patient reported feeling somewhat better, with an easier movement of the arms and legs.

She returned with some difficulty the next day, again requiring an analgesic injection. The same treatment was repeated. She returned again three days later, reporting that her condition had improved considerably. However, she expressed concern about her finances and her ability to maintain treatments. At this time, bloodletting was applied in the same regions, with moxa applied to HT-9, LR-1, KI-7, and BL-23.

Following this treatment, bloodletting was applied two to three times a month, and she performed moxibustion therapy on herself at home. Over a period of six months of therapy in this manner, her condition gradually improved to the point that she was able to function much better.

Case 33[12]

PATIENT:

Female, age 4.

MAIN COMPLAINT:

Otitis media.

OBSERVATION AND EXAMINATION:

The girl had been visiting doctors for about two years for the treatment of otitis media, but without any improvement. Examination revealed that she was rather skinny, and fussy about what she ate. At night she would suffer from pain in the right auricle; the pain disturbed her considerably. While she was suffering from her auricular pain, a three-edged needle was inserted so as to barely penetrate the skin at TB-1 and GB-44. A few drops of blood were carefully squeezed out of each point. Within two minutes of applying the technique, the pain stopped. Next, needle techniques using skin contact and light rubbing were applied to supplement

---

[12]This case comes from S. Okabe, *Shinkyū Keiraku Chiryō (Acupuncture and Moxibustion Meridian Therapy)*, p. 317.

the diagnosed liver vacuity. Following the application of the blood-letting, her pain was relieved and did not return. To strengthen her condition, the light needling treatments were applied daily over a two-month period. On a two-year followup, the otitis media had not recurred. The bloodletting was applied only once—at the initial visit.

MANAKA WOODEN HAMMER & NEEDLE TREATMENTS[13]

Case 34

PATIENT:

Female, age 79.

MAIN COMPLAINT:

Rheumatoid arthritis.

OBSERVATION AND EXAMINATION:

The patient had suffered from rheumatoid arthritis for many years; she had severe deformation and pain of the spine and feet, with lesser deformation and pain of most other joints. She had to be helped into the treatment room by members of her family. Aside from the pain, she was very fatigued, partly as a result of her age. She came periodically to Manaka for treatment to relieve her dis-comfort.

TREATMENT METHOD:

The *yin qiao–ren mai* was treated with ion-pumping cords as the first step (KI-6 black clip, LU-7 red clip). In order to help with the spine and foot discomfort, the wooden hammer and needle tech-nique was employed. GV-14 was tapped at a rate of 112 beats per minute for about 20 taps; then again GV-14 was tapped at a rate of 120 beats per minute for about 20 taps; once more GV-14 was tapped at a rate of 132 per minute for about 20 taps.

The patient remarked that she felt a dulling of the discomfort in the feet and legs, and that she had a very comfortable warm sensation spreading throughout her legs and eventually across her torso. GV-14 was used because it is the meeting point of the yang chan-nels. The tapping was applied at rates of 112, 120, and 132 because those are the rates of the three leg yang channels: bladder, gall-bladder, and stomach.

In very elderly patients it is important to carefully regulate the doses of stimulation that you give. In this case, the wooden ham-mer and needle was able to deliver a sufficient low-dose treatment.

---

[13]The following anecdotal cases (#34–#36) were observed in Yoshio Manaka's Odawara clinic in the summer of 1986. They illustrate treatments where the wooden hammer and needle was successfully employed.

Case 35

PATIENT:
Male, age 25.

MAIN COMPLAINT:
Following a tracheotomy surgery for cancer, the patient was unable to flex or rotate his neck, and had severe neck pain.

OBSERVATION AND EXAMINATION:
The patient had strong pressure pain at right LU-1 with some at both KI-11, and pressure pain on the bladder–lung reflex point on the calf.[14] This confirmed a bladder–lung polar channel diagnosis.

TREATMENT METHOD:
Treatment was applied by using the wooden hammer and needle with metronome. BL-65 were tapped bilaterally at a rate of 112 beats per minute for about 20 taps to each side. Then right LU-9 was tapped at a rate of 126 beats per minute for about 20 taps.; then the lung point in the right auricle was tapped at a rate of 126 beats per minute for about 20 taps.

Following this, the patient reported decreased neck pain and slightly increased range of motion. GV-12 was then tapped at a rate of 126 beats per minute, and *jōsen* at a rate of 112 beats per minute, both for about 20 taps each.[15] With the arms abducted to the sides, GB-21 was tapped bilaterally at a rate of 120 for 20 taps. Following these last points, the patient again reported less pain and greater range of motion. The treatment finished with the placement of an intradermal needle to the neck point in the right auricle.

Case 36

PATIENT:
Female, age 69.

MAIN COMPLAINTS:
Chronic knee pain; obesity.

OBSERVATION AND EXAMINATION:
The patient had a long history of right knee pain and pain on the lower portions of the right leg. While it had improved somewhat over time with therapy, it had not been cured, probably due to the obesity problem. On the day that the patient came for treatment, she complained that she had not been able to bear weight on her

---

[14]See Y. Manaka, K. Itaya, and S. Birch, *Chasing the Dragon's Tail*, pp. 162–165.

[15]112 is the bladder rate, 126 the lung rate, and 120 the gallbladder rate. For more details of this kind of treatment, see *Ibid.*, where Manaka's general step-by-step treatment protocol is detailed.

right leg comfortably and without limping for around three months. The patient was observed limping into the clinic.

Examination revealed an abdominal pattern of upper right and lower left abdominal quadrant reactions, characteristic of Manaka's "cross-syndrome" diagnosis.

TREATMENT METHOD:

The ion-pumping cords were used as follows: right PC-6 (black clip), right SP-4 (red clip), left TB-5 (black clip), left GB-41 (red clip). After the cords were removed, the patient was asked to step off the treatment bed and try walking; she still had difficulty and was clearly limping. The patient was then asked to sit on the side of the treatment bed. Manaka palpated the lower portions of the right leg, finding strong pressure pain along the three leg yang channels. He treated GV-14 with the wooden hammer and needle as follows: first he tapped at a rate of 112 beats per minute for about 20 taps. He palpated the bladder channel again on the right calf and found it less sensitive. Then he tapped GV-14 again at a rate of 120 beats per minute for about 20 taps. On checking the gallbladder channel on the right calf he found it less reactive as well. Then he tapped GV-14 at a rate of 132 beats per minute for about 20 taps, after which he found the sensitivity along the stomach channel on the right calf to be reduced. The patient was asked to walk, and to her delight, she had no more pain in the right knee or lower leg, and was clearly able to walk without limping and could walk up and down stairs without pain. This degree of mobility had not been possible before.

ROOT SYMPTOM-CONTROL TREATMENT METHODS[16]

Case 37

PATIENT:

Male, age 64.

MAIN COMPLAINT:

Bleeding gums due to pyorrhea alveolaris.

OBSERVATION AND EXAMINATION:

The patient had a somewhat weakened constitution, and when younger had suffered from pulmonary tuberculosis. For several years he had experienced bleeding gums from pyorrhea alveolaris, and was unable to chew hard things. Examination revealed a primary diagnosis of lung vacuity with secondary liver involvement.

---

[16]The following two cases (#37–#38) were presented by Kōdō Fukushima in a special issue of the Tōyōhari journal, *Keiraku Shinryō*, March, 1988, pp. 5–20, which focussed especially on treatment by bloodletting.

TREATMENT METHOD:

After administering the appropriate treatment for this diagnosis, bloodletting was applied. Slightly deep "wiggler-like" vascular spiders were found on both the left and right ST-4 and ST-6 regions. Each of these were bloodlet using the squeezing method (rather than cupping), and 7 to 10 drops of relatively dark blood was removed from each. The squeezing was stopped when the blood became lighter in color at each site.

His second visit was two weeks later, at which time he reported that he had experienced no further gum bleeding. Since the vascular spiders appeared unchanged, the same treatment was applied. At the third visit two weeks later, the patient reported that not only had there been no gum bleeding, he had been able to start eating hard foods again. The same treatment was applied again.

Fukushima recommended the utility of bloodletting for disorders of the oral cavity, especially dental disorders such as dental caries, pyorrhea alveolaris, and stomatitis. He also reported that since vascular spiders appear relatively easily on the facial regions, implying that qi and blood stagnate there easily, bloodletting can be useful for a variety of other disorders, such as facial palsy, facial spasm, trigeminal neuralgia, eye disorders, and nasal disorders.

Case 38

PATIENT:

Male, age 6.

MAIN COMPLAINT:

Asthma.

OBSERVATION AND EXAMINATION:

The patient had been having acupuncture therapy for his chronic asthma condition, with good results. One day he came for treatment in the middle of a moderately bad attack, the first he had suffered in many days. His constitution was slightly weak, and he was thin-chested. Rattling sounds could be heard in his chest and he looked very uncomfortable. The pulse quality was floating, fast, and big. The primary diagnosis was of lung vacuity with secondary liver involvement.

TREATMENT METHOD:

Treatment was administered according to this diagnosis, then inspection was made of the area around GV-14 and a very clear superficial vascular spider was found on the right side of it.

The vascular spider was bloodlet and cupped, showing a strong spouting of dark blood; the cup was about half full. Because the blood did not become lighter in color, the cup was placed a second time, with less spouting of blood. Altogether, a great deal of dark blood (a clear indication of blood stasis) was removed, and the pulse became slower and firmer around the "middle pulse." His face seemed to return to a more normal color, and he could inhale more easily. However, while trying to insert intradermal needles on the child after the bloodletting, his face suddenly became pale and he vomited. This was immediately recognized as a reaction to the bloodletting, and cone moxa was applied to the navel and direct moxa to ST-36. The child then reported feeling better and the color returned to his face. The next day the child's parents were called to determine how the child was doing. They reported that his attack had gradually subsided.

This case is given not only to emphasize the usefulness of bloodletting in the treatment of asthma, which should focus primarily in the C7 to T4 area, but also in order to draw attention to the hazards of overdosing the patient. In this case, because of being distracted by the darkness of the blood and rate at which it came out, the subtle changes that indicate sufficient treatment were missed and excessive doses of bloodletting were given to the child. Such reactions are temporary, and easily countered with prompt moxa therapy. It is important to pay careful attention to the changes in the color of the blood, and to carefully note all signs other than the patient's symptoms. In this case it would have been more prudent to apply the bloodletting in smaller doses over a number of treatments, rather than all at once.

MIXED CASE STUDIES[17]

Case 39

PATIENT:

Male, age 37.

MAIN COMPLAINT:

Upper back spasm and pain.

OBSERVATION AND EXAMINATION:

The patient had suffered from upper back problems of tightness and pain on and off for about three years but, about ten days before the first visit, he had seen a chiropractor who had adjusted the region, leaving the patient with a significant increase and focalization of spasm and pain from C7 down to T7.

---

[17]The following cases (#39–#47) are selected from the clinical caseload of Stephen Birch. The first is illustrative of the simple combined uses of Manaka's general treatment procedure with the *chishin* (leaving needle) and intradermal needle techniques comprising the extent of the local treatment options.

Pressure pain was found on the upper right and lower left quadrants of the abdomen, a pattern indicative of Manaka's "cross-syndrome."

TREATMENT METHOD:

Based on this finding, the first treatment was to use the ion-pumping cords on right PC-6 (black), SP-4 (red), and left TB-5 (black), GB-41 (red). While the cords were attached, a silver *zanshin* was used with light tapping techniques on the regions of the supraclavicular fossa. *Kyūtōshin* (moxa on the handle of the needle) was then applied to BL-18, with simultaneous *chishin* applications to pressure pain points, GB-20, SI-11, and the *huato* point of BL-15. To finish the treatment, intradermal needles were placed at right BL-43, left SI-11, and on the right auricle at the neck point.

When he returned a week later, he reported an overall improvement of between 70% to 80%. He had a mild headache and was tired from a stressful work week. The first step of treatment was the same, with the exception of adding *chishin* at left SP-60. The second step was the same, except that *chishin* was applied to GB-21 instead of SI-11. Intradermal needles were applied to right BL-43 and left SI-11 again, with two more to the left auricle at the *shenmen* and neck points.

When he returned the following week, his back had been good, although there was some stiffness in forward flexion. The first step of treatment was the same as the first visit, the second step was the same as the second visit. *Chinetsukyū* (cone moxa) was also added at BL-13 and BL-17, while the needles were left during step two. Intradermal needles were applied to BL-15 and on the right auricle at the *shenmen* and neck points.

At his next visit one week later, he reported that his neck had not been bothersome at all. Since he was doing very well, a little more fine-tuning was applied. The first step was the same as the first and third visits. *Kyūtōshin* (moxa on the handle of the needle) was applied to BL-18, with *chishin* at GB-21 and BL-15 and *chinetsukyū* at GV-3 and BL-23. Then using a *teishin*, supplementation techniques were applied to CV-12, ST-25, and left LU-9. Next, intradermals were applied to BL-15 and on the left auricle at *shenmen*.

When the patient returned a week later he reported that his neck and back had been very good. However, he had strained his lower back slightly lifting something during the week, and was also very tired, having just come off a 36-hour work shift. This time the first step of treatment was the use of the ion-pumping cords at BL-62 (black) and SI-3 (red). *Chishin* was applied to GV-14 and to right BL-23, BL-52, and BL-25, with moxa on the handle of the needle at right BL-18 and BL-58, and at left BL-23 and BL-25, all points having been selected by palpation. Intradermals were then applied to an *ashi* point on the right lower back, to the right hand at the low-back area, to the right auricle at *shenmen,* and on the posterior and anterior surfaces at the low-back points; a total of five needles.

Eleven days later the patient reported that the acute back problem had completely resolved itself within two days of the last treatment, and that the upper back and neck problem seemed resolved. Treatment was discontinued.

Case 40

This next case history illustrates how the simple use of Manaka's general treatment protocol, using ion-pumping cords, moxa on the handle of the needle, and intradermal needles, can be effective for the treatment of pain.

PATIENT:

Female, age 68.

MAIN COMPLAINT:

Back pain and sciatica.

The patient had thrown her back out two weeks before, from which condition she had recovered with bedrest. After feeling better, she reinjured the back with a simple stretching exercise, and was confined to bed again. She had risen two days before her first visit, and still suffered from low-back pain with left sided sciatica. She had experienced similar problems 37 and 5 years before. Her medical history included slightly low blood pressure, tinnitus, and mild stress incontinence, for which she had undergone surgery 15 years before; recurrent mild costochondritis of the lower sternal region; a hysterectomy 36 years before; and a prolapsed uterus at the age of 22 which had been surgically corrected at that time.

OBSERVATION AND EXAMINATION:

There was a clear *yin qiao–ren mai* pattern.

TREATMENT METHOD:

Treatment used the ion-pumping cords to LU-7 (red) KI-6 (black) bilaterally, followed by *chishin* to BL-23 and BL-25. Intradermal needles were left at *jōsen,* and on the sciatic and low-back points of the left auricle.

She returned four days later, reporting that her back had been bad on the day after the treatment but had been much improved since then. The severe low-back pain was gone, mobility was much improved, and the sciatica was reduced, but she felt discomfort in her left knee. Ion-pumping cords were used on the same points, with moxa on the handle of the needle at BL-23 and BL-25. Intradermal needles were then placed at *jōsen* again, and on the low-back point of the right auricle and knee point of the left auricle.

When she returned five days later, she had noted improvements all week, but felt some pain due to overworking mid-week. Overall everything was much improved. The first two steps of treatment were the same with the addition of moxa on the handle of the needle at left GB-30. Intradermals were left at *jōsen,* left GB-30, and on the knee and low-back points of the left auricle.

The patient returned one week later, reporting no problems, except for some minor discomfort from overworking the day before. The first two steps of treatment were the same, with the addition of *chishin* at left TB-17. Intradermal needles were left at *jōsen* and on the neck and low-back points of the left auricle.

Case 41

This next case illustrates the effectiveness of Manaka's general step-by-step treatment protocol for the treatment of both fatigue and pain.

PATIENT:

Female, age 31.

MAIN COMPLAINT:

Extreme fatigue; right-sided shoulder and neck pain.

The patient had been diagnosed as having mononucleosis six weeks earlier, and had spent three weeks in bed with it. She had hepatomegaly, but with normal liver enzyme blood levels. Her main complaint from mononucleosis was extreme fatigue. She also had right-sided neck and shoulder pain which had been persistent over the last ten years. As an adolescent, she had suffered pneumonia yearly for three to four years, and was given regular prescriptions of antibiotics for the condition. She was still somewhat susceptible, catching colds easily, especially when stressed. She was allergic to penicillin. She also seemed allergic to alcohol. She had a slight menstrual irregularity, and suffered from occasional urinary tract infections and heartburn. She had some pain of the knees and of the left big toe. The patient was a pianist who performed on a very regular basis. She had several performances scheduled in the near future.

OBSERVATION AND EXAMINATION:

There was a clear liver-related pattern on the abdomen, with pressure pain and tightness in the right subcostal region and to the right side of the navel. The liver and kidney pulses were weak.

TREATMENT METHOD:

Treatment involved the application of Manaka's special hepatitis treatment. Ion-pumping cords were attached with a silver needle (black clip) at right PC-7, and a gold needle (red clip) at right LR-3. Then *chishin* was applied to BL-17, BL-18, and BL-25, with intradermal needles to left BL-18, right GB-21, and the liver and shoulder points in the right auricle.

The patient returned one week later, reporting a 70% to 80% improvement in her overall energy and fatigue problem, with decreased pain levels in the shoulder. A similar treatment was administered, with the exception of using touch-needle supplementation techniques on CV-12, CV-4, and ST-25 following the ion-pumping cords treatment.

The patient returned the following week, reporting that she was a little more tired from overworking, and that she had a little more shoulder pain and some mild stomach upset from stress. The treatment was similar to the last one, with the exception that moxa on the handle of the needle was used on BL-20 and right BL-27, in place of the *chishin* techniques.

The patient returned again one week later with no improvements, commenting that she had been very busy and stressed from work. Virtually the same treatment was administered. She returned again eight days later, reporting a much improved week. She had really overworked and not gotten too tired; she now felt that she had energy reserves to call on. The treatment shifted to an ion-pumping cord on right LU-7 (red), left KI-6 (black). This was followed by supplementing needle and moxa techniques on CV-12, CV-6, and ST-25. Moxa on the handle of the needle was applied to BL-20, with *chishin* to right BL-43 and intradermal needles to left BL-20, right BL-43, GB-21, and the stomach point on the left auricle.

She returned three more times in the next three weeks. Except for some digestive upset, from excessive consumption of holiday food, she was doing very well, with much improved energy and shoulder discomfort. Similar treatments were applied on each occasion.

After these seven visits, treatment was discontinued, because the condition was rectified.

PRESS-SPHERE TREATMENTS

Case 42

The next two cases illustrate how the use of press-spheres as part of the local treatment armamentarium can be very useful.

PATIENT:

Female, age 55.

MAIN COMPLAINT:

Insomnia and anxiety. The patient had been diagnosed 15 years before as having a mild case of Parkinson's syndrome, which affected the right side of the body. She was taking various medications that caused the side effect of insomnia, which disturbed her greatly. She had suffered from insomnia for about the last seven months. She suffered also from other less disruptive problems such as low blood pressure, clogged ears, hair loss, and prolapsed mitral valve.

OBSERVATION AND EXAMINATION:

She showed a considerable amount of blood stasis, with the classic abdominal signs of upper right and lower left abdominal quadrant reactions. These symptoms suggested Manaka's approach focussing on the liver channel, typically using the "cross-syndrome" treatment, and administering bloodletting techniques. She also had very stiff muscles in the neck and shoulder regions.

TREATMENT METHOD:

The first treatment used ion-pumping cords on right PC-6 (black) and SP-4 (red), with left TB-5 (black) and GB-41 (red). After this, *chishin* technique was used at GB-20, with moxa on the handle of the needle at BL-23 and right BL-58. Intradermals were then left on the right auricle at the *shenmen* and brain points.

The patient reported ten days later that her neck had been looser, but that her symptoms were not really much improved. Treatment at this and the next treatment expanded upon the basic treatment protocol by adding:

> 1. The use of the *zanshin* with tapping technique on the neck, while the ion-pumping cords were in place.

> 2. The use of bloodletting and cupping alternating on the upper back and lumbosacral regions.

> 3. The use of *chishin* at *anmien* instead of GB-20.

> 4. Intradermals at the kidney, heart, *shenmen,* and heart auricle points, alternating auricles each treatment.

By the fourth treatment, it became clear that the sleep disturbance was most likely due to very frequent night urination. The same treatment was administered, with the addition of a press-sphere at CV-3. The patient reported at the next treatment that she had been able to sleep better for the first four nights following treatment, with fewer night urinations.

The same treatment tactics were employed at each of the next seven treatments over a period of six-and-a-half weeks. By the end of the treatments, the night urination and insomnia were much improved. At a follow-up two months later, the patient was still doing much better.

In this case, the simple addition of a press-sphere to a reactive point in the region of CV-3 seemed to have a significant impact on the patient's night urination and associated insomnia problems.

Case 43

PATIENT:

Male, age 8.

MAIN COMPLAINT:

Hearing difficulties and poor concentration that had recently been labeled as "Attention Deficit Disorder." The patient was somewhat obese, and suffered from excessive mucus production, which caused nasal stuffiness, postnasal drip, and blocked eustachian tubes. On two occasions he had suffered ear infections and the blockage of the eustachian tubes had left him with decreased hearing abilities. The decreased hearing ability seemed to relate to his poor concentration in the classroom. Treatment was therefore directed to the excessive mucus production and impaired hearing.

OBSERVATION AND EXAMINATION:

According to traditional Keiraku Chiryō methods, his condition was lung vacuity.

TREATMENT METHOD:

Because it was his first visit, no needles were inserted, and the general *shōnishin* (children's treatment methods) were employed. First, using a silver *teishin*, left LU-9 and SP-3 were supplemented, and right LR-3 was drained. Then using a silver *enshin*, the general body treatment was applied across the abdomen, chest, back, arms, and legs. Next, a silver *zanshin* was employed on the neck region, using a tapping technique. To finish the treatment, cone moxa or *chinetsukyū* was used at BL-43, GV-12, BL-20, CV-12, CV-6, and ST-25. He was sent home with press-spheres on GV-12, BL-43 and TB-16, all of which were quite reactive. The treatment took less than 30 minutes.

He returned 10 days later, reporting a 10% improvement in hearing and some improvement with the mucus production problem. The same treatment pattern was employed, with the exception that 00 gauge needles (0.12mm) were inserted painlessly and very shallowly at TB-16 and ST-6, before the lung channel was supplemented. This same general approach was used on the next treatment a week later, leaving the press-spheres on the reactive points around the auricles, i.e., TB-17 and TB-18. At this third treatment, his parents were taught how to use the *ibuki* moxa and press-spheres, and were instructed to use the moxa and press-spheres daily.

He returned 15 days later with further improvement in his condition. His parents reported that they had managed to attend to some kind of treatment at home about every other day. The same treatment was administered, and a similar regimen of home therapy was recommended.

He returned six days later reporting that his hearing was "like new." The same kind of treatment protocol was employed, leaving a few more press-spheres in an effort to have a stronger impact on his mucus production problem, which was still irritating, and to try and help him lose some weight. The press-spheres were left at GV-12, BL-20, TB-17, CV-9, left auricle, stomach, and *shenmen*.

After this treatment, he no longer complained of impaired hearing. His hearing remained normal, and he showed slow improvement in his classroom attention and grades. Further treatment began to focus much more on weight loss and mucus production.

In this case, the press-spheres served a useful role in the relief of the patient's hearing problems with subsequent improvement in concentration, classroom performance, and school grades. It also seemed that their recommended use at home was very beneficial in the treatment of his general condition.

BLOODLETTING AND CUPPING TREATMENTS

The following case histories illustrate how the use of the bloodletting and cupping techniques within Manaka's general treatment framework can be helpful for some rather stubborn problems.

Case 44

PATIENT:

Female, age 66.

MAIN COMPLAINT:

Atrial fibrillation; back problems.

The patient was suffering from a chronic atrial fibrillation problem for the last three years or so which, despite numerous tests, was of unclear etiology; she was being treated with a host of medications including the bloodthinner COUMADIN™. The problem left her unable to do rigorous work and very short of breath. Her back problem was quite severe, going back more than thirty years. Currently she was suffering from back pain and pains that radiated down the left leg and to the right side of the body; if she raised her arms over her head, she would lose strength in the left leg. This problem was due to a joint condition of spinal stenosis and lumbar disc problems. The patient had a significant history of surgeries. Thirty years before, she had undergone surgery for a herniated disc. She had also undergone a right knee joint replacement surgery, a total hysterectomy, and surgery on both feet for Morton's neuroma. She suffered from osteoarthritis that affected both her hands and knees and for which she was taking anti-inflammatory medications. She had suffered from irritable bowel syndrome in the past, and had poor posture with fused cervical vertebrae. The patient also described being quite stressed. Her mother had passed away recently and she was also having a hard time adjusting to retirement.

OBSERVATION AND EXAMINATION:

Examination revealed tightness and pain in the subcostal regions, and extensive clusters of vascular spiders on both the upper and lower back.

TREATMENT METHOD:

Treatment in Manaka's style was applied using ion-pumping cords to PC-6 (black) and SP-4 (red) bilaterally. Since it was the first treatment, *chishin* only was applied to BL-25, SI-14, BL-15, BL-18, BL-23, BL-28. Intradermal needles were applied to *jōsen*, and to *shenmen* and low-back points on the left auricle.

The patient returned a week later, reporting less pain in the back and leg, a more localized pain in the back, and fewer disturbing symptoms when she raised her arms. Overall she felt "more nimble." On this occasion, treatment was applied with ion-pumping again to bilateral PC-6 (black) and SP-4 (red). Then bloodletting and cupping was applied to both the upper and lower back regions, with very dark blood coming out in the lower back region. Great care was taken when applying the bloodletting technique because of the atrial fillibration and the fact that she was on a blood-thinning medication. Next, *chishin* was used at left BL-43, both BL-17, and the *huato* point of BL-15. Moxa on the handle of the needle was applied to BL-25. Intradermal needles were applied to *jōsen*, the left *huato* point of BL-14, and the left auricle heart point.

The patient returned a week later reporting continued improvement in her back and leg symptoms. The same treatment protocol was applied with intradermal needles instead to *jōsen* and to left PC-4, left BL-15 (the latter two points for the atrial fibrillation).

The patient returned a week later with more improvements in the leg and back. However, at this point, no changes had been seen in the atrial fibrillation problem. Thus, for this and the next three treatments, ion-pumping was used instead at LR-3 (red) and HT-5 (black), in an effort to affect the heart problem. The rest of the treatment was much the same on each occasion.

The patient reported continued improvement in the back and leg, and that she was now able to start exercising more. As a result of being more agile, and virtually pain-free with no more restrictions in the mobility of the arms and left leg, she was exercising more. But her heart was not improving, and she started becoming slightly more fatigued. Because of this, the first step of treatment was changed, applying the ion-pumping cords at LU-7 (red) and KI-6 (black), with the rest of treatment the same. Over the next two months this same protocol was used three more times. She had been able to go on an extended canoeing trip with no problems with her back or leg.

After a total of eleven treatments, the heart problem had not changed. Her back and leg problems were greatly improved, her ability to exercise and carry out daily tasks was greatly improved, and she was coping much better. Bloodletting in this case was a significant factor in her remarkable improvements. It is typical to develop problems of blood stasis following surgical procedures or any traumatic injuries. She had undergone many surgical procedures over the years, and her condition when she first presented for treatment exhibited extensive blood stasis. Bloodletting can be very helpful in such cases.

Case 45

This next case history is not as remarkable, but demonstrates how the addition of the bloodletting and cupping procedures at the correct juncture can change a stubborn and resistant pain problem.

PATIENT:

Female, age 30.

MAIN COMPLAINT:

Right hip pain. The hip pain had started about one month before. She had a history of mild constipation, vaginal yeast infections, abdominal bloating, and some premenstrual symptoms, all of which were relatively mild.

OBSERVATION AND EXAMINATION:

Her abdomen was overall soft and cool to the touch; she had weak kidney and lung pulses. This particular pattern is usually a sign of relative vacuity, and often presages slower than normal progress in healing.

TREATMENT METHOD:

Initially, and for a number of later treatments, ion-pumping cords were used at KI-6 (black) and LU-7 (red). This was followed usually with moxa on the handle of the needle at BL-23, the right GB-30 area ,and on the right buttock, e.g., BL-28 and BL-53. As a last step, intradermal needles were left at points such as *jōsen*, right GB-30, right auricle, and hip point. These treatments were beneficial, and the pain improved but did not go away. The pain would return easily if extended periods of time occurred between treatments. Eleven treatments were administered over a four-month period. While the patient was frustrated, but not discouraged, it seemed puzzling that a simple hip pain had not disappeared after this many treatments.

On the twelfth visit, it was decided that different treatment tactics were required. Bloodletting and cupping were applied to vascular spiders around the right hip joint and on the right buttock, and bloodletting was applied to right BL-67, along with a typical Manaka-style treatment protocol. The pain abated considerably and remained greatly improved after this treatment.

It is easy to become overconfident and not tap the full repertoire of techniques that are available to us. At later sessions, with this patient, issues of physical abuse surfaced and it became clear why the bloodletting would be useful. Traumatic injuries often cause blood stasis, and until the bloodletting treatment, the focus had been only the general vacuity problem.

Case 46

The next case illustrates how Manaka's general treatment procedure, combined with *chishin* needling, intradermal needles, and bloodletting, was very effective in the treatment of a chronic pain disorder with neurologic involvement.

PATIENT:

Male, age 28.

MAIN COMPLAINT:

Pinched nerve in the neck.

The patient had sustained trauma to the neck while he was athletically active in college, and at the age of 23 had started having symptoms of loss of strength in the left arm, with numbness and radiating burning pains down the upper back and across the chest on the left side of the body. The pain was continuous, and was worsened by certain postures. He had undergone a number of tests which revealed a pinched nerve due to "a mild to moderate overgrowth of the left C6/7 facet joint encroaching on the neural foramen." Aside from these complaints, he was relatively healthy, with mild digestive symptoms which improved with a better diet, and some night urination. His cholesterol was somewhat elevated. At the age of 5 weeks, he had undergone surgery for "twisted intestines."

OBSERVATION AND EXAMINATION:

There was a clear liver channel involvement, with strong tension in the subcostal regions, especially the right, with tightness of the rectus abdominus muscles and both ASIS (anterior superior iliac spine). A polar-channel diagnosis of liver–small intestine involvement was determined.

TREATMENT METHOD:

Following Manaka's polar-channel therapy for liver–small intestine, ion-pumping cords were applied to left LR-2 (black), LR-8 (red) and left SI-3 (red), SI-8 (black). Moxa on the handle of the needle was then applied to left SI-11, right BL-18, and left BL-27, with *chishin* at left GB-12 and both GB-21. Intradermal needles were left around left BL-42, and the left auricle, neck, and muscle relaxant points.

When he arrived for treatment five days later he reported that he had felt better for a while after the previous treatment, but that the improvement was short-lived. For this and the next two treatments, a variety of first-step treatment options were tried. These included bilateral BL-62 (black), SI-3 (red); GB-41 (red), TB-5 (black); left PC-6 (copper), right BL-62 (zinc); left SP-4 (zinc), right SI-3 (copper).

These treatments yielded some improvements, but nothing lasted very long. At the fifth treatment very careful inspection for vascular spiders was made on the upper back and neck regions. This had not been done before because the patient had relatively dark skin, which made searching for vascular spiders more difficult. What appeared to be vascular spiders were found. After another ion-pumping treatment to the liver–small intestine channel pair, bloodletting and cupping techniques were applied on the left upper back. This was followed by moxa on the handle of the needle at left BL-43, right BL-18, and *chishin* at both GB-20 and GB-21. Intradermal needles were left at GB-21 and the left auricle neck point.

The patient returned eight days later. His neck had felt good until the day before. His left arm had been good, much stronger with no numbness, and he had not experienced the burning pain down the chest and upper back. (These symptoms had been virtually continuous for several years.) Essentially the same treatment was repeated. After this, no further treatments were administered because of financial considerations. But, in a follow-up with him the next week, he reported feeling much better.

This was another case where bloodletting and cupping seemed to make a significant difference in the change of symptoms and the duration of treatment effects. Fortunately, not too many treatments passed before the bloodletting procedure was used. The problem was the hesitation in looking for vascular spiders, because they were so difficult to discover.

Case 47

The next case history illustrates how a simple Keiraku Chiryō treatment approach, combined with simple uses of *chinetsukyū* or cone moxa, intradermal needles, press-spheres, occasional direct moxa, and a single use of bloodletting was very effective in the treatment of fatigue and poor concentration.

PATIENT:

Female, age 43.

MAIN COMPLAINT:

Daily fatigue and poor concentration.

The problem had started about two months previous, with extreme fatigue setting in daily between 11am to 1pm, and lasting until the early evening. Symptoms accompanying this fatigue were feelings of "foggy-headedness," heavy eyes, dizziness, poor appetite, and occasional flushing. Various tests had been done with no clear results. The patient had a history of grinding her teeth at night accompanied by soreness of the jaws and neck tension. She also had cervical dysplasia, and had been treated three times before with laser or cryosurgery; she was several months away from her next checkup which would determine whether or not further surgery was required. She had a recurrent tendinitis problem of the right wrist which she treated by wearing a support brace.

OBSERVATION AND EXAMINATION:

There was a clear lung vacuity pattern, with corresponding reflex reactions on the right side of the navel. The lung and spleen pulses were the weakest pulses. Pressure pain was also found on the *yin qiao–ren mai* and *yang qiao–du mai* points, LU-7, KI-6, SI-3, BL-62, with signs and symptoms confirming their use in the Toyohari method of treatment.

TREATMENT METHOD:

To begin treatment, zinc and copper plates were applied as follows: right LU-7, copper; left KI-6, zinc; left SI-3, copper; right BL-62, zinc. After these had been left on for the proper length of time, judging from the pulses, supplementation and draining techniques were applied in the Tōyōhari "touching-needle" style, using a number one silver needle, as follows: supplementation: CV-12, left and right ST-25, CV-6, right LU-9, right SP-3; draining: left LR-3; sup-plementation: left and right TB-4; draining: right ST-40, left GB-37. All these techniques involved no insertion of needles, and after the GB-37 point, the pulses and abdomen were considerably improved. The region of the supra-clavicular fossa was then treated with a light touching-needle technique, and then with a tapping tech-nique, using a silver *zanshin*. Next, left and right BL-13 and BL-20 were supplemented. *Chinetsukyū* was applied to GV-14 and points either side of it, and to left and right *pigen*. Moxa was applied to GV-12, and intradermal needles to CV-12 and *shenmen* in the left auricle. (The intradermal needles were the only inserted needles.)

The patient returned a week later. She had been fatigued the day after the treatment, but had felt more energetic since then and had a better appetite. On this occasion, the zinc and copper plates were used only on LU-7 and KI-6. The same points were treated in the same manner, with the exception that left SI-7 was supplemented instead of TB-4, and left BL-58 and right TB-5 were drained instead of right ST-40. *Chinetsukyū* was also used on the supraclavicular region and at *yintang*. Intradermal needles were placed at right BL-13 and left BL-20, with a press-sphere at GV-12.

The patient returned two weeks later. She had been feeling much better. An almost identical treatment as the second treatment was applied. At this visit, she mentioned that she was scheduled to undergo oral surgery in two weeks, and wanted to use acupuncture to help with the anesthesia, and to alleviate the post-surgical pain and healing.

She came two weeks later for a brief visit, at which intradermal nee-dles were placed at left and right ST-44, LI-4, ST-7, and the tooth extraction point in the auricle.

She returned three days later following the oral surgery. She had some mouth and jaw pain, and constipation from the anesthetic, but had experienced no problems with fatigue since the third treat-ment. At this time, treatment nearly identical to the second and third treatments the exception being that copper was used at right and left LI-4, and zinc at ST-43. At the end of treatment, intrader-mal needles were placed at right and left LI-4 and ST-7.

She returned nineteen days later. Her fatigue problem was com-pletely cured, her mouth was residually a little sore, and her neck and shoulders were stiffer and more sore than usual. A nearly iden-tical procedure was administered as the last treatment, with the exception that *chishin* needling was used at GB-12, and intrader-mal needles were left at left BL-13, right BL-20, and the upper-back point on the left auricle.

The patient returned for a final visit about two-and-a-half months later, more as a "tune-up" than because of any particular complaints. Since the third treatment she had encountered no problems with the fatigue or poor concentration. She was still grinding her teeth, and had some shoulder stiffness associated with it. A very similar treatment protocol was again used, with the addition of bloodletting and cupping at GV-14 to relieve the shoulder stiffness and help her stop grinding her teeth.

The therapeutic outcome in this patient was very positive, and it illustrates very well the principle that "less is better." For this patient, with the exception of a few intradermal needles on each visit, *chishin* on the next-to-last visit, and bloodletting on the last visit, no needles were inserted. Clearly, positive results can be obtained with careful, well directed, mild stimulation techniques.

Appendix 1
Education and Practice in Japan

ACUPUNCTURE DEMOGRAPHY AND CURRICULA

It is difficult to develop a precise and accurate account of the numbers of practitioners of acupuncture and moxibustion, because there is no authoritative statistical source. We consulted several recent studies and discussed these with knowledgeable Japanese practitioners to assure that there were no particular, known biases on the parts of the inquirers or their sponsors. The following data seem reasonably accurate.

Acupuncture and Moxibustion Practitioners			
Source	**Year of Study**	**Acupuncture**	**Moxibustion**
Matsunaga (1983), p 13	1978	42,720	42,393
Lock (1980), p. 65[1]	1980	40,000	
Sonoda (1988), p. 78[2]	1984	52,794	51,433
[1]Lock's estimates make no distinction between acupuncture and moxibustion. [2]Sonoda's numbers represent the total number of licensees; the number of licensees actually practicing is fewer.			

In a recent study (16, 1987)[1] the same figure of about 52,000 licensees is given, but from analysis of phone books, the number actually practicing is closer to 41,000. Estimates from 1993 put the number at over 60,000 licensees.[2] This number makes no distinction between acupuncturists and moxibustionists. No mention is made of the other 11,000 or so licensees in the Nakagawa study (16, 1987). It may be assumed that they have given up practicing, or have moved to other countries to practice. This same study estimates that given the population of Japan (120 million people), the ratio of practitioner to population is 1:2924. Of this total number of practitioners, somewhere between 21% and 29% use acupuncture and moxibustion exclusively in their practice, while the rest combine *anma* massage, *shiatsu*, or both. There are roughly 10,000 licensed and moxibustionists inJapan who use these methods exclusively to earn a living, and about 30,000 who combine their practices with *anma* massage or *shiatsu* to be able to earn a sufficient living.

---

[1]See endnotes for Appendix 1 on p. 317.

[2]K. Tsutani, personal communication.

Western-trained physicians are permitted to practice acupuncture and moxibustion without additional licensure, but we do not know of any records available citing the number of physicians practicing acupuncture or moxibustion. It is likely there are a reasonably large number of physicians practicing acupuncture and moxibustion, since many medical associations research and practice acupuncture and moxibustion side-by-side with biomedicine. This puts the total number of people practicing acupuncture and moxibustion in Japan in excess of 42,000.

It is estimated that about 35–40% of these practitioners (excluding physician practitioners) are blind (15, p.13). Sonoda (23, p.78) breaks down the number of sighted and blind licensees as follows:

Sighted and Blind Licensees			
License	Total	Sighted	Blind
Acupuncture	52,794	33,562	19,232
Moxibustion	51,433	33,339	18,092

Since acupuncture and moxibustion are socially accepted professions for the blind, it is probable that the majority of the 11,000 or so licensees who no longer practice are not blind since it is easier for one who can see to find alternative employment. Thus, of those remaining, 40–50% are blind. While there are a few specialists in each field, most moxibustion licensees also hold acupuncture licenses. It is thought that most blind moxibustion licensees practice acupuncture only and rely on spouses, assistants, or students for moxa application.

While acupuncture and moxibustion are looked on with relatively high favor by laity in Japan (23, pp. 92 *passim*), it is estimated that only between 2% and 5% of the population will visit a traditional medical specialist such as an acupuncturist, moxibustionist, or massage therapist (23, p.100). While over 35% will use *kampo.* traditional herbal medicine (23, pp 92-93, 100), perhaps the main reason for the discrepancy between the percentages of the population interested in manual traditional medical practices and the percentages of the population actually visiting such practitioners is the fact that while *kampo* and modern medicine are covered under Japan's national health insurance scheme, acupuncture, moxibustion, and massage are not covered (23, p. 79).

At present, health care in Japan is following trends in the West, and is becoming very expensive, as it is in most industrialized nations. Most people opt for a system covered by insurance. The current situation with medical care in Japan, we can state quite emphatically, is predominantly Western; traditional medicines co-exist.

However, recent changes in the laws that govern the practice of acupuncture and moxibustion and the curricula of acupuncture and moxibustion schools in Japan will allow for changes in this situation. Insurance reimbursement is now allowed for acupuncture treatment of low-back pain, whiplash, 50-year shoulder, neuralgia, arthritis, and knee pain.

EDUCATION, EDUCATIONAL REQUIREMENTS, AND SCHOOL CURRICULA

There are 37 schools that teach acupuncture and moxibustion to non-blind students in Japan (23 p.78). These schools have either three- or four-year programs. The four-year program is actually an undergraduate bachelor's program, and only a few schools, such as the Meiji school in Kyoto, have this status. Many of the remaining schools are equivalent to at least two years of junior college as well as three years of acupuncture school.

There are 17 schools for blind students (23 p.78). The programs for blind students take up to five years. However, in prefectures throughout Japan, many vocational schools within institutions for the blind have shorter programs in acupuncture and moxibustion. Thus the number of places available for blind students to study is actually greater than 17.

The following tables summarize the required courses in the three-year programs in Japan and compare these with the proposed four-year program currently under legislative review (7). The proposed changes are designed to allow the National Insurance program in Japan to begin covering acupuncture. If this amendment is accepted, it is likely to greatly increase the number of acupuncturists and moxibustionists, and the demand for their services, as currently no insurance policies cover the cost of therapy. Patients must pay out of their own pockets, unless the therapy is performed by a physician.

These tables cover four categories of student: (1) those who study only acupuncture; (2) those who study only moxibustion; (3) those who study both; and (4) those who study both and additionally *anma* massage and *shiatsu*. This last category is probably the most typical of the schools in Japan. The numbers in the columns are the number of hours of study in each subject. Entrance requirements are that the applicants be high school graduates.

THE CURRENT THREE-YEAR PROGRAM

SUBJECT	(1)	(2)	(3)	(4)
Civic Studies				
Mathematics				
Science	180	180	180	180
Physical Education				
Psychology				
SUBTOTAL	180	180	180	180
Medical History	30	30	30	30
Hygenics	90	90	90	90
Medical Laws & Regulations	30	30	30	30
Anatomy	210	210	210	210
Physiology	165	165	165	165
Pathology	75	75	75	75
Introduction to Diagnosis	105	105	105	105
Clinical Studies	240	240	240	240
SUBTOTAL	945	945	945	945
Introduction to Kampo	135	135	135	135
Introduction to Acupoints	105	105	105	105
Theory of Anma, Shiatsu	–	–	–	60
Acupuncture Theory	60	–	90	90
Moxibustion Theory	–	60	same	same
Practice Anma, Shiatsu	–	–	–	480
Acupuncture Practice	555	–	780	780
Moxibustion Practice	–	345	same	same
SUBTOTAL	855	645	1110	1650
TOTAL	1980	1770	2235	2775

THE PROPOSED FOUR-YEAR PROGRAM				
Cultural Science (2 subjects)	60	60	60	60
Social Science (2 subjects)	60	60	60	60
Natural Science (2 subjects)	60	60	60	60
Health & Physical Education	60	60	60	60
Foreign Language	60	60	60	60
SUBTOTAL	300	300	300	300
Introduction to Medicine[1]	45	45	45	45
Hygienics & Public Hygienics[2]	90	90	90	90
Laws & Regulations	45	45	45	45
Anatomy	210	210	210	210
Physiology	165	165	165	165
Introduction to Pathology	75	75	75	75
Introduction to Clinical Medicine[3]	105	105	105	105
Clinical Medicine Studies[4]	195	195	195	195
Rehabilitative Medicine[5]	75	75	75	75
SUBTOTAL	1005	1005	1005	1005
Introduction to Oriental Medicine	135	135	135	135
Introduction to Meridians & Acupoints	105	105	105	105
Anma, Shiatsu Theory	-	-	-	-60
Acupuncture Theory	60	-	90	90
Moxibustion Theory	-	60	same	same
Clinical Theory, Oriental Medicine	90	90	90	90
Anma, Shiatsu Practice	-	-	-	1290
Acupuncture Practice	570	-	840	same
Moxibustion Practice	-	360	same	same
SUBTOTAL	960	750	1260	1770
Selective Required Subjects	300	300	300	90
TOTAL	2565	2355	2865	3165

1. Includes medical history.
2. Includes sterilization procedures.
3. Includes clinical psychology and physical therapy.
4. Includes orthopedics & neuroanatomical medicine.
5. Includes introduction to rehabilitative medicine and kinematics.

Examination of the tables above reveals that only for those in the fourth category, i.e., studying acupuncture, moxibustion, *anma* massage and *shiatsu*, is the curriculum at least half concerned with traditional concepts and techniques (with an emphasis on hands-on practical training). In the other three categories, less than half of the curriculum is traditionally related.

Many schools are already in conformity with the proposed four-year curriculum. The 1990 catalog of the Waseda school, in the Shibuya district of Tokyo, is an example of such a school. Some schools, such as the Meiji school in Kyoto, have been run as undergraduate colleges for a number of years, and have thus had four-year programs in place for some time.

Very few of the 37 schools currently have clinical programs where students treat under supervision. Estimates put the number at less than 5 (we know of only 3, such as the Meiji schools and Mori's Osaka school.) The numbers of hours in acupuncture and moxibustion practice represent extensive needle and moxa labs; the same is true of the hours of *anma* massage and *shiatsu* practice.

Beyond these required courses each school teaches its own specialities and techniques. For example, a school that has a senior instructor well-versed in certain techniques will teach those techniques while other schools, without such an instructor, will not. This allows an important variety among the schools, giving interested students a range of schools from which to choose. Some schools completely de-emphasize traditional theories, teaching them only as historical theories, and instead focus practical and clinical skills on methods that are given entirely scientific rationales. Other schools make their practical and clinical focus the traditional literature, playing down the scientific approaches.

For example, students attending the Tōyō Shinkyū Senmon Gakkō (a more traditionally oriented school in Tokyo) from 1983 to 1986[3] encountered a different emphasis from the standard three-year requirements. The following table summarizes and compares the two.

COURSE	THREE-YEAR REQUIREMENTS	TŌYŌ SHINKYŪ SENMON GAKKŌ
Introduction to Kampo	135	270
Acupuncture & Moxibustion Theories	90	720
Anma and *Shiatsu* Theory	60	90
Medical History	30	180
Introduction to Acupoints	105	175
Acupuncture & Moxa Practice	780	545
Anma and *Shiatsu* Practice	480	190

Overall, the total number of course hours for the Tōyō Shinkyū Senmon Gakkō was the same as the three-year course requirements. The night courses offered had fewer hours than day courses, but more intensive presentation. The day program included more classroom hours than required by law.

A review of transcripts for a student graduating from the Tokyo Therapeutic Institute in 1979 shows that for all but one course, the number of hours studied were the same as those required in the three-year course. The one case in which a difference was found was that the course "Introduction to the Acupoints" was replaced by "Principles of Chinese Medicine" and allotted over twice as many hours.

Students are technically well-prepared, which is important if they are to pass the difficult practical components of the licensure exams, but most do not gain clinical experience in actual treatment during school. Clinical learning comes through assistantships and apprenticeships which comprise a large (but variable) amount of a student's training. Assistantships and apprenticeships are completed during both undergraduate and postgraduate study. They are typically arranged privately by the student in agreement with a clinician. These arrangements range from a minimal commitment involving visits to a practitioner's clinic to observe and assist, to a more extensive program which would include rigorous, systematic training. The most comprehensive are the apprenticeships, which are often residential and last for as many as five years or occasionally more. Japanese clinical training is very dependent on the aptitude and dedication of the student.

---

[3]This information is taken from the transcripts of Masahiro Kurita, who attended the Tōyō Shinkyū Senmon Gakkō from 1983 to 1986.

Students are not legally required to pursue this clinical training, but the most important apprenticeships are hotly contested, and students who fail to secure significant clinical training often never enter practice, or fail to establish a viable practice. The availability of assistantships and apprenticeships is quite good. There are many clinics around the country. Most are small, typically run by an individual practitioner and often located in his or her own house. Recently, there are increasing numbers of larger, centralized clinics where several practitioners work together, often under the supervision or tutelage of a more advanced practitioner. Apprenticeship-type training is often emphasized in these larger clinics. This is especially so in the more traditionally-oriented clinics. Historically and thus traditionally, apprenticeship-type training was the predominant method of education. In Kōdō Fukushima's Tōyōhari Center Clinic in Tokyo, for example, as many as four or five practitioners treated patients under his guidance with as many as three assistants providing supportive techniques and methods.

There are also clinics run by physicians, who have access to hospitals, thus allowing acupuncture apprentices access to a mainstream medical situation. The most successful practitioners enjoy the same economic advantages one expects to see in the West. Dr. Manaka, for example, owned his own small hospital and had his acupuncture clinic within that hospital. Dr. Hyōdō ran his pain clinic in a hospital in Osaka.

In such situations, non-physician acupuncturists work in hospital clinics under the supervision of their physician supervisor-teachers. Recent estimates put the number of hospitals in Japan that have some form of acupuncture clinic in them as high as 60%.

Often there are practitioners many years beyond graduation who undertake assistantships or apprenticeships to attain greater clinical skill. We encountered several such students performing apprenticeships and assistantships in Japanese clinics. In Mr. Fukushima's clinic, for example, there were two acupuncturists who had already been practicing for ten or more years and who were now engaged in five-year apprenticeships with a master practitioner. This attitude towards studying and the refinement of skills is an important strand in the continued development of acupuncture and moxibustion in Japan.

PRACTICE IN JAPAN

Two significant factors contribute to the scope and nature of practice in Japan. The first factor we must consider is social custom in Japan, which promotes belonging to groups rather than remaining an isolated individual in one's chosen field (11). The second factor is the fierce economic and ideological competition that is engendered by the "turf-sharing" of East Asian and Western medical practice in Japan. This in turn fosters an extensive and varied continuum of research within the different medical professions (10, p. 259.)[1]

---

[1]We agree in principle with Lock that the pluralistic nature of East Asian and Western medicine in Japan is important to the overall success of the healthcare system.

PROFESSIONAL ASSOCIATIONS

In Japan, the social group is often seen as more important than the individual, and individuals often find their identity through the groups they join. This partly explains the diversity and large numbers of associations.

Many associations hold meetings on a regular basis, from three times a month to two times a year. The following table shows the frequency for national association annual conferences in Japan for the years 1987, 1988, 1989, and 1990.[2]

Many associations are too small to make such national announcements, and some announced for one or two years but did not announce in all the years surveyed. Though this analysis is incomplete, the comparison does give something of the flavor of what is happening in Japan.

FREQUENCY OF ANNUAL ASSOCIATION MEETINGS, BY MONTH								
MONTH	1987		1988		1989		1990	
	T	P	T	P	T	P	T	P
January					1			
February	2		1		1		1	
March	1	5		6	3		7	
April	2	10		9	1	7	1	9
May	2	7	1	9	1	7	1	15
June	4	6	2	6	1	4	2	13
July	3	4	2	4	3	3	1	7
August		1		2	2	2	1	3
September	4	2	5	5	4	3	5	6
October	3	5	5	2	4	6	5	6
November	4	7	4	4	6	7	4	8
December				1				1
TOTAL	25	47	20	48	23	43	20	76

T = licensed acupuncturists and moxibustionists
P = physicians using and researching acupuncture and moxibustion

It is estimated that there are more than fifty Western medical subspecialities having physician-members who research and practice acupuncture and moxibustion.[3] In addition, there are easily one hundred or more non-physician associations of acupuncture and moxibustion in Japan. Many are relatively unknown with small memberships. There are at least 25 well-established groups with large memberships.

In a 1982 study (1), 53 different associations were listed. This list clearly did not include all the associations since some of the associations described above were not listed. Of these 53 associations, 1982 estimates of the numbers of members for 50 associations were given. These are summarized in the following table.

---

[2]These tables are summaries of calendars published in *Idō no Nippon Magazine* (6.) The numbers here are by no means complete because many associations do not announce their meetings in the *Idō no Nippon Magazine*.

[3]These include the Japanese Cardiovascular Association, the Japanese Obstetrics and Gynecology Association, the Japanese Internal Medicine Association, the Japanese External Medicine Association, the Japanese Pediatric Association, the Japanese Ophthalmology Association, the Japanese Otorhinolaryngology Association, and the Japanese Physiology Association.

ASSOCIATION MEMBERSHIP	
MEMBERS	NUMBER OF ASSOCIATIONS
3000+	1
2000+	1
1000+	1
700-800	2
400-700	2
300-400	4
200-300	3
100-200	5
50-100	10
8-50	21

There are a vast number of non-physician associations of acupuncture and moxibustion in Japan. Many are relatively unknown with small memberships. Several teachers and practitioners with whom we consulted in Japan estimated that 20% of practitioners practice traditional Keiraku Chiryō acupuncture, 20% practice according to scientific principles, and the remaining 60% combine techniques regardless of origin. The provided numbers of members for each association are 1990 estimates, or are derived from a 1982 study [1] or are estimates derived from information gathered in numerous discussions with Japanese colleagues.

Often, practitioners may belong to more than one association, so the numbers of members are only approximate. Many associations have their own specialized approaches. In other associations, ideas, rather than a particular set of techniques, bind members together. In such associations, a great variety of techniques and treatment methods are represented. This is clearly reflected in Manaka's association, the Shinkyū Topology Gakubukai, where diversity of ideas and treatment methods have been highly regarded.

As well, there are many strong-minded individuals who practice their ideas and techniques outside of accepted groups. We have met several individual practitioners with highly unusual treatment ideas and methods.

There are several extremely specialized associations, some of which are not listed. There are also associations that specialize in and research *shōnishin* (children's needle therapies), cupping, bloodletting, and other refinements of needle therapy. For instance, the Nippon Akabane association specializes in the use of *hinaishin* (intradermal needles). Some moxibustion associations study and practice according to the requirements for the separate licensure for moxibustion.

The following table displays information on the larger non-physician associations:

NON-PHYSICIAN ASSOCIATIONS OF ACUPUNCTURE AND MOXIBUSTION

NAME OR AFFILIATION	STYLE	MEMBERS	SOURCE/DATE
Keiraku Chiryō Gakkai	†	2500	1*
Tōyōhari Igakukai	†	1100	2*
Meishinkai	†	1300	1*
Tōhōkai	†	80	3*
Nikkaidō Juku	†	~100	
Koten Shinkukai Kenkyūkai	†	<100	
Shimada Rinjii Genjuku	†	<100	
Myakushin Kenkyūkai	†	>500	4*
Jingei Myakukai	†	>300	4*
Kyūshū Keiraku Gakkai	†	350	4*
Nippon Dento Keiraku Shimpōkai	†	<100	
Tōyō Igaku Kenkyūkai Kyūshū Konwaki	†	100	4*
Fukuokaken Keiraku Chiryō Kenkyūkai	†	104	4*
Nippon Kyūkakuho Kenkyūkai	†	<100	
Koten Shinkyū Kenkyūkai	†	61	4*
Washinkai	†	<100	
Gensai Juku	†	<100	
Kampōhari Dōjinkai	†	<100	
Rinshō Shinkyū Kenkyūkai	†	<100	
Zen Nippon Shinkyū Gakukai	†	2900	4*
Nippon Rinshō Shinkyū Konwakai	‡	>100	
Kurashima Sōji	‡	<100	
Shinkyū Topology Gakubukai	¥	>100	
Kōshinkai	¥	211	4*
Ōsaka Jichi Ika Hari Rinshō Kenkyukai	‡	156	4*
Shinkyū Sawada Ryū Keishōkai	¥	80	4*
Akabane Shihō Chubū Kenshūkai	‡	30	4*
Nippon Akabanekai	‡	1730	4*
Tokyo Shinkyū Ikagaku Tōzaijiku Kenkyūkai	‡	386	4*
Tōyō Igaku to Pain Clinic Kenkyūkai	‡	800	4*
Nippon Shinkyū Hiden Gakkai	‡	385	4*
Nippon Denkishin Kenkyūkai	‡	424	4*
Nakajimashiki Gendai Kikei Chiryō Kenkyūkai	¥	266	4*
Kikei Igaku Kenkyūkai	¥	<100	
PIA	‡	<100	
AMI Group	‡	<100	
Nippon Shinkyū Ryōdōraku Igakkai	‡	800	4*

<100 signifies estimates of less than 100 members.
>100 signifies estimates of more than 100 members.

† signifies a group that focuses exclusively on traditional techniques and ideas.
‡ signifies a group that focuses on modern techniques and ideas.
¥ signifies a group that mixes and matches traditional and modern techniques.

1* Meiyu Okada, personal communication.
2* *Tōyōhari Igakukai Ka n Meibo (Tōyōhari Association Membership)*, 1990.
3* Bunkei Ono, personal communication.
4* *Harikyū ni Kansuru Gakkai Kenkyūkai Ichiran*, 1982.

Three of the largest specialist associations in Japan, the Keiraku Chiryō Gakkai, the Meishinkai, and the Tōyōhari Igakukai, are strictly traditional in their approaches. The Tōyōhari Igakukai is probably the best-organized association in the country. 1996 estimates (2) put the fully-trained membership at around 1000, with about 60 students in training at any one time. Of this 1000, about 750 or 75% practice acupuncture and moxibustion exclusively, with no *anma* or *shiatsu*. Thus, about 5% of all non-physician practitioners in Japan who practice only acupuncture and moxibustion belong to this association, and about 2% of all practicing licensees in Japan belong to this association.

One reason the Tōyōhari Igakukai is so popular stems from its politically active stance on behalf of the many blind practitioners in Japan. At least half of its members are blind, as are most members of the board of directors. The late president, Kōdō Fukushima, was also blind and was active in associations for the blind around the country. Another reason for the success of this association is the degree of educational organization it has achieved and the relative sophistication it has developed for teaching simply explained ideas and techniques that are particularly difficult to master technically. The organization has an academic department which meticulously researches and reviews all proposed changes or additions in the standard curriculum or technical methods that the association teaches and promotes.

ONGOING STUDY AND CONTINUING EDUCATION

Almost all the various associations have annual meetings to which the whole membership is invited. Many meet semi-annually or more often, many have meetings once a month or more. As a consequence, on any single weekend, there might be twenty different associations having some form of meeting for their whole or partial membership; probably there are more than this. When we add to this the numerous seminars and workshops run by individuals or sponsored by particular groups or associations, the total number of educational occasions available on a typical weekend around Japan is considerable. Estimates put the number at 20 in or around Tokyo alone.

The Tōyōhari Igakukai retains an approved group of teachers who are groomed and qualified by the headquarters in Tokyo and sent to each of the branches around Japan. The members of each branch are required to study from at least one qualified teacher every year. The membership is divided into 60 branches, with each member required to attend one meeting a month and, depending on the branch to which he belongs, one, two, or three additional meetings every month. These meetings focus on educational themes and the continued development and refinement of techniques. In 1991 the first U.S. branch was opened in Boston, Massachusetts. Today there are four branches in the U.S.—in Boston, Seattle, Connecticut/New York, and Washington, DC. Recently a European branch has been undertaken in the Netherlands.

This emphasis on continuing education and the importance attached to it is a significant factor in the growth and development of acupuncture in Japan.

ECONOMIC AND IDEOLOGICAL COMPETITION

Economic and ideological competition in the practice of acupuncture and moxibustion in Japan is particularly fierce. Success for the practitioner usually depends on multiple factors.

First, good results must be obtained. This pushes practitioners into developing their skills and arts as much as possible. Such development can be achieved partly through participation in study groups, where feedback, exchange, and friendly competition is very useful, and partly by means of their own clinical research and trials, where they can investigate and refine new or learned techniques.

Second, it is useful to be able to point to or demonstrate scientific models of how a particular therapist's treatments work. Many practitioners will adhere to the theory of some scientific group or be involved in some form of scientific validation or investigation themselves. In their practice and within their associations, the practitioners carry out a gread deal of investigative and scientific work, which parallels the wider social trend in Japan—the 95% of the general population who prefer a scientific biomedical system for their primary health care.

Third, survivability in the clinical setting is often enhanced by uniqueness of approach. Having something new or different to try is often appealing to patients, and many practitioners work in earnest to refine and develop their techniques and skills in order to showcase new treatment techniques and ideas. This too probably parallels wider social trends where we see biomedical research on the cutting edge.

Fourth, a high level of specialization is often necessary. This is clear in the physician medical subspecialities, but this also often occurs in the non-physician groups. Many groups have specialized by using narrowly defined techniques and methods. To treat successfully and survive, members of these groups have developed almost unbelievably detailed knowledge concerning the rationale and use of these specific techniques so that effectiveness of the techniques and ideas can be enhanced and expanded (11).

This process has been fostered in the clinical setting by the strong emphasis on palpation diagnosis. The use of touch and pressure as the primary method of diagnosis allows immediate assessment of both the condition of the patient and the efficacy of treatment. This in turn allows for very rapid reassessment and redesign of treatment when necessary, and it gives the practitioner a reasonably detailed and rapid feedback system. We saw above how this emphasis developed in Japan with influences from various massage techniques. There is a large and diverse body of literature concerning the use of palpation.[4]

---

[4]A representative example of this literature can be seen in the 500th special edition of the *Idō no Nippon* magazine, which is devoted entirely to papers contributed by authors from many clinical backgrounds (8) on the nature, functions, and uses of pressure pain. Sophisticated investigative and clinical techniques utilizing palpation can be found in Y. Manaka, K. Itaya, and S. Birch, *Chasing the Dragon's Tail.*

While these four factors probably are not the only factors involved in survivability, they represent the most obvious and important. In effect, there is an openness and creativity in the study and research of acupuncture and moxibustion in Japan that is perhaps unparalleled in the rest of the world. The attention to detail, the refinement of technique, the creative and investigative tendencies, are all furthered by the current status and structure of the system in Japan—they exist in a very fertile framework. The fact that over 10,000 practitioners make a living from the use of these techniques, that over 30,000 more do so with supplemental massage practices, and that an unknown number of physicians also practice, attests to the success of this process.[5]

SCIENTIFIC AND CLINICAL RESEARCH

Scientific and clinical research into acupuncture and moxibustion in Japan has a very broad base of activity. First, there are the usually less specialized researchers who come from the ranks of the practitioners and who are associated with specific associations. There are the institutional researchers. Institutional research into acupuncture and moxibustion in Japan is quite advanced, certainly much further than any Western country. Very little of this work has yet been translated into English or other European languages.

Aside from the many acupuncture schools in Japan having research departments, some of which are very high-tech and sophisticated (for example, the Osaka School, or the Meiji school in Kyoto which has a state-of-the-art research facility with hospital connections), there are university-level, medical school-level, and hospital clinic-level facilities that have research departments in acupuncture and moxibustion. Dr. Manaka was the head of the acupuncture research department at the Kitazato Institute in Tokyo and Dr. Hyōdō was the head of the pain clinic in the hospital attached to the Osaka medical college. Dr. Toda runs a small physiology lab at the Tokyo Medical and Dental University.

The quantity and sophistication of research coming from these institutions far surpasses the total from the U.S., U.K., and Europe. Additionally, there is much more specific research conducted by physicians who specialize in particular areas of practice. All this work is important for both the scientifically-minded practitioners and the traditionally-minded, since it creates a wider base of social acceptance for acupuncture and moxibustion in general.

20TH CENTURY PRACTITIONERS

The following is a list of well-known 20th-century acupuncturists and moxibustionists in Japan. It is by no means a complete list; it is mostly comprised of the names of those practitioners and authors with whom we are familiar or who came up in discussion with Japanese colleagues. Those whose names have a (D) next to them are no longer alive,

---

[5]For references to the equivalent statistics on practitioners in China, the United States and the United Kingdom, see the original version of this essay, published in the journal *Review*. (3)

those whose names have a (P) next to them have published books or articles in Japanese, and those whose names have an (E) next to them have had works published or translated in English or other European languages as well as in Japanese. The names are sorted by group specialties.

Keiraku Chiryō—Traditional Meridian Therapy

Sorei Yanagiya	(D) (P) (E)	Meiyu Okada	(P)
Sōdō Okabe	(D) (P) (E)	Masabumi Inoue	(P)
Keiri Inoue	(D) (P) (E)	Harumichi Ogawa	(P)
Bunkei Ono	(P) (E)	Denmei Shūdo	(D) (P) (E)
Kōdō Fukushima	(D) (P) (E)	Takio Ikeda	(P)
Shōhaku Honma	(D) (P) (E)	Masakazu Ikeda	(P)

Okyū—Moxibustion Therapy

Isaburo Fukaya	(D) (P) (E)	Takeshi Sawada	(D) (P) (E)
Seiji Irie	(P) (E)	Bunshi Shirota	(D) (P) (E)

Ion-Pumping Cord Therapies

Yoshio Manaka	(D) (P) (E)	Tadashi Irie	(P)
Kazuko Itaya	(P) (E)		

T. C. M. School (Acupuncture and Moxibustion)

Akira Hyōdō	(P) (E)

M. P. School Minus-Plus Needle Therapy (including magnets)

Tsugio Nagatomi	(D) (P) (E)	Masahiro Nawahune	(D) (P)
Osamu Itō	P) (E)	Tada Kono	(P)

Hinaishin—Intradermal Needle Therapy

Kobe Akabane	(D) (P) (E)	Teiken Shimizu	(P) (E)

Shiraku—Bloodletting Therapy

Masao Maruyama	(D) (P) (E)	Kunimasa Kudō	(D) (P) (E)

Shōnishin Children's Needle Therapy

Hidetaro Mori	(P) (E)	Hirohisa Yoneyama	(D) (P) (E)

A.M.I. Electrodiagnostic Therapy

Hiroshi Motoyama	(P) (E)

Ryōdōraku Electrodiagnostic Therapy

Yoshio Nakatani	(D) (P) (E)	Masayoshi Hyōdō	(D) (P) (E)
Tsuneo Kobayashi	(P)	Hirohisa Oda	(P) (E)

Auricular Acupuncture

Yoshihide Kobayashi	(P)

Acupuncture Using Purely Scientific Rationale

Yoshio Nagahama	(D) (P)	Katsusuke Serizawa	(P) (E)
Haruto Kinoshita	(D) (P) (E)	Sōji Kurashima	(P) (E)
Akio Debata	(P)	Yukio Kurosu	(P)

It is interesting to note that bloodletting is a treatment method that only physician-acupuncturists may use legally. During the Meiji Restoration in the late 1800s, the practice of bloodletting was prohibited for non-physician practitioners. Today, non-physician practitioners use it, but typically they will conceal the fact that they do. To date, no test cases have been made of the ruling.

ENDNOTES FOR APPENDIX 1

(1) Anon. *Harikyū ni Kansuru Gakkai, Kenkyūkai Ichiran (List of Acupuncture and Moxibustion Associations and Study Groups)*. Tokyo: All Japan Acupuncture Association, 1982.

(2) ———. *Tōyōhari Igakukai Kaiin Meibo (Tōyōhari Association Membership)*. Tokyo: Tōyōhari Association, 1990.

(3) Birch, S. "Acupuncture in Japan: An Introductory Survey." *Review* 1989 6:12–13; 1990 7:16–20; 1990 8:21–26; 1991 9:28–31, 39–42.

(4) Bischko, J. *Intermediate Acupuncture vol II*. Heidelberg: Karl F. Haug Publishers, 1986.

(5) Hillier, S. M. and J. A. Jewell. *Health Care and Traditional Medicine in China; 1800–1982*. London: Routledge Kegan Paul, 1983.

(6) *Idō no Nippon Magazine*. Editorials 46, 2, 510:115–117, 1987; 47, 2, 522:136–138, 1988; 48, 2, 534:148–150, 1989. 49, 2, 546:142–145, 1990.

(7) ———. Editorial, 48, 5, 537:101–103, 1989.

(8) ———. 500th special edition, 45, 4, 500, 1986.

(9) Itaya, K. "Essays on the History, Nature, Functions, Methods and Research of Moxibustion in Japan." *Medical Encyclopedia of Kōdansha*. Tokyo: Kōdansha, 1985.

(10) Lock, M. M. *East Asian Medicine in Urban Japan*. Berkeley: University of California Press, 1980.

(11———. "Organization and Practice of East Asian Medicine in Japan: Continuity and Change." *Social Science and Medicine* 148:245–253, 1980.

(12) Lu, Gwei–Djen and J. Needham. *Celestial Lancets*. Cambridge: Cambridge University Press, 1980.

(13) Manaka, Y., K. Itaya, and S. Birch. *Chasing the Dragon's Tail*. Brookline, MA: Paradigm Publications, 1995.

(14) Matsumoto, K. and S. Birch. *Hara Diagnosis: Reflections on the Sea*. Brookline, MA: Paradigm Publications, 1988.

(15) Matsunaga, T. "Socio–cultural Transformation of Japanese Medical Systems." Ph.D. thesis. Western Michigan University, 1983.

(16) Nakagawa, Y. "The Present Situation for Acupuncture and Moxibustion Clinics and Practitioners in Japan." *Idō no Nippon Magazine* 46, 7, 515:02-107, 1987; 46, 8, 516:91-95, 1987.

(17) Norbeck, E. and M. M. Lock, eds. *Health, Illness and Medical Care in Japan: Cultural and Social Dimensions*. Honolulu: University of Hawaii Press, 1987.

(18) Ohnuki-Tierney, E. *Illness and Culture in Contemporary Japan*. Cambridge: Cambridge University Press, 1984.

(19) Omura, Y. *Acupuncture Medicine*. Tokyo: Japan Publications, 1982.

(20) Rosenthal, M. M. *Health Care in the People's Republic of China: Moving Toward Modernization*. Boulder: Westview Press, 1987.

(21) Serizawa, K. and M. Kusumi. *Clinical Acupuncture*. Tokyo: Japan Publications Inc., 1988.

(22) Sivin, N. *Traditional Medicine in Contemporary China*. Ann Arbor, MI: Center for Chinese Studies, University of Michigan, 1987.

(23) Sonoda, K. *Health and Illness in Changing Japanese Society*. Tokyo: University of Tokyo Press, 1988.

(24) Unschuld, P. *Medicine in China: A History of Ideas*. Berkeley: University of California Press, 1985.

(25) Unschuld, P. *Medicine in China: Nan Ching, the Classic of Difficult Issues*. Berkeley: University of California Press, 1986.

(26) Unschuld, P. "Traditional Chinese Medicine: Some Historical and Epistemological Reflections." *Social Science and Medicine* 24, 12:1023–1029, 1987.

Appendix 2
Chinese Studies Using Seeds Taped to Auricular Points

Published studies from China indicate that application of various types of seeds to auricular points is useful for the treatment of cholelithiasis, i.e., encouraging contraction of the gallbladder and the elimination of small calculi. Other studies that we have come across indicate efficacy in the treatment of enuresis, neurasthenia, abnormal fetal position, and weight loss.

A number of studies have been published showing how the taping and subsequent pressing of seeds in the auricles can cause the gallbladder and common bile duct to contract, sometimes expelling calculi of up to one centimeter in diameter. On occasion the calculi are as big as two to four centimeters. Some of these studies were controlled,[1] and therefore seem more reliable. Others were not controlled[2]. A recent review[3] summarized the findings, with remarkable claims of effectiveness.

Different practitioners and researchers used different points in the auricles, but the most commonly used were the bile-pancreas, liver, *sanjiao,* spleen, duodenum, stomach, kidney, sympathetic, *shenmen,* and small intestine points. Points are selected by finding pressure pain at the loci and using a probe such as the *teishin* to pinpoint the exact locations. Often from six to eight points were selected and treated. Treatment consisted of taping the seeds to the chosen points and then applying pressure to them for certain periods of time at fixed intervals. For instance, pressure might be applied after meals for about twenty to thirty minutes. The points were pressed until they caused some discomfort. The seeds were changed every other day. Alternating auricles is a relatively safe way of preventing excessive irritation at the treatment points. All researchers

---

[1]Dang Shaorong *et al.* (1986); Guo Qintang *et al.* (1987); and Guo Qintang *et al.* (1991).

[2]Du Daiyi *et al.* (1987); Zhang Ren *et al.* (1986).

[3]Wang Tianjun *et al.* (1990).

recommend wiping the points thoroughly with alcohol before applying the seeds and some even sterilize the seeds before application.

A controlled study in the treatment of primary hypertension comparing auricular point pressure to the use of hypertensive medications purported to demonstrate comparable results between the two groups. The group using auricular points experienced no side effects.[4] It further claimed to show a lowering of blood lipids, blood plasma viscosity, and erythrocyte sedimentation rate in the auricular point pressure groups. The primary treatment points were heart, *shenmen,* adrenal gland, and sympathetic. The auxiliary treatment points were ear dorsal center, labyrinthine root, pulvinar, kidney, and endocrine. The points were massaged three times a day for 3 to 5 minutes each time.

A recent controlled study on the effectiveness of taping and then massaging seeds in the auricles for the treatment of abnormal fetal position claimed very good results.[5] Treatments involved palpating and selecting sensitive points from among uterus, sympathetic, subcortex, liver, spleen, kidney, and abdomen points in one auricle. The points were wiped first with alcohol, then seeds were taped to the points. Pressure was applied to each point with a to-and-fro movement for about five minutes, three times a day before meals. After two days, the seeds were removed and the procedure repeated on the other auricle. This procedure was repeated until the fetal position moved to normal.

A recent uncontrolled study claimed reasonably good success in the treatment of obesity.[6] Two groups of points were selected and used alternately. The first was the spleen and *shenmen* points, the second the lung and sympathetic points. After palpating for tender points and placing the seeds, the patients were instructed to rub the points for five minutes before every meal, employing enough pressure to cause pain.

An uncontrolled study on the use of the taping and pressing of seeds in the auricles for the treatment of neurasthenia claimed good therapeutic effectiveness.[7] According to this study, neurasthenia involves the following set of symptoms: insomnia, dream-disturbed sleep, dizziness, and headache. Treatment involved placing seeds at the heart, kidney, and *shenmen* points on one auricle for one day, and then on the other auricle the next. Placement was on alternate auricles daily for ten days. Pressure was applied at each point several times daily until discomfort and heat were felt at each point.

An uncontrolled study claimed good clinical effectiveness using this method in the treatment of enuresis.[8] The treatment points were kidney, bladder, spleen, and brain. Seeds were placed in one auricle, with instructions that they be pressed two to three times daily, especially before sleep. Seeds were removed and placed at the opposite auricle every three or so days.

---

[4]Yu Peng *et al.* (1991).

[5]Qin Guangfeng *et al.* (1989).

[6]Gu Yueshan *et al.* (1989).

[7]Sun Guixia *et al.* (1987).

Another uncontrolled study claimed to show good clinical effectiveness in the treatment of "competitive syndrome." Competitive syndrome is "exhibited by students or candidates sitting for examinations." The symptoms are insomnia, palpitations, headache, dizziness, hypomnesia, dysphoria, thirst, anorexia, nausea, vomiting, diarrhea, constipation, and menorrhagia, among others. These occur prior to or during exams due to overstrain and worry. The symptoms usually handicap the students in their examination and affect their health.[9]

Clearly, if these results are valid, this treatment approach might be good for stressed, anxious patients in general. The primary treatment points were *shenmen*, heart, kidney, liver, brain point, and endocrine, with three to five points selected for each treatment. Other points were added according to the symptoms:

palpitations	heart
hypomnesia	forehead
dysphoria and thirst	gallbladder, throat
anorexia	stomach
diarrhea	lower rectum
constipation	large intestine
menorrhagia	uterus, sympathetic, abdomen

Pressure was applied to each point about 60 times during each of three to five sessions each day. Therapy was started about two weeks prior to the start of the exams, and terminated at the end of the exams.

---

[8]Zhou Kongyu (1987).

[9]Zhu Jisheng *et al.* (1991).

Bibliography

Akabane, K. *Chinetsukando Niyoru Shinkyū Chiryōhō (Acupuncture and Moxibustion Therapy by the Heat Sensitivity Method)*. Yokosuka: Idō no Nippon Sha, 8th edition, 1985.

———. *Hinaishin Hō (The Method of Intradermal Needle)*. Yokosuka: Idō no Nippon Sha, 12th edition, 1986.

———. *Kyūtōshin Hō (The Moxa on the Handle of the Needle Method)*. Yokosuka: Idō no Nippon Sha, 6th edition, 1986.

Anon. *Harikyū ni Kansuru Gakkai, Kenkyūkai Ichiran (List of Acupuncture and Moxibustion Associations and Study Groups)*. Tokyo: All Japan Acupuncture Association, 1982.

———. "One in Five Canadians is Using Alternative Therapies, Survey Finds." *Canadian Medical Asociation Journal* 144, 4:469, 1991.

———. *Tōyōhari Igakukai Kaiin Meibo (Tōyōhari Association Membership)*. Tokyo: Tōyōhari Association, 1990.

Auteroche, B. *et al. Acupuncture and Moxibustion: A Guide to Clinical Practice*. Edinburgh: Churchill Livingstone, 1992.

Birch, S. "Acupuncture in Japan: An Introductory Survey." *Review* 1989 6:12–13; 1990 7:16–20; 1990 8:21–26; 1991 9:28–31, 39–42.

Birch, S. and R. Felt. *Understanding Acupuncture*. Edinburgh: Churchill Livingstone, at press.

Bischko, J. *Intermediate Acupuncture vol II*. Heidelberg: Karl F. Haug Publishers, 1986.

Cheng, X. N., ed. *Chinese Acupuncture and Moxibustion*. Beijing: Foreign Languages Press, 1987.

Cui J. and Zhang G. Q. "A Survey of Thirty Years of Clinical Applications of Cupping." *Journal of Traditional Chinese Medicine* 9(2):151–154, 1989.

Dang, S. R. *et al.* "Clinical Analysis of Therapeutic Efficacy in 365 Cases of Cholelithiasis Treated by Pressure over Ear Points." *Journal of Traditional Chinese Medicine* 6, 1:1–5, 1986.

Du, D. Y. *et al.* "Clinical Observation on 95 Cases of Cholelithiasis by Pressing Auricular Points." *Selections from Article Abstracts on Acupuncture and Moxibustion*. Beijing: China Association of Acupuncture and Moxibustion, 1987, pp. 114–115.

Eisenberg, D. M. *et al.* "Unconventional Medicine in the United States: Prevalence, Costs and Patterns of Use. *New England Journal of Medicine* 326, 4:246–252, 1993.

Epler, D. C. "Bloodletting in Early Chinese Medicine and its Relation to the Origin of Acupuncture." *Bulletin of the History of Medicine* 54: 337–367, 1980.

Fukaya, I. *Kadenkyū Monogatari (Family Recipes in Moxa Therapy)*. Tokyo: Sankei Publishing Company, 1982.

Fukushima, K. *Meridian Therapy: A Hands–on Text for Traditional Japanese Hari based on Pulse Diagnosis*. Tokyo: Tōyōhari Medical Association, 1991.

———. "Clinical Cases of Bloodletting Therapy." *Keiraku Shinryō*, March, 1988, pp. 5–20.

Fulder, S. J. and R. E. Munro. "Complementary Medicine in the United Kingdom: Patients, Practitioners and Consultations." *Lancet* 542–545, September 1985.

Gu, Y. S. *et al.* "Clinical Observations on Weight Reduction by Pressing Auricular Points with Semen Vaccariae." *Journal of Traditional Chinese Medicine* 9, 3:166, 1989.

Guo, Q. T. *et al.* "Clinical and Experimental Observations of Gallstone Treated by Herbal Seeds Sticking and Pressing Method on Ear Points." *Selections from Article Abstracts on Acupuncture and Moxibustion.* Beijing: China Association of Acupuncture and Moxibustion, 1987, pp. 111–112.

———. "Clinical and Experimental Observation on Treating Cholelithiasis by Ear–Point Pressing." *International Journal of Clinical Acupuncture* 2, 1:29–35, 1991.

Hillier, S. M. and J. A. Jewell. *Health Care and Traditional Medicine in China; 1800–1982.* London: Routledge Kegan Paul, 1983.

Hosho, K. "Effects of the *Enpishin.*" *Idō no Nippon Magazine* 55,4, 428:61–62, 1980.

Hyodo, M. *Itami no Atarashii Chiryōhō (New Treatments for Pain).* Tokyo: Chugai Igaku Company, 9th edition, 1983.

——— *Shiranakatta Itami no Hanashi (Unknown Stories of Pain).* Tokyo: Kenkyukan Publishing Company, 1987.

Idō no Nippon Magazine. Editorials 46, 2, 510:115–117, 1987; 47, 2, 522:136–138, 1988; 48, 2, 534:148–150, 1989. 49, 2, 546:142–145, 1990.

———. Editorial, 48, 5, 537:101–103, 1989.

———. 500th special edition, 45, 4, 500, 1986.

Imagawa, M. "Peripheral *Kyūtōshin* Techniques." *Idō no Nippon Magazine* 44, 10, 494:45–53, 1984.

Itaya, K. "Essays on the History, Nature, Functions, Methods and Research of Moxibustion in Japan." *Medical Encyclopedia of Kōdansha.* Tokyo: Kōdansha, 1985.

Kinoshita, H. *Illustration Af acupoints.* Yokosuka: Idō no Nippon Sha, 1970.

Kobayashi, Y. and K. Cho. *Zusetsu Jishingaku (Illustrated Ear Acupuncture Study Guide).* Tokyo: Shizensha, 1980.

Kosoto, T. and T. Hamada. *Ishaku Kōtei Daikei Reisu (An Explanation of the Yellow Emperor's Nei Jing Ling Shu).* Tokyo: Tsukiji Publishing Company, 1972.

Kudō, K. *Zusetsu Shiraku Chiryō (Illustrated Guide to Bloodletting Therapy).* Tokyo: Shizensha Publishing Company, 1983.

Lock, M. M. *East Asian Medicine in Urban Japan.* Berkeley: University of California Press, 1980.

———. "Organization and Practice of East Asian Medicine in Japan: Continuity and Change." *Social Science and Medicine* 148:245–253, 1980.

Lu, Gwei–Djen and J. Needham. *Celestial Lancets.* Cambridge: Cambridge University Press, 1980.

Manaka, Y. *Hiratashi Junihannōtai Nesshin Shigeki Ryōho (Hirata-style Hot-needle Therapy).* Yokosuka: Idō no Nippon Sha, 1982.

———. *Ika no Tameno Shinjutsu Nyūmon Kōza (Introductory Lectures on Acupuncture for Medical Doctors).* Yokosuka: Idō no Nippon Sha, revised 2nd edition, 1980.

———. *Kyū to Hari (Moxibustion and Acupuncture).* Tokyo, Shufu no Tomo Publishing Company, 8th edition, 1983.

———. *Okyū no Kenkyū (Moxibustion Studies). Tokyo: Goma Sha, 1976.*

———, and K. Itaya. "Wooden Hammer and Needle Therapy, Which Even the Layperson Can Perform." Reprinted by the Shinkyu Topology Association office in Kyoto, n.d.

———, K. Itaya, and S. Birch. *Chasing the Dragon's Tail.* Brookline, MA: Paradigm Publications, 1995.

———, and H. Okusada. "Wooden Hammer and Needle Therapy." Unpublished manuscript, 1986.

Maruyama, M. *Shinkyū Igaku to Koten no Kenkyū (Research Book of Acupuncture and Moxibustion Medicine and the Classics).* Osaka: Sogen Sha, 1979.

———, and K. Kudō. *Shimpan Shiraku Ryōho (Bloodletting Therapy).* Tokyo: Seki

Bundo Publishing Company, 1982.

Matsumoto, K. and S. Birch. *Five Elements and Ten Stems.* Higganum, Connecticut: Paradigm Publications, 1983.

———. *Extraordinary Vessels.* Brookline, Massachusetts: Paradigm Publications, 1986.

———. *Hara Diagnosis: Reflections on the Sea.* Brookline, MA: Paradigm Publications, 1988.

Matsunaga, T. "Socio–cultural Transformation of Japanese Medical Systems." Ph.D. thesis. Western Michigan University, 1983.

Meguro, A. *Kyūkaku Ryōhō (Cupping Therapy).* Tokyo: Midori Shōbō Publishing Company, 5th edition, 1991.

Mizutani, J. "Practical Moxibustion Therapy 1–12," *North American Journal of Oriental Medicine.* Special Issue, Spring 1998.

Nagahama, Y., H. Kinoshita, and R. Nakamura. *Shinkyū Chiryō no Shinkenkyū (New Studies on Acupuncture and Moxibustion Therapies).* Osaka: Sogen Publishing Company, 1983.

Nakagawa, Y. "The Present Situation for Acupuncture and Moxibustion Clinics and Practitioners in Japan." *Idō no Nippon Magazine* 46, 7, 515:02–107, 1987; 46, 8, 516:91–95, 1987.

Norbeck, E. and M. M. Lock, eds. *Health, Illness and Medical Care in Japan: Cultural and Social Dimensions.* Honolulu: University of Hawaii Press, 1987.

O'Connor, J. and D. Bensky. *Acupuncture: A Comprehensive Text.* Seattle: Eastland Press, 1981.

Ohnuki-Tierney, E. *Illness and Culture in Contemporary Japan.* Cambridge: Cambridge University Press, 1984.

Okabe, S. *Shinkyū Keiraku Chiryō (Acupuncture and Moxibustion Meridian Therapy).* Tokyo: Sekibundō Publishing, 8th edition, 1989.

Omura, Y. *Acupuncture Medicine.* Tokyo: Japan Publications, 1982.

Ono, B. *Keiraku chiryō: Shinkyū rinshō nyūmon (Meridian therapy, an introduction to clinical acupuncture).* Yokosuka: Idō no Nippon Sha, 1988.

Qin, G. F. and H. J. Tang. "413 Cases of Abnormal Fetal Position Corrected by Auricular Plaster Therapy." *Journal of Traditional Chinese Medicine* 9, 4:235–237, 1989.

Rosenthal, M. M. *Health Care in the People's Republic of China: Moving Toward Modernization.* Boulder: Westview Press, 1987.

Serizawa, K. and M. Kusumi. *Clinical Acupuncture.* Tokyo: Japan Publications Inc., 1988.

Shimizu, K. "Pressure Pain Points, Diagnosis and Treatments." *Idō no Nippon Magazine* 45, 4, 500:315–324, 1986.

Shiozawa, F., "Treatment Effects of the *Empishin.*" Yokosuka: *Idō no Nippon Magazine* 35, 11, 387:36–40, 1976.

———."Effects of the *Empishin.*" *Idō no Nippon Magazine* 36, 9, 397:51–54, 1977.

Shirota, B. *Kyūryō Zatsuwa (Miscellaneous Lectures on Moxa Therapy).* Yokosuka: Idō no Nippon Sha, 6th edition, 1982.

———. *Shinkyū Chiryō Kisogaku (Fundamentals of Acupuncture and Moxibustion Therapy).* Yokosuka: Idō no Nippon Sha, 16th edition, 1986.

———. *Shinkyū Shinzui (Basics of Acupuncture and Moxibustion).* Yokosuka: Idō no Nippon Sha, 14th edition, 1986.

Shūdo, D. *Japanese Classical Acupuncture: Introduction to Meridian Therapy.* Seattle: Eastland Press, 1990.

Sivin, N. *Traditional Medicine in Contemporary China.* Ann Arbor, MI: Center for Chinese Studies, University of Michigan, 1987.

Sonoda, K. *Health and Illness in Changing Japanese Society.* Tokyo: University of Tokyo Press, 1988.

Sun, G. X. and Zhong L. "The Clinical Effect of Auricular pressure Therapy of Vaccaria Pyramidata for Neurasthenia." *Selections from Article Abstracts on Acupuncture and Moxibustion.* Beijing, China: Association of Acupuncture and Moxibustion 1987, pp. 52–53.

Takaoka, M. *Ika no Tameno Itami no Hari Chiryō: Hinaishin Chiryōno Hiketsu (Acupuncture Treatment of Pain for Physicians: Key Points for Intradermal Needle Therapy).* Yokosuka: Idō no Nippon Sha, 5th edition, 1988.

Tanaka, H. "Introduction to *Kyūtōshin* (1)." *Idō no Nippon Magazine* 43, 6, 478:57–59, 1984.

———. "Introduction to *Kyūtōshin* (2)." *Idō no Nippon Magazine* 43, 8, 480:50–52, 1984.

———. "Introduction to *Kyūtōshin* (3)." *Idō no Nippon Magazine* 43, 9, 481:78–83, 1984.

———. "Introduction to *Kyūtōshin* (4)." *Idō no Nippon Magazine* 43, 11, 483:48–50, 1984.

———. "Introduction to *Kyūtōshin* (5)," *Idō no Nippon Magazine* 44, 11, 495:69–71, 1985.

———. "Introduction to *Kyūtōshin* (7)," *Idō no Nippon Magazine* 45, 10, 506:56–58, 1986.

———. "Introduction to *Kyūtōshin* (8)," *Idō no Nippon Magazine* 45, 11, 507:55–58, 1986.

———. "Introduction to *Kyūtōshin* (9)," *Idō no Nippon Magazine* 45, 12, 508:38–43, 1986.

Tsutani, K. "The Evaluation of Herbal Medicines: An East Asian Perspective." *Clinical Research Methodology for Complementary Therapies,* ed. Lewith G.T. and D. Aldridge. London: Hodder and Stoughton, 1994.

Unschuld, P. *Medicine in China: A History of Ideas.* Berkeley: University of California Press, 1985.

Unschuld, P. *Medicine in China: Nan Ching, the Classic of Difficult Issues.* Berkeley: University of California Press, 1986.

Unschuld, P. "Traditional Chinese Medicine: Some Historical and Epistemological Reflections." *Social Science and Medicine* 24, 12:1023–1029, 1987.

Visser, J. "Alternative Medicine in the Netherlands." *Complementary Medical Research* 4, 2:28–31, 1990.

Wang, F. Y. and Ren H. Z. *"Kyūgyoku Ryōhō (Cupping Therapy),"* ed. Fumihiko Shiroda and trans. Kaname Asakawa. Ichikawa City: Tōyō Gakujutsu Publishing Company, 1985.

Wang, T. J. et al., "Auricular Acupoint Pellet Pressure Therapy in the Treatment of Cholelithiasis." *Journal of Traditional Chinese Medicine* 10, 2:26–131, 1990.

Yu, Peng et al. "Clinical Study on Auricular Pressure Treatment of Primary Hypertension." *International Journal of Clinical Acupuncture* 2, 1:36–40, 1991.

Zhang, Ren et al. "The Effect of Auricular-Plaster Therapy on Gallstone Expulsion and on Expansion-contraction Function of the Biliary System." *Journal of Traditional Chinese Medicine* 6, 4:263–266, 1986.

Zhou, K. Y. "Treatment of Enuresis by Ear-Pressing of Traditional Chinese Medicine, Report of 143 cases." *Selections From Article Abstracts on Acupuncture and Moxibustion.* Beijing: China Association of Acupuncture and Moxibustion, 1987, pp. 161–162.

Zhu, J. S. et al. "Auricular-Plaster Therapy for Competitive Syndrome: An Observation of 210 Cases." *International Journal of Clinical Acupuncture* 2, 1:41–43, 1991.

Index

Other quality books on Japanese Acupuncture

CHASING THE DRAGON'S TAIL

Yoshio Manaka, Kazuko Itaya, Stephen Birch
P, 7x10", 453 pp; ISBN: 9780912111322

Index ~ Bibliography ~ Footnotes ~ Appendix ~
~ Photographs ~ Illustrations.

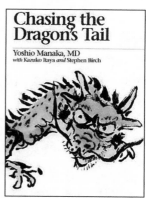

This seminal work introduces the major clinical and theoretical accomplishments of Dr. Yoshio Manaka's impressive career as one of the most distinguished acupuncture physicians of his era. It begins by describing how the "X-signal system" is the foundation of human topology, function, and response. In essence, the X-signal system defines qi, yin-yang, and the five phases as clinical events, just as traditional Oriental thinkers recognized these ideas through right-brain pattern recognition. While Dr. Manaka references some of the most advanced scientific thinking of our era — information theory, holographic models and new paradigms — his explanations are full of practical tests which readers can use to confirm his ideas for themselves. The core of the text is a complete description of Dr. Manaka's treatment system. It is thus a clinical manual of unique value because it describes Dr. Manaka's most important techniques: ion pumping and other root treatments, as well as his distinctive use of fire needles, channel stimulation techniques, sotai, moxibustion, and other modern Chinese and Japanese clinical developments. Beginning with a step-by-step template for formulating and confirming a diagnosis, this work provides the instructions necessary to apply these techniques quickly and with confidence. The text concludes with case histories and appendices that provide supporting technical details.

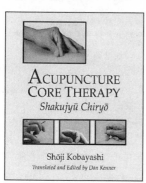

ACUPUNCTURE CORE THERAPY

Shoji Kobayashi

P, 7x10", 212 pp; ISBN: 9780912111896

Index ~ Bibliography ~ Footnotes ~ Glossary ~
Appendix ‒ Photographs ~ Illustrations

Shakujyu Chiryo a popular acupuncture methodology in Japan that is increasingly taught in the academic schools and colleges. *Shaku* is a concept that refers to fullness or repletion, and *jyu* is a concept that refers to emptiness or vacuity. "Acupuncture Core Therapy" is the author's English language term for his *shakuju chiryo* method. "Core" refers to the innermost essence of something. Both the concept and the methodology of the system of Acupuncture Core Therapy combine three fundamental elements of the body's vital energy system: the hara, which is the abdominal center of physiological vital force; the spinal energy system, which is the original source of our being and our link with other realms of consciousness; and qi gong, which is the development of the body's ability to intentionally store, concentrate, and distribute vital force. Kobayashi has refined the essence of this technique from his study of classical teachings on the vital energy system and has developed a unique method of acupuncture root treatment. Using the flexibility of yin-yang, the five phases, the eight principles, and other basic tenets of acupuncture, he applies these to clinical situations. He has reassembled the fragments of transmitted teachings and condensed them to their intrinsic core significance. Acupuncture Core Therapy is a reliable and significant methodology for achieving remarkable clinical results using these classical patterns and directing the body's energy with the intention of the needle and the choice of point selection.

~ Order from ~
Redwing Book Company
202 Bendix St, Taos, NM USA 87571 ~ tel 575 758 7758 ~ fax 575 758 7768
online at **www.redwingbooks.com**